WOMEN'S HEALTH

WOMEN'S HEALTH

Intersections of Policy, Research, and Practice

SECOND EDITION

edited by

PAT ARMSTRONG and ANN PEDERSON

Women's Press

Toronto

Women's Health: Intersections of Policy, Research, and Practice, Second Edition
Edited by Pat Armstrong and Ann Pederson

First published in 2015 by
Women's Press, an imprint of Canadian Scholars' Press Inc.
425 Adelaide Street West, Suite 200
Toronto, Ontario
M5V 3C1

www.womenspress.ca

Library and Archives Canada Cataloguing in Publication

Women's health : intersections of policy, research, and practice / edited by Pat Armstrong and Ann Pederson. —Second edition.

First edition edited by Pat Armstrong and Jennifer Deadman, Toronto
: Women's Press, 2008.
Includes bibliographical references and index.
Issued in print and electronic formats.
ISBN 978-0-88961-570-0 (paperback).--ISBN 978-0-88961-571-7 (pdf).—
ISBN 978-0-88961-572-4 (epub)

1. Women--Health and hygiene—Canada. 2. Women's health services—Canada. 3. Minority women—Health and hygiene—Canada. 4. Medical policy—Canada. 5. Medicine—Research—Canada. 6. Gender mainstreaming—Canada. I. Armstrong, Pat, 1945-, editor II. Pederson, Ann P., editor

RA564.85.W678 2015 613'.042440971 C2015-904672-6 C2015-904673-4

Text design by Susan MacGregor
Cover design by Em Dash Design

15 16 17 18 19 5 4 3 2 1

Printed and bound in Canada by Webcom

Canadä

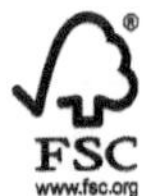

MIX
Paper from
responsible sources
FSC® C004071

Contents

Acknowledgements

As is the case with all books, this one would not have been possible without the contributions of many others. First, we would like to thank the authors of the chapters. Some wrote entirely new chapters, others substantially revised earlier ones, but all worked with patience, efficiency and good humour in response to our many requests. They all produced accessible, critical contributions to our understanding of women's health. Second, we would like to thank Jane Springer. Once again, she quickly provided an expert and sympathetic edit of our messy collection. Third, we would like to thank all of the wonderful people at Women's Press, especially Emma Johnson, Natalie Garriga, and Keriann McGoogan. They continue to offer professional and sympathetic support for progressive work, so important in these times of major cutbacks in women's health.

Introduction

Pat Armstrong

That only women menstruate, get pregnant, and breastfeed are just some of the factors that usually provide the basis for talking about the female sex, understood as being about biological characteristics and often equated with what is natural. However, no bodies are conceived, develop, or live outside their physical, social, and economic environments. Relationships, often based on inequalities, are critical components in those environments. Moreover, some transgender people who live as men still menstruate, and some of the people who live as women never do, just as some women never become pregnant or breastfeed. Such influences have led to the term "gender," which is usually understood to refer to the ways lives are lived and thus is often equated with nurture. They have also contributed to the recognition that there is no simple dichotomy between male and female bodies, or masculinity and femininity. Indeed, there are multiple gender identities and classifications. As biology professor Fausto-Sterling (2005, p. 1516) shows with her research on bone density: "sex-gender or nature-nurture accounts of difference fail to appreciate the degree to which culture is a partner in producing body systems commonly referred to as biology—something apart from the social." In other words, sex and gender are inextricably integrated even if they can be distinguished analytically.

A focus on sex implies an emphasis on what women share, although this includes recognizing differences related to such factors as age. A focus on gender is more likely to emphasize differences among women, although acknowledging that women often face similar conditions and share similar fates. It may be important to group women together in research and policy whether sex, gender, or sex/gender is the starting point. Treating women as a category can tell us, for example, if women are more likely than men to suffer from arthritis, to smoke, to experience domestic violence, or to lack secure employment. What is defined as female can be real in its consequences, consequences that are felt in the body. And women are usually defined as a distinct group with particular traits and capacities. With information on women as a group we can then work for changes in policy and practices for women collectively. At the same time, however, it is always important to ask which women are more likely to experience these problems, under what conditions, so that we can develop strategies for particular groups of women and for individuals, recognizing inequalities not only between women and men but also among women. In doing so, it is important to recognize the intersection of racialization, class, sexual orientation, age, and other social relations.

Biomedical approaches, primarily found in the health sciences, tend to focus on anatomy, physiology, genes, and hormones: on sex. The gold standard in such research is the double-blind randomized clinical trial. Neither researchers nor participants know who is receiving the intervention, and as much of the other social relations as possible are controlled by strategies such as matching the characteristics of participants. While this method does recognize that the values of researcher and participant can shape both results and their interpretation—hence the double-blind approach that randomly selects participants to receive or not receive the intervention—it also assumes that biology can be studied in isolation from environments and social relations. Similarly, Cochrane-style (Cochrane Collaboration, 2014) systematic reviews are designed to assemble "original studies (predominantly randomised controlled trials and clinical controlled trials, but also sometimes, non-randomised observational studies)" based on specific scientific criteria. Although the website does note that the reviews take specific patient groups and settings into account, the emphasis tends to be on stripping context and on research that controls for or ignores the social. Moreover, Doull et al. (2010) found that the reviews rarely disaggregated data by sex or gender and when they did, often used the terms interchangeably. Nevertheless, such research can provide valuable information on biological processes even though we need to approach the results with caution, asking for whom the intervention worked, under what conditions, and when, and to recognize that bodies cannot be removed from their environments.

Social determinants of health approaches are more common in social science and health services research. According to Raphael (2009, p. 2), the social determinants of health are "the economic and social conditions that shape the health of individuals, communities, and jurisdictions as a whole." The list of what is included as a determinant varies somewhat, but usually includes education, income, early childhood, nutrition, housing, personal practices, social support, and health services. A York University conference on the determinants (Raphael, 2009, p. 7) lists 12 determinants, adding Aboriginal status, the social safety net, unemployment and employment security, and gender. The Public Health Agency of Canada (2014) provides a somewhat different list of 12, but also includes gender as a separate category. There are two ways of seeing gender as a social determinant. On the one hand, gender has a profound influence on health and access to care. There are health issues specific to women, most common in women, or experienced in specific ways by women. On the other hand, listing gender as a separate variable can mean that it is not recognized as a factor in all the other variables.

A population health approach uses large databases to move away from an individual focus to look at patterns in specific populations, often exposing significant inequalities and the importance of locations. It can reveal overall patterns for women. But as Robertson (1998) argues, this approach gives equal weight to various causal factors and fails to locate these patterns within their social, economic, and political context. A health-promotion approach, which also recognizes the various determinants of health, tends to focus more on the structural factors that contribute to health and illness (Rootman, Dupéré, Pederson, & O'Neill, 2014).

A feminist political economy approach shares a great deal with a social determinants of health approach (Armstrong, Armstrong, & Scott-Dixon, 2008), especially as described by Raphael. However, it differs in that it understands all these determinants as interrelated and shaped by the political economy at the global, national, regional, and local level. The political economy refers to the complex of institutions and relations that constitute not only what is usually referred to as the political and economic systems but also the social, physical, ideological, and cultural systems. It thus encompasses the private and public sectors of the formal economy, as well as households. The feminist aspect means both working for change from women's perspectives and understanding gender as a component in all these integrated systems. Like the social determinants of health approach, however, it runs the risk of ignoring or underestimating the parts that bodies play.

Together these approaches have contributed to the development of gender-based analysis of health and health care. Such analysis is increasingly recognized and supported as crucial to the effective investigation of the complex health issues faced by all people—whatever their gender. The differences in causes, experiences, and outcomes of health and health care among genders are exposed in the process and further analyzed in order to better understand the patterns and contradictions that underlie and perpetuate inequalities in health and care.

The importance of a gender lens emerged with the women's health movement in the 1960s for multiple reasons. Research demonstrated women's greater use of the health care system for themselves and others, the often dismissive treatment they received in health care services, their absence from research, and their limited numbers in medical practice and in policy-making, combined with their dominance in other health care work, to name only the most prominent patterns exposed. Such evidence further justifies a women-specific focus in research, policy, and practices. Although gender-based analysis emerged from the women's movement, it has neither excluded men nor been irrelevant to men. A gender-based analysis looks at issues unique to women, more common in women, experienced in particular ways by women, or less understood in women. It develops these issues in relation to the full range of policies, research, and practices in health and care. And it can do the same for men. But such an analysis also means looking at gender influences that not only shape relations between women and men, boys and girls, but also at the way health and care are constructed for all of them in their multiple forms.

We can identify common patterns, even while recognizing that the categories *women* and *men* do not capture the experiences of everyone. Women's lives are in many ways different from those of men and these differences are reflected in, and reinforced by, their bodies. At the same time, there are significant differences among women that must be taken into account. That is why we need a text on women's health.

Intersections of Policy, Research, and Practice

This book about women's health is unique in a number of ways. First, in keeping with the aim of bridging the gap between research, health care management, and policy, it brings together women writing from a range of disciplines as well as women writing from a range of workplaces. There are medical doctors who teach and practise and a midwife who also does policy and managerial work. The social scientists who teach in universities or work in research institutes have long been involved in working across communities; there are those who have worked as nurses and those who do full-time policy work; there is a woman who runs a clinic who also teaches and does policy work, and one who makes films intended to bring about change. There is a woman who spends most of her time sharing research with the community, and one who works with communities to make their voices heard through photography. There are graduate students and senior academics. There are authors with extensive publications in peer-reviewed journals and authors who write primarily for community groups. And this only touches on some of their relevant and impressive expertise. All these women cross boundaries that move from research to policy, to other action, and back. They have a wealth of knowledge and a range of experiences to draw on for their chapters, making this a rich collection that goes well beyond most academic texts to talk about making a difference in shared knowledge and in daily practices.

Reflecting their many starting points and diverse experiences, there is no single way of seeing, no particular theory or paradigm that unites the chapters. Indeed, one of the strengths of this collection is the exposure to different questions and different ways into questions. What those writing here do share is a commitment to rigorous, gender-based research that is made accessible in a manner intended to empower women and improve women's health. They bring their particular perspectives to bear in ways that illustrate their academic preparation and their workplaces. You will not find here a single standard in terms of length, theoretical approach, style, methods, or evidence. Instead, you will find articles that bear the stamp of disciplines, philosophies, and workplaces, albeit ones that challenge many of the traditional approaches and assumptions in those fields. The collection, in one book, of these different voices is designed to provoke discussion not only about the specifics that are the focus of each piece but also about thinking and working across boundaries both of disciplines and workplaces. It is very much in keeping with the latest talk in health research, where interdisciplinary or transdisciplinary sharing and links among research, policy, and practices are promoted. It insists on extending this talk in that it insists on taking gender into account in all aspects of health research and health work.

Second, the chapters in this book are original. Some chapters began as presentations to an intensive, one-week course organized as part of the Ontario Training Centre (OTC) focused on the intersections of research, policy, and practice. The OTC was a six-university consortium that offered a graduate diploma in health services and policy research, funded by the Canadian Health Services Research Foundation. The emphasis was on interdisciplinary and intersectoral work, as well as on shared learning and exchanges with policy-makers. Each spring, students in the program came together for a week of intensive study. In 2006, the course was on women's health and the lineup of presenters was the product of consultations with an advisory group that included those from policy, practice, and research circles. It was led by Pat Armstrong, whose Chair in Health Services and Nursing Research was focused on taking gender into account in research, policies, and practices. The material was presented for discussion and debate in ways that allowed the authors to benefit from the exchange. The very positive response of participants was the motivation for transforming the presentations into a book so others could benefit from the rich, diverse knowledge in the course. The chapters that appeared in the first edition have been revised and updated, and some basically rewritten. In addition, in response to comments by reviewers, we have added new chapters to fill what were perceived as important gaps or the need to address emerging issues.

Third, this book is about women in Canada. Although there is a rapidly growing body of literature on women's health, much of it focuses on women in other countries. Given that we know environments shape women's health and care, it is crucial to have research and writing that locates women in this country. The chapters here emphasize research and experiences in Canada, with some references to the literature from other countries to situate the Canadian experiences. Much of the data reported on in the various chapters are based on original research by these authors. In concentrating on Canada, the authors take into account differences among women as well as conditions they share, emphasizing the intersection of gender with other physical and social locations and relations.

In sum, this book brings together gender-based knowledge about women's health by academics, health-care professionals, and government decision-makers. Rather than attempting to provide a compendium of issues women face, it blends the work of these experts into a text that directs the reader through various complexities and gaps, advancements, and possibilities for women as well as for health and health care, and it ties them together in ways that emphasize the importance of a gender analysis and of differences among women.

This second edition of *Women's Health: Intersections of Policy, Research, and Practice* examines women's health issues from multiple perspectives, drawing upon research and practices that include both qualitative and quantitative methodologies in data collection and knowledge formation. It incorporates work that has been produced from grassroots investigations of women's health issues and from large-scale, quantitative studies; it touches upon specific health issues and diversity issues, and a variety of issues unexplored in most texts of this genre. In an effort to exemplify alternative forms of methodologies and to emphasize the importance of recognizing the differences that are too often combined with inequality, this book also highlights the work of women whose voices may not normally be heard or recognized as viable sources for understanding issues in health in a way that stretches beyond the traditional parameters of knowledge-sharing practices.

It also points to work still to be done if we are to understand health issues for women in general and for particular groups of women, and if we are to develop strategies to ensure that women have access to health and health services that are appropriate and effective. Indeed, as many of the authors in this new edition make clear, there is a real risk that women's health issues are falling off agendas along with the disappearance of money to support work on research and reform.

References

Armstrong, P., H. Armstrong, & K. Scott-Dixon. (2008). *Critical to Care: The Invisible Women in Health Services*. Toronto: University of Toronto Press.

Cochrane Collaboration. (2014). Cochrane Reviews. Retrieved from http://www.cochrane.org/cochrane-reviews.

Doull, M., V. Runnels, S. Tudiver, & M. Boscoe. (2010). Appraising the Evidence: Applying Sex and Gender-Based Analysis (SGBA) to Cochrane Systematic Reviews on Cardiovascular Diseases. *Journal of Women's Health* 19(5): 997–1003.

Fausto-Sterling, A. (2005). The Bare Bones of Sex: Part 1—Sex and Gender. *Signs* 30(2): 1491–1527.

Public Health Agency of Canada. (2014). *What Determines Health?* Retrieved from http://www.phac-aspc.gc.ca/ph-sp/determinants/index-eng.php#What.

Raphael, D. (2009). *Social Determinants of Health* (2nd ed.). Toronto: Canadian Scholars' Press Inc.

Robertson, A. (1998). Shifting Discourses on Health in Canada: From Health Promotion to Population Health. *Health Promotion International* 13(2): 155–166.

Rootman, I., S. Dupéré, A. Pederson, & M. O'Neill (Eds.). (2014). *Health Promotion in Canada: Critical Perspectives on Practice* (3rd ed.). Toronto: Canadian Scholars' Press Inc.

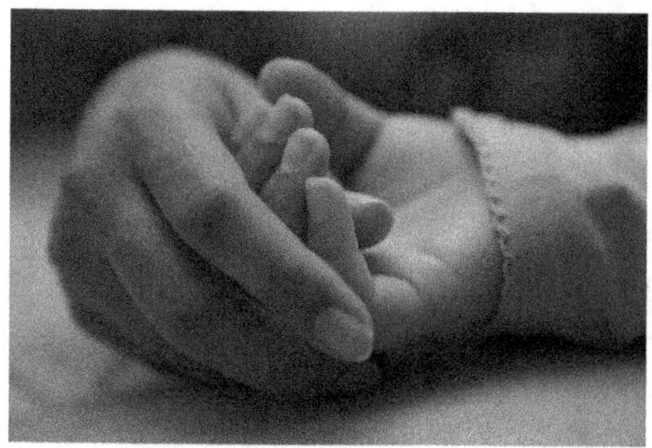

Setting the Stage for Women's Health Research

This section establishes a broad base for understanding women's health. It traces some of the history of the women's health movement and some of the links between women's health advocacy and research, policy, and practice. It introduces the challenges of fostering change within the bureaucracy of government and the tools of gender-based analysis and gender mainstreaming. And it illustrates aspects of the debates about the meanings and usefulness of differentiating between the concepts of "sex" and "gender" from the perspective of evidence and of action for change.

The first chapter, by sociologist Lorraine Greaves, grounds the importance of gender-based research with an analytical review of the history of the women's health movement and women's health research within the context of discussions about gender. As executive director of the BC Centre of Excellence for Women's Health for more than a decade and the recipient of an honorary degree from the University of Ottawa in recognition of her extraordinary contribution to women's health, she is particularly well placed to set the stage for the examinations of women's health issues in policy, research, and practice that follow. In Chapter 2, former senior policy analyst Sari Tudiver offers reflections on the federal government role in fostering women's health. It complements and expands on the introduction in Chapter 1 by exploring the highest public policy level in Canada. Chapters 1 and 2 raise concerns about changes in Canada to the resources allocated to women's health research and the development of women-specific health information and what they may mean for women's health in the future.

The third chapter ties the previous two together through the application of a gender-based analysis (GBA) to a specific area of government policy, namely, wait times for hip and knee replacements. This chapter extends the analysis of wait times offered in the first edition by describing a review of key concepts and evidence in the gender and wait times literature. It illustrates how gender-based analysis begins with disaggregation of data by sex but necessarily moves beyond it to locate those data within the evidence and research on the lives of women and men or of each alone that is absent from most research and from systematic reviews of the research. Gender-based analysis requires multiple methods, often used together, as well the development of new methods, as is evident in other chapters in this book. Yet most systematic reviews, and the research on which they are based, fail to integrate a range of methods. This chapter, co-authored by Ann Pederson and Pat Armstrong, is a shorter version of a paper written by a team from Women and Health Care Reform and the BC Centre of Excellence for Women's Health. It raises significant questions about how to study "gender" using existing methods for systematic review.

The next chapter illustrates the value of paying close attention to "sex" in women's health research and health care. Karin Humphries, who holds of the UBC Heart and Stroke Foundation Professorship in Women's Cardiovascular Health, is an epidemiologist with training in biochemistry, kinesiology, and experimental pathology. She applies a critical lens to the specific issue of heart disease in women.

Together, these four chapters provide an outline of women's health issues and illustrate both the methodology and importance of a gender-based analysis through the application to specific health issues for women. As you read this section, you might consider the following questions:

1. Is the women's health movement as relevant today as it was over the past four decades when it established women's health as a separate medical, social, and political area of research, policy, and care?
2. What are the strengths and weaknesses of a gender-based analysis approach? Of gender mainstreaming? Of intersectionality?
3. What are the benefits and limitations of distinguishing between "sex" and "gender"?
4. How might we account for differences in health outcomes and health care utilization between women and men and between various groups of women?

CHAPTER 1

Women, Gender, and Health Research

Lorraine Greaves

Introduction

This chapter is about women's health, women's health research, gender and health, and the women's health movement. It is about both science and politics. The many opportunities for doing women's health research available in 2015 were hard won, based on 50 years of advocacy, research, and writing. They have been achieved in the context of feminist activism and a recognition of the importance of population health and the determinants of health, particularly gender. Together, these activities have identified the key factors that influence health and the uneven opportunity for health and health equity. During these decades, a range of theoretical approaches incorporating politics, economics, sociology, rights, and ethics have defined health as going well beyond the body and the presence or absence of disease (Raphael, Bryant, & Rioux, 2006). But in 2015, women's health in Canada is in an unstable place, diminished by funding cuts, in a field splintered by diverted attention to men's health, gender and health, equity, and intersectional factors.

Women's health was not always on the agenda. Or, if it was, it was drenched in sexism, inaccuracy, or social control. Crucial services such as the provision of contraception services were only decriminalized in 1969, and restricting abortion was declared unconstitutional in 1988 as it violated women's rights to life, liberty, and the security of the person. Midwifery was reintroduced in Canada after 1960, but its availability is still uneven across Canada, well below utilization in other countries, leaving low-risk normal childbirth often controlled by specialists (Bourgeault, 2006). All of these advances occurred only after intense activism, legal challenges, criminal convictions, and social pressure. Women's self-knowledge was typically privately shared until books such as *Our Bodies, Ourselves* emerged in 1973, providing women with frank and useful information about any subject pertaining to their health, and igniting a North American women's health movement (Boston Women's Health Collective, 2011).

Clearly, gender matters to women's health. So does sex. Gender refers to the social and cultural and economic influences that affect women and men, and is among the determinants of health, signalling the importance of being female or male or transgender for one's health, and of and experiencing life with these labels. It is a key influence on people's access to health and health care, and their experiences of life in general. Sex refers to our biological and genetic characteristics. Our designated sex signals the specific capacities of our bodies, and affects the propensity and trajectory of diseases and health conditions. This chapter describes how both sex and gender came to matter to women's health research, and what some of the conceptual issues are in understanding women's health. While it is a story of science, it is also a story that invokes values, politics, policy, and opportunity.

The History of Women's Health in Canada

In 1970, the *Report of the Royal Commission on the Status of Women* was released with 167 recommendations for improving the status of Canadian women, only five of which were linked to women's health. Nonetheless, the release of this report set the stage for improving services for women, more research on women's issues, and more equity-based legislative improvements. An emergent women's health movement was to become a key part of these activities, which has, since 1970, identified numerous issues to improve women's health and increase the control women have over their health.

The issues and concepts of importance to women's health have evolved considerably in the intervening years. The story rolled out in stages, dependent upon political and strategic opportunities, as well as broader intellectual shifts in understanding health and health research. Initial approaches to women's health coalesced around a *reaction* to the health care system, health care professions, and societal norms and values that led to negative outcomes for women's health. Some of the initial topics were against such prevailing forces as over-medicalization, paternalism, lack of information, lack of consent, lack of inclusion, or, more generally, the widespread sexism embedded within societal norms and values that expressed itself in health care and access to health information. This phase was aimed at raising awareness of women's health issues, and getting women inserted into the debates about health, health care, and health research.

In subsequent decades, the framework for activity in women's health became more *proactive*, developing women-specific responses to health concerns, women-centred care, women's programming, and more inclusive policy-making. This built upon awareness raised in the reactive phase and manifested in many new women's health enterprises such as health centres, magazines, journals, as well as government strategies and programs devoted to women's health. These activities were underpinned by a conceptual understanding of what went into being "women-specific" and "women-centred," and using these principles to build new versions of services and knowledge about women's health.

Box 1.1
Initial Themes

Some of the initial important topics and themes in women's health were against prevailing forces such as over-medicalization, paternalism, lack of information, lack of consent, lack of inclusion, or, more generally, sexism embedded within societal norms and values that expressed itself in health care and access to health information. Later on, a more proactive approach began to define and request women-specific and women-centred responses to women's health, and more inclusive policies and programs.

In time, there was a push to integrate or mainstream women's health issues into more general health-related activity, care provision, or policy-making. The goal of mainstreaming was to build capacity and knowledge among non-women's health specialists, and to spread the recognition that being female was an important component of almost all health and health care issues. This effort also made attempts to mainstream awareness of gender, and affected the status quo in health research, health care, and our understanding of what affects health. Gradually, gender began to get much wider play and recognition across health research, and was rigorously employed to promote the women's health agenda.

At the same time, the population health movement (Public Health Agency of Canada, 2004) and assessment of the impact of the determinants of health (Commission on Social Determinants of Health, 2008; Public Health Agency of Canada, 1999) gained global prominence and were seen as fitting frameworks for advancing women's health concerns. Not coincidentally, Canada was a leader in these domains, housing the birth of the important 1986 Ottawa Charter, which drove a view of health and health promotion that incorporated social context and social determinants (including gender) in the examination of health and health care. Despite continuing widespread support for such an approach in 2015, an analysis of subsequent charters and documents in the intervening decades indicates that gender has been almost completely ignored in health promotion in the intervening years (Gelb, Pederson, & Greaves, 2011).

During the 1990s, the women's health movement often converged with other movements to promote a broader view of health for women. At the advocacy level, the women's health movement formed alliances with anti-poverty, anti-racism, and other equity-based movements, enlarging the base of support for women's health as well as integrating a range of diverse issues into women's health. These developments set the stage for an important debate during the 1990s about women's health research, and how knowledge about women's health could best be generated. While concerns about specific research-related issues such as clinical trials inclusion criteria, or safety issues related to treatment and drug testing had been simmering among women's health advocates and researchers for decades, it was in the 1990s that opportunities arose for making headway in more radically changing the health research landscape.

As an "inequities" framework evolved, there was marked and increased attention to both social and economic concerns in women's health and identifying gender as a key divide in understanding the population's health. On a political level, this approach also implied that "redress" was required to right historical imbalances and to rapidly evolve new knowledge about women's health to meet a variety of research, advocacy, care, and policy concerns. The women's health agenda ultimately became embedded in discussions of "gender"; indeed, in this phase, "women" and "gender" were often used synonymously in health discussions, not just in Canada but globally.

This shift to including equity (and sometimes equality) concerns was reflective of an increasingly complex discourse surrounding women's rights, gender oppression, and a search for options for improving women's lot. However, the presence of biological factors and their impact on health raised key questions about whether health outcomes and access to health in and among women were reflections of biological or social factors. Reflecting on this with respect to health matters, Sen, Östlin, and George (2007) state: "Thus, gender equity in health cannot be based only on the principle of sameness but must stand directly on the foundation of absence of bias" (p. 7). In short, disentangling sex and gender and describing the interactions of sex and gender and their effects, as well as planting this analysis in the context of other, intersecting oppressions became increasingly important to understanding women's health.

During the 1990s, numerous government initiatives to improve women's health emerged in Canada, ranging from provincial advisory councils on women's health to the development of numerous women's health strategies, outlining both provincial and federal priorities for action. This decade was an active phase of institutionalizing the women's health movement and supporting it with government funding. However, these government initiatives have mostly now come and gone, reflecting political shifts and changing priorities. Even the Women's Health Bureau (later renamed the Bureau of Women's Health and Gender Analysis), established in 1993 in Health Canada as the focal point for women's health within the federal government (Health Canada, 2007), was gradually dismantled by 2013. Its mandate was to address how sex and gender affect women's health across the lifespan, determine the health and health care issues pertinent to women, and to carry forward the gender-based analysis policy of Health Canada, which was released in 1999. The Bureau was the lead on Health Canada's Women's Health Strategy, Health Canada's Gender-Based Analysis Policy, the Women's Health Indicators Project, and the Women's Health Contribution Program. The latter program housed and supported five federally funded Centres of Excellence for Women's Health, the Canadian Women's Health Network, Women and Health Care Reform, the Aboriginal Women's Health and Healing Research Group, and Women and Health Protection.

In short, between 1970 and 2000, many health issues were advanced by a strong Canadian women's health movement in the context of increasing public and financial support for research, policy, and programming. These activities added to knowledge and practices regarding both women's health and gender and health. The community-based sector identified issues such as access to health and health care for various subpopulations of women, such as women with disabilities, immigrant and refugee women, Aboriginal women, women with low incomes, girls, and lesbians, among others. Specific issues affecting women's health that were unknown in 1970, such as reproductive technologies, prenatal testing, emergency contraception, and genetic and epigenetic knowledge, were added to the agenda along the way. In addition, many issues that had long affected women's health but were under-acknowledged in 1970, such as sexual assault and violence against women, effects of child sexual abuse and trauma, tobacco use, alcohol and drug use, postpartum depression, the over-prescription of psychotropic drugs, and the effects of the environment on women's health, became priorities. Indeed, as Ratcliffe states, "the topic of women's health is a cornucopia of questions" (2002, p. 2).

This vast agenda was daunting, but the key to advancing this agenda, and keeping it alive, is research. One site was in the Centres of Excellence for Women's Health, which pushed forward a wide research agenda on women's health that elaborated on themes of population health, gender as a social determinant of health, and the impact of policy. This included promoting the development and usage of concepts such as sex and gender, as well as substantive research on a myriad of issues to expand, build, and translate the knowledge base about women's health. Further, as mandated, the Centres did policy research and offered policy advice to all levels of government on women's health issues. In 2000, the Institute for Gender and Health (IGH) at the Canadian Institutes of Health Research (CIHR) came into being, and the Canadian government began to fund knowledge development from biomedical to population health for both males and females.

However, the years since 2000 have seen a dilution of a focus on *women's* health in Canada. Significantly, federal government support for, and investment in, women's health programs waned, culminating in the end of funding for the Women's Health Contribution Program in 2013. This lack of investment arrived in an environment of changing conceptual understandings of health and shifting government priorities. An initial indicator was the establishment of the Institute of Gender and Health in the CIHR in 2000, which reflected a political compromise. Instead of establishing an Institute for Women's Health as was advocated by a large coalition of Canadian women's health scientists and advocates (Grant & Ballem, 2000; Greaves et al., 1999), the government chose to focus on gender and health, embracing a territory that included men's and boys' health, diluting the investment and emphasis on women's health, erasing the feminist inspiration for this initiative, and burying the rationale of redressing historical deficits in women's health research. This would herald a decade of diminishing emphasis and investment in women's health as a clear and discrete government priority.

Evolving Concepts in Women's Health Research

Alongside these shifts, there was a growing community of scholars in a wide range of disciplines that began to develop a new language for investigating and understanding women's health. Feminist academics, often in league with health providers and advocacy organizations, built more complex theories and conceptual frameworks that were ultimately applied to health, identifying both sex and gender, along with other factors, as key components of understanding women's health. Debates about these theories, concepts, and measures continue, promising to become even more complex and refined in the years to come.

Other conceptual advances influence women's health as well. In the 1990s, a growing literature had begun to describe the "opportunity for health" as an equity issue where women, in particular, had fallen short. This approach extended the recognition of gender to also count a range of determinants affecting diverse groups of women in the context of their economic status, culture, and ethnicity. While this equity-based health approach has (re)introduced and sharpened the concepts of status and equality, which had motivated the women's health movement in its earlier days, it also gave rise to a growing interest in the interactions and intersections of determinants as a defining direction for understanding and researching the health of women. In other words, differences *among* women became an important dimension of women's health. This approach not only added an important complexity to women's health research, it also signalled that the comparison of "women" to "men" was not the only or, indeed, always even the most salient approach to determining what mattered in women's health research. Indeed, the concept of "differences" between men and women became secondary to a wider and more fluid understanding of the intersecting influences of gender and other social determinants and factors on and among both women and men, and gender-diverse people.

A tension emerged, however. These shifts in complexity of thought about women's health gave governments in particular a chance to highlight health equity over gender equity, and use the discourse on intersecting influences on health to support this view. After 2000, it became increasingly difficult to keep women's health or even gender on the agenda as both equity and gender mainstreaming supported rationales for advancing both women and men in health, especially those experiencing inequity. Indeed, between 2000 and 2010 numerous provincial and federal initiatives, investments, and strategies on women's health were gradually eroded, ignored, or erased, or had their titles changed, diminishing targeted activity and funding on women's health.

Internationally, human rights became more visible as a driving conceptual framework for defining health and the rights to health. This approach utilized legal and treaty-based precedents to argue that health is a human right. When these treaties are read in the context of women's equality treaties, women-specific rights to health are able to be highlighted. This has had a defining impact on the direction of action and policy in tobacco control, reproductive rights, sexual health, violence, and maternity care, among other issues. It has set the stage for examining the effects of global processes on women's health such as globalization, migration, urbanization, and conflict. Within Canada, similar rights- and equity-based arguments have been mounted to frame the health issues of Aboriginal women, low-income women, and women with disabilities. Almost 50 years after the Royal Commission, a status-oriented, rights-based framework is still extremely relevant to promoting action on health issues of concern to women.

Sex, Gender, and Women

By the 1990s the concepts of sex, gender, and women's health had become a focus of discussion within health research communities in particular, but interdisciplinary research on women's health quickly revealed discipline-specific differential uses of these terms. For example, "sex" and "gender" were often used interchangeably (Davidson et al., 2006). However, in some cases, usages developed that were discipline-specific. Gender, for example, is still used in some biological science or medical circles to indicate what social scientists refer to as sex, a biological concept. Although the distinction between sex and gender has been made within the social sciences, this is not necessarily the case for biomedical sciences, which have often merged the usages of these terms. This problem is compounded by linguistic issues, where some languages do not have parallel or adequate terms to describe the emerging conceptual differences.

These debates are more than "academic." Indeed, U.S. observers suggest that the frequent amalgamation of these terms can have serious implications for health research, since failing to differentiate these concepts can have an impact on the quality and understanding of research results with subsequent impacts on health and health care for both women and men. Without a strong understanding of the definitions of "sex" and "gender," confusions are replicated, ultimately impacting the equitable treatment of women and men in health research and practice (Fishman, Wick, & Koenig, 1999). In Canada, some key documents have influenced the usage of terminology in women's health research. For example, *CIHR 2000: Sex, Gender, and Women's Health* (Greaves et al., 1999), which was written to inform the development and design of the Canadian Institutes of Health Research, highlighted the importance of examining sex, gender, and women's health in a systematic and effective way in order to transform and integrate Canadian health research.

The document *Better Science with Sex and Gender* (Johnson, Greaves, & Repta, 2007), produced by the Women's Health Research Network in British Columbia, argues that including the concepts of sex and gender in research leads to a variety of benefits such as increased rigour and validity of research, cost savings, greater social justice, and the potential to save lives. Further, it offered suggestions to researchers on how sex (the combination of biological factors that are different for each individual, body size, genitalia, hormones) and gender (the socially prescribed and experienced dimensions of being "male" or "female" in a society) can be incorporated into research in a variety of ways. Following this, efforts were made to instruct researchers how to apply these concepts, and a 2012 methods book supported this movement with a range of detailed approaches (Oliffe & Greaves, 2011).

These documents were important political as well as scientific advocacy instruments. The arguments embedded reflect values of inclusiveness and equity, and are ultimately inspired by historical claims for redress for women. In these documents, these values and claims are applied to science, specifically health research, even when applying to men's health or gender and health. The arguments evoked long-standing power issues inherent in defining knowledge and accumulating evidence. The naming of inclusiveness and equity issues as scientifically relevant reflects a generation of thinking about what constitutes "evidence," recognizing it to be a very fluid concept, reflective of power and vested interests. Indeed, as Evelyn Fox Keller stated over 30 years ago in explaining her work on gender and science, "[i]t's not women I am learning about so much as men. Even more, it is science" (Keller, 1985).

Gender-Based Analysis and Change

The concept of gender was introduced into health research by social philosophers and social scientists. However, it has over the past few decades become increasingly central to research, policy, and program and service development in women's health as it fit with the increased prominence of the social and population models of health. As the determinants of health approach grew and gained support, gender was identified as a key determinant and used to support a gendered view of women's health. This trend was evident not only in Canada, but across the world.

The adoption of the concept and term demanded changing practices in policy development and health planning as well as research. In order to build capacity for using gender, the notion of applying a tool and process called "gender-based analysis" (GBA) was established and developed. GBA is a government policy in Canada, is supported by training and resources led by Health Canada and other federal departments, and in 2009 was the subject of the chief auditor's report (Auditor General of Canada, 2009).

The document *Exploring Concepts of Gender and Health* (Health Canada, 2003) was one of the first Canadian documents outlining how GBA can be integrated into every step of the health research and policy development process by assessing the differential impact of proposed or existing policies and programs on women and men. It suggests that not incorporating these steps can lead to significant shortcomings. Consideration of sex and gender enhances understanding of all the determinants of health, their interaction with other determinants, and the effectiveness of policies, programs, and treatments. More recently, *Rising to the Challenge* offered examples of how to apply GBA to a range of issues, with detailed case examples (Clow, Pederson, Haworth-Brockman, & Bernier, 2009).

It is suggested that GBA promoted better research and better scientific knowledge by asking wider questions and using comprehensive analytic methods, thus providing more accurate and relevant health information. This is aimed at enhancing health outcomes and strengthening health care. Therefore conducting health research in a manner that is sensitive to manifestations of sex and gender (Health Canada, 2003) and incorporating sex and gender into research will assist in producing more rigorous findings. Indeed, Health Canada suggests that excluding gender and sex from health research is a serious omission that can lead to problems of validity and generalizability (Health Canada, 2003). Implicit in GBA is an understanding that, in addition to gender, both sex and a range of diversity issues are also addressed.

Since 2000, the CIHR has officially promoted research that systematically inquires about biological (sex-based) and socio-cultural (gender-based) influences on and differences between women and men, boys and girls, without presuming the nature of any differences that may exist. They use the term "SGBA" (sex- and gender-based analysis) and state that their purpose is to promote rigorous sex- and/or gender-sensitive health research that expands an understanding of health determinants in both sexes to provide knowledge that can result in improvements in health and health care (CIHR, 2006). They request that all applicants for research funding indicate how they are addressing sex and gender in their applications, and offer assistance on how to do this in a range of documents (CIHR, 2014b; CIHR IGH, 2012). The CIHR now operates as part of the "Health Portfolio," a cluster of health-related departments or agencies of the federal government, and increasingly coordinates its priorities and resources in concert with each other and with government.

Box 1.2
Sex and Gender Matter

Both sex and gender relations influence the risk of contracting infectious diseases and their outcomes. For example, women face specific sex- and gender-based inequities when it comes to contracting HIV and seeking medical care for HIV infection. First, the vagina is physiologically more susceptible than the penis to contracting sexually transmitted infections (STIs) (Darroch & Frost, 1999). In addition, because of gender relations, women usually have less power in and control over sexual relationships, putting them at greater risk of contracting HIV (Amaro & Raj, 2000). Finally, due to gender roles, women may delay seeking treatment for HIV/AIDS due to family and child-care obligations.

Source: J. Johnson, L. Greaves, & R. Repta, 2007, *Better Science with Sex and Gender: A Primer for Women's Health Research* (Vancouver: Women's Health Research Network), p. 10.

Sex, gender, and diversity analyses were meant to be pursued at the same time. Sex and gender interact to produce health or disease and both intersect with cultural, ethnic, and socio-economic characteristics. These more complex intersections have particular and increasing importance for investigating and responding to the diversity of women's health concerns in Canada as the population is increasingly multicultural, and where discrimination and socio-economic status interact with gender and sex to affect health. These intersectional-type analyses have been used to supersede GBA at times on the basis that other factors in addition to gender may matter as much or more than gender in assessing and improving health. This theoretical approach has, as a consequence, unfortunately diverted interest and investment from women's health research and practice. The interest in health equity in governments has added to this dilution by suggesting that equity and inequities in health are caused by a myriad of factors and determinants in addition to, or instead of, or more important than, gender.

Indeed, the global health equity movement has moved forward without a gender analysis in most cases, reflected in the often gender-blind fields of health impact assessments or health in all policies (Health Canada, 2004). These new dimensions in theoretical and conceptual thoughts have often served as platforms for those in government or practice who want to avoid redressing women's health issues and deficiencies, or who ignore gender as a determinant of health, or, most importantly, think that every other determinant of health is gendered. This gender-blind approach can slow down the process of improving the science of sex and gender as it often ignores and fails to measure the impact of gender on equity or on the gendered elements of all the diverse factors that intersect to produce health.

Gender Mainstreaming

Gender mainstreaming is a process whereby gender concerns are integrated horizontally into health research and policy development in order to minimize the inequalities that exist between men and women (Health Canada, 2003). Gender mainstreaming has been identified by some as the most effective strategy to achieving gender equity (Bekker, 2003). It asserts that gender needs to be considered in every phase of research and policy development in order to respond adequately to problems caused by gender inequality. Internationally, Canada was a leader at incorporating gender into policy and research. Health Canada's publications, policies, and models aimed at integrating gender into the health research and policy development process are widely regarded.

Others however, suggest that an assessment of the practice of gender mainstreaming is at a crossroads (Mehra & Gupta, 2006). Since its adoption in the mid-1990s, when it was introduced to bring women's issues more firmly into the machinery and operations of policy and program development, there has been considerable emphasis on training and capacity building. But a decade later, there was still a gap between policy goals and implementation, with variable assessments of comprehensiveness and effectiveness (Mehra & Gupta, 2006). In Canada, the auditor general assessed the use of the gender-based analysis policy across the government of Canada in 2009, 10 years after its inception, and found it spotty and, when done, wanting. Without political will and effective leadership, transformative processes are unlikely to develop through gender mainstreaming. Gender mainstreaming was and still is often used as a cover for paying attention to women, especially in development where attending to women was even more politically fraught than in Canada.

Despite the uneven results of gender mainstreaming and GBA, or perhaps because of them, recent shifts in gender and health have begun to focus on improving women's health via shifting gender norms. This more radical approach is often critical for addressing issues such as HIV infection, sexual and domestic violence, as well as reproductive health and contraception planning, but it is also relevant to tobacco and alcohol use (Bialystok, Greaves, & Poole, 2014; Bialystok, Poole, Greaves, & Thomas, 2014; Durey, 2014; Greaves, 2014; Hemsing & Greaves, 2014). These initiatives address not only the influence of gender, but also gendered norms, roles, cultural practices, and legislative initiatives, and aim to reverse negative impacts on women and girls and their health and well-being. Gender-transformative health promotion, planning, and initiatives are the most recent manifestations of integrating gender into health in ways that also enhance gender equity at the same time (Greaves, Pederson, & Poole, 2014). This dual and multi-layered approach is now at the forefront of integrating gender into health initiatives, policies, and programs.

Methodological and Measurement Issues

The conceptualization of sex and gender has evolved considerably over the past 20 years. Contemporary thinking about these terms indicates that both sex and gender are important in health research, but they ought not to be considered binary concepts (Johnson et al., 2007; Oliffe & Greaves, 2011). Indeed, it is helpful to understand these concepts as continua, not dichotomous, and graded, each with various strengths of influences on a person or a body system. Hence, referring to sex and/or gender "differences" is generally less useful than sex and gender "influences," or even "sexes and genders," indicating that there is a multiplicity of conceptual understandings and fluid realities attached to both sex and gender. This move to a more nuanced and accurate view of sex and gender not only improved science, but also makes space for understanding the health and experiences of gender-diverse people. The Institute for Gender and Health has made important inroads in this domain for researchers, recognizing gender diversity in science, and simultaneously generating more complex views of the concepts of sex and gender in health (CIHR, 2014a).

These evolutions raise difficult methodological and measurement issues. While sex is somewhat easier to identify and measure, gender is less so. Measurements of sex typically include anatomy (body size, body shape, and reproductive organs), physiology (hormones, biochemical pathways, organ function, and metabolism), and genetics (sex chromosomes). Meanwhile, measurements of gender are less concrete and, by its very definition, shifting. Further, there are multiple levels of gender. Gender can include gender identity (dress, roles, behaviours, values, masculinity/femininity), institutionalized gender (rules, structures, policies), and gender relations (cultural scripts, generational structures, opportunities) (Johnson et al., 2007). All of these aspects of gender are cultural and temporal, and therefore dependent upon a range of other influences.

Adding another layer of complexity to measurement is the interaction of sex and gender with each other and with other determinants in producing health outcomes. Social experiences can affect brain processes, or genetics and biological endowments can affect behaviour. For example, gendered occupational participation may put women and men in different parts of the labour force, exposed to different environments, which interact with (sex-based) biological susceptibilities to the elements of those environments, such as exposure to chemicals or patterns of activity. In short, sex can not only affect gender and vice versa, but also interacts with gender to produce health and health conditions (Johnson et al., 2007). Complicating this is that gender and sex are subject to change, not just in individual bodies over a life course, but also in societies over time. Gender in particular is regarded as a fluid social construct that is determined by the systems and cultures that surround us. As a result, this fluidity allows gender roles to be challenged in order to address inequity. However, it is increasingly recognized that the concept of sex is also dynamic in that variable amounts of sex hormones may be present in a body, may be ambiguous, or indeed may be manipulated by individuals or society to create specific changes in sex. Indeed, the notion that two sexes or two genders "are not enough" has now been increasingly accepted as fundamental to the development of these concepts (Devor, 1989; Preves, 2000).

Improved and expanded methods and measurement are key issues facing both the fields of women's health research and gender and health research in 2015. Improving the utility of these concepts and accuracy in measurement will lead to better research, more accurate treatments, and ultimately improved health outcomes, programs, and policies for women and girls. Measurement issues also apply to what is not measured. The history of exclusion of women from health research is well established (Laurence & Weinhouse, 1994). Females have been excluded not only in human but also animal research. This has often been based on assertions that cycles and reproductive issues complicate research models and designs. But failing to incorporate females and/or women in health research has clearly prevented certain knowledge about women from being gained, and left female-specific manifestations of disease, health, and treatment undiscovered.

There are several stops along this process. First, specific questions do not get asked. Second, inclusion criteria and appropriate methods and measures do not get applied. If and when results are achieved, they may be misapplied. For example, male-specific knowledge can be masqueraded as gender-neutral, and can lead to treatments and policies that do not reflect women and femaleness. In some cases, this can lead to misdiagnosis and mistreatment. The history of heart disease research and treatment is a good case in point, where ignoring sex and gender has led to unbalanced and incomplete medical responses to women. Neglecting to include sex and/or gender as a variable within health research can lead to bias, problems of validity and generalizability, and inadequate treatment and health care. Clearly, gender bias in research reduces the quality of evidence-based medicine (Holdcroft, 2007).

Minorities and children have also often been excluded, and the United States introduced a policy in 1993 to remedy this in health research funded by the National Institutes of Health (NIH), with recent calls for inclusion of sex-specific cell lines and rodents in preclinical research (NIH, 2014). In Canada, we have addressed these concerns most recently through clinical trials policy at the CIHR and through requesting that GBA considerations be included in research proposals for some funding agencies and in some strategic calls. Practical suggestions for rectifying these issues in research include critiquing and reanalyzing previous research results, creating a research plan that includes sex, gender, and diversity analyses, or, ideally, incorporating sex and gender from the beginning to minimize and remedy the measurement issues mentioned above (Johnson et al., 2007; Oliffe & Greaves, 2011).

Interdisciplinarity and Transdisciplinarity

The push for interdisciplinarity in health care practices and in health research has both encouraged more sex and gender considerations in health research and created some of the difficulties in measurement and conceptual congruence discussed above. The disciplinary nature of health care and health research perpetuates a fragmented understanding of the concepts of sex and gender, and interdisciplinarity and multidisciplinarity have been seen as solutions to this, especially in health care. Indeed, it may be that transdisciplinarity is the better practice vis-à-vis women's health. Transdisciplinarity is seen to transcend multiple disciplines in ways that integrate and synthesize content, as well as theory and method (Russell, 2000). This sets the stage for new methods, concepts, language, and measurement tools to be created and to draw all health researchers to a higher level of analysis that truly reflects the broad and fluid impacts of sex, gender, and diversity on women's health. It also sets a parallel goal in health care—that of endorsing multidisciplinary teams or shared care models for health care providers. The growing complexity of sex and gender and health will require more transdisciplinary research and professional training (Greaves, Poole, & Boyle, 2015), setting the stage for a broader understanding of what evidence and practices are required for policy and program improvements in women's health. It is possible that the calls for a holistic, integrated approach to women's health, long made by the women's health movement, may be addressed through adopting these new approaches.

Why Women's Health?

Despite 50 years of activism, research, and policy-making, the politics of women's health remain salient. "Why women's health?" remains a tired and familiar question. There are specific arguments for pursuing women's health research that are different from those for pursuing gender and health research. In 2000, a Canada-wide group of women's health researchers worked together to develop a proposal entitled *Women's Health Research Institute in the CIHR* (Grant & Ballem, 2000). The proposal built upon *CIHR 2000: Sex, Gender, and Women's Health*, and outlined the importance of establishing a Women's Health Research Institute (WHRI) in CIHR, as well as integrating sex and gender across all institutes within CIHR (mainstreaming). The proposal outlined the specific contributions that the WHRI would bring to CIHR and health research in general. Specific categories within women's health research were outlined, including health issues that are unique to women, more common among women, or less understood in women.

Since 2000, even more knowledge has been generated that lengthens the list of health issues unique to women that have heretofore gone unrecognized (Wizemann & Pardue, 2001). Issues such as the trajectory of lung cancer, the links between breast density and breast cancer, women's lower utilizations of joint-replacement surgeries, or the higher utilizations of health care by women with breast implants are but a few of many, many examples. Biologically based differences alone are enough to warrant increased attention to women-specific health research in order to pursue both better science and political redress. Dedicated women's health research and policy programs will continue to advance science by addressing these gaps in knowledge and understanding, many of which we have still not identified.

Why Gender and Health?

As this question refers to both men and women, and the benefits will accrue to both men and women, there is often more openness and less resistance to asking it. Both women and men are subject to the health effects of gender (CIHR IGH, 2012; Phillips, 2005). Research examining men's health has been fragmented by the various lenses (i.e., psychological, anthropological, medical) through which it has been examined, which has led to an understanding of specific health issues experienced by men, but has neglected to provide insight into masculinities and men's experiences more broadly (Courtenay, 2002). However, given the historical exclusion of females and women from much health research and from most clinical trials, there is arguably more information about men and men's health than about women's. Indeed, a key learning of GBA is that most research and policy efforts have used males or maleness *as the norm*, and assumptions and subsequent policies and programs have been developed on that basis. Indeed, there is evidence from multiple fields that broad responses to health issues (i.e., tobacco control policies, heart health diagnostics and treatment) have been aimed at the (male) majority, and only later are subpopulations, women, or other groups considered as "special populations" needing specific attention.

These illustrations point to the necessity for assessing gender and health as a separate field of work. Indeed, gender and health research will reveal comparisons and relationships between males and females that are of intrinsic importance to setting the agenda for women's health research, policy, and programming. However, a strict gender and health approach will not identify the many yet-to-be-discovered women-specific knowledge gaps that will form the agenda for women's health research, or help to develop the field of women's health research and practice into a fully fledged specialty and approach. Nor will it pursue the issues related to policy, redress, and equity that are of intrinsic importance to women's health due to women's ongoing inequitable position in society, both in Canada and globally.

What Does the Future Hold?

Over the past few decades, there has been a growth in awareness, a phase of high activity, and government support, followed by a denouement of women's health initiatives in Canada. Conceptual and theoretical advances in gender, intersectional- and equity-oriented approaches to health have removed women's health from the agenda in research and policy and replaced it with gender, or in some cases, men's health. "Women" as a category can also be further diluted in the context of gender fluidity and diversity, and in strategies to jockey for attention in a crowded and underfunded health research domain. As we go forward, politics, pressures, and new needs will undoubtedly continue to affect the future of women's health and women's health research in Canada, but there is no doubt that the story of women's health will continue to be more than a story of science. Indeed, the history of women's health and women's health research reinforces the political nature of the development of knowledge, and the fact that knowledge is never neutral, value-free, or static, but rather the result of a constellation of forces that defines "evidence" and continues to distribute the "power to know" in unequal ways across a society.

There will be increasing pressure for better science in the years to come. A focus in women's health research on improving methods, measurement, and concepts will hopefully rectify the shape and breadth of evidence currently available and add more sources of information to the women's health enterprise. The lack of a comprehensive approach to women's health research (in both biomedical and social sciences) has left significant gaps in knowledge about health, particularly among various subpopulations of women, as well as between different groups of women. Examining sex, gender, equity, and diversity in health research leads to better science and is a better reflection of the comprehensive vision of health as supported by many governments and international health organizations.

There will be an increased need for the integration of diversity into health care and research. Within the changing context of health in Canada, there are several issues. The aging of the Canadian population will mean that higher rates of chronic disease and cancer will be of concern to women. In some subpopulations, however, such as Aboriginal peoples, the shape of the population is aging less quickly as fertility rates are higher than in the general population, demanding a focus on girls' and reproductive health. Urbanization and migration patterns in Canada have resulted in intensification of multicultural populations in urban areas, which highlight many women's health issues in a diversity context. A general pressure on the health care system and a health human resource shortage has specific effects on the female-dominated health labour force. Health technology improvements will put pressure on women's health in areas such as assisted reproduction, genetic testing, and prenatal testing. All of these trends will create opportunities for women's health to become subspecialized and to develop into an increasingly complex and progressive endeavour, including personalized medicine. These trends also raise the issue of data gaps or data reporting that currently mask the situations of subgroups, and highlight the lack of adequate surveillance and indicator development to accurately address the full range of women's health issues in Canada.

Some of these subpopulations of women need redress. Despite the presence of legislation, policies, and programs dealing specifically with women's health, many Canadian women still experience inequalities (Health Canada, 2006). There are increasingly strong calls to reduce the health gap between Aboriginal and non-Aboriginal women, for example. Within Canada, the impact of health inequalities are most acutely experienced by various subpopulations of women, including single mothers, Aboriginal women, elderly women, women with disabilities, women of colour, and immigrant women (Day, 1998). There are also clear gaps of both knowledge and care for women with addictions and women who are under-housed, among many others.

Continued and increased emphasis on the fields of women's health and gender and health will reveal these and more specific issues. Within gender and health, a gender and diversity lens identifies the needs and differences between different groups of men and women. All of these analyses are important and must be developed simultaneously, but not at the cost of women's health. It is still vital that evidence about women's health becomes a requirement for medicine, programs, and policy development in order to bring better science to bear on the lives of all women.

There is a need for better training to increase capacity for women's health research in Canada. But further building and fostering of capacity is required and stronger integrated and transdisciplinary approaches to researching health issues are of key importance for women's health. This will require a clear capacity to train, offer practice, and build interest in research and policy development in women's health. Of particular importance to women's health is the training of community-based researchers in conjunction with academics to continue to broaden the base of evidence. All of these changes will lead to better research findings that will advance health promotion and care.

Old Values, Long Horizons

The values identified by the Royal Commission on the Status of Women in 1970 remain pertinent. Almost 50 years later, the need for more services for women and more equity are just as pertinent to women's health. Until historical inequities are corrected, the pursuit of two mutually reinforcing tracks—one centred on women, the other on gender—is required. In March 1999, at the 43rd Session of the UN Commission on the Status of Women, member states called for governments to adopt this two-pronged approach, endorsed by the UN General Assembly on April 1, 1999: "[to] … continue to take steps to ensure that the integration of a gender perspective in the mainstream of all government activities is part of a dual and complementary strategy to achieve gender equality. This includes a continuing need for targeted priorities, policies, programmes, and positive action measures for women" (Health Canada, 2000).

In order to continue to advance women's health, both within Canada and internationally, we must also address the equity and redress needs of various groups of women. There are several international health initiatives addressing health as a human right (i.e., the tobacco control movement, anti-violence movement, sexual and reproductive health movements), all of which offer opportunities for learning how to advance the health of women and girls. Women's health must be pursued in the context of women's rights as well. The Convention on the Elimination of All Forms of Discrimination Against Women (CEDAW), an international policy adopted by the United Nations, outlines rights for women and 30 articles relating to the elimination of discrimination against women. Article 12 is specifically related to health and states that, in order to eliminate discrimination against women, they must have equal access to health care services, family planning, and services related to pregnancy and postnatal health.

Despite the basic right to the highest standard of health, health and well-being are not a reality for the majority of women globally (Gijsbers Van Wijk, Van Vliet, & Kolk, 1996; United Nations, 1995). Inequalities result from a variety of factors, including women's

Box 1.3

Effects of Women's Health Activism

Both the fields of gender and health and men's health are positive by-products of the feminist theory, activism, and policy-making of the past 40 years. But going forward, gender-transformative approaches are key to advancing women's health and reducing gender inequities and to counter ongoing negative gender roles, stereotypes, and socio-economic inequities that affect women's health.

child-bearing roles, sex preference (discrimination against female children in health and general care), women's workloads, access to quality health care, and lack of autonomy (Gijsbers Van Wijk et al., 1996; Okojie, 1994). Further, ongoing sexism inspires anti-health practices such as female genital mutilation (FGM), "honour" killings, female infanticide, selective abortion, child and forced marriage, and woman abuse, none of which can be deemed "cultural" or seen through a culturally relativistic lens. For these reasons, the specific issues in women's health and the driving need to make advances in women's health research will remain a reality for a very long time to come.

Conclusions and Directions

In 1999, a group of Canadian women's health researchers proposed three separate approaches to improving health research: to do research addressing sex and gender in women's health, gender mainstreaming sex and gender concerns into all health research, or a combined approach. (Greaves et al., 1999). However, the intervening period has shown these are false choices and that all three are required to advance women's health. There are more knowledge gaps in 2015 than in 1999. We did not know then the extent of what we did not know about women's health. We did not know how more science and more sophisticated measures would foster a wider agenda, not reduce our agenda. We did not know how the erosion of support for women's health could quickly occur under the guise of gender and health or under the banner of resolving health inequity. To ensure continued progress, to respect the long roots of the women's health enterprise in so many sectors, and to reset goals for women's health, it is time for a more robust and refreshed plan for addressing women's health in Canada. In research, continued and increased attention to evidence gaps is required, utilizing a broader range of methods that challenge the very nature of evidence. In care, more fully evidenced women-focused care is a must to meet modern standards of accountability, safety, and quality. The policy arena requires a clearer understanding of how gender and women both need attention, and how attending to equity does not meet our domestic or international obligations to advance women's health. Renewed action in all of these domains will assist in creating a better system that more efficiently and effectively meets the needs of all women in Canada.

Alongside this, the field of gender and health remains a very necessary enterprise to advance health research and policy. The concept of gender is constantly developing and being made more complex to more fully incorporate issues of both biological and social science that affect health. These scientific developments will demand that the processes of gender-based analysis must be improved and made more reflective of gender(s) and other diversities within the Canadian population and that gender transformative health be incorporated into Canadian planning (Clow et al., 2009; Greaves et al., 1999). In addition, the growing interest in men's health is a positive trend in that various issues for men need addressing in a unique manner, and some need addressing in the context of improving gender norms in ways that benefit both women and men. Both the fields of gender and health and men's health are positive by-products of the women's health movement, feminist theory, activism, and policy-making of the past 40 years.

In short, there has been a lot accomplished in women's health in Canada through the efforts of many groups and individuals in a wide variety of sectors. This work has been cumulative and organic, political and scientific, research-oriented and practical. It has led to some key achievements and improvements in women's health and spawned the areas of gender and health and men's health. It led to internationally recognized approaches and enterprises and reflected a spirit in Canada to advance women's health and women's status in ways that led the world. To keep this momentum going will need equally tenacious efforts to refresh the approach, in a more nuanced and collective way and to continue to push the political as well as the scientific aims of advancing women's health. Everyone will likely benefit.

References

Amaro, H., & A. Raj. (2000). On the Margin: Power and Women's HIV Risk Reduction Strategies. *Sex Roles* 42(7): 723–749.

Auditor General of Canada. (2009). *The Spring 2009 Report of the Auditor General of Canada to the House of Commons: Chapter 1 Gender-Based Analysis.* Ottawa: Office of the Auditor General of Canada.

Bekker, M. H. J. (2003). Investigating Gender within Health Research Is More Than Sex Disaggregation of Data: A Multi-Facet Gender and Health Model. *Psychology, Health and Medicine* 8: 231–243.

Bialystok, L., L. Greaves, & N. Poole. (2014). Rethinking Preconception and Maternal Health: A Prime Opportunity for Gender-Transformative Health Promotion. In L. Greaves, A. Pederson, & N. Poole (Eds.), *Making It Better: Gender-Transformative Health Promotion* (pp. 178–193). Toronto: Canadian Scholars' Press Inc.

Bialystok, L., N. Poole, L. Greaves, & G. Thomas. (2014). Recalculating Risk: An Opportunity for Gender-Transformative Alcohol Education for Girls and Women. In L. Greaves, A. Pederson, & N. Poole (Eds.), *Making It Better: Gender-Transformative Health Promotion* (pp. 93–110). Toronto: Canadian Scholars' Press Inc.

Boston Women's Health Collective. (2011). *Our Bodies, Ourselves.* New York: Simon and Schuster.

Bourgeault, I. L. (2006). *Push! The Struggle for Midwifery in Ontario.* Montreal & Kingston: McGill-Queen's University Press.

Canadian Institutes of Health Research (CIHR). (2006). *Grant and Awards Guide.* Retrieved from http://search-recherche.gc.ca/cgi-bin/query?mss=cihr%2Fenglish%2Fsimple&pg=q&what=web&filter=cihr&enc=iso88591&site=main&q=grant+and+awards+guide&kl=XX.

CIHR. (2014a). *Definitions of Sex and Gender.* Ottawa: Author.

CIHR. (2014b). *Gender, Sex, and Health Research Guide: A Tool for CIHR Applicants*. Ottawa: Author.

CIHR IGH. (2012). *What a Difference Sex and Gender Make: A Gender, Sex, and Health Research Casebook*. Vancouver: Author.

Clow, B. N., A. Pederson, M. Haworth-Brockman, & J. Bernier. (2009). *Rising to the Challenge: Sex- and Gender-Based Analysis for Health Planning, Policy, and Research in Canada*. Halifax: Atlantic Centre of Excellence for Women's Health.

Commission on Social Determinants of Health. (2008). *Closing the Gap in a Generation: Health Equity through Action on the Social Determinants of Health: Final Report of the Commission on Social Determinants of Health*. Geneva: World Health Organization.

Courtenay, W. (2002). A Global Perspective on the Field of Men's Health: An Editorial. *International Journal of Men's Health* 1(January): 1–13.

Darroch, J. E., & J. J. Frost. (1999). Women's Interest in Vaginal Microbicides. *Family Planning Perspectives* 31(1): 16–23.

Davidson, K. W., K. J. Trudeau, E. Van Roosmalen, M. Stewart, & S. Kirkland. (2006). Gender as a Health Determinant and Implications for Health Research. *Health Education and Behavior* 33(6): 731–743.

Day, S. B. D. (1998). *Women and the Equality Deficit: The Impact of Restructuring Canada's Social Programs*. Ottawa: Status of Women Canada.

Devor, H. (1989). *Gender Blending: Confronting the Limits of Duality*. Bloomington: Indiana University Press.

Durey, R. (Ed.). (2014). *Taking a Stand: A Gender-Transformative Approach to Preventing Violence against Women*. Toronto: Canadian Scholars' Press Inc.

Fishman, J. R., J. G. Wick, & B. A. Koenig. (1999). The Use of "Sex" and "Gender" to Define and Characterize Meaningful Differences between Men and Women. In National Institutes of Health, Office of the Director, Office of Research on Women's Health, *Agenda for Research on Women's Health for the 21st Century* (Vol. 2, pp. 15–20). NIH Publication No. 99-44385. Bethesda, MD: U.S. Department of Health and Human Services.

Gelb, K., A. Pederson, & L. Greaves. (2011). How Have Health Promotion Frameworks Considered Gender? *Health Promotion International* 27(4): 445–452.

Gijsbers Van Wijk, C. M. T., K. P.Van Vliet, & A. M. Kolk. (1996). Gender Perspectives and Quality of Care: Towards Appropriate and Adequate Health Care for Women. *Social Science and Medicine* 43(5): 707–720.

Grant, K., & P. Ballem. (2000). *A Women's Health Research Institute in the Canadian Institutes of Health Research*. Vancouver: British Columbia Centre of Excellence for Women's Health.

Greaves, L. (2014). Can Tobacco Be Transformative? Reducing Gender Inequity and Tabacco Use among Vulnerable Populations. *International Journal of Environmental Research and Public Health* 11(1): 792–803.

Greaves, L., et al. (1999). *CIHR 2000: Sex, Gender, and Women's Health*. Vancouver: BC Centre of Excellence for Women's Health, British Columbia Women's Hospital and Health Centre.

Greaves, L., A. Pederson, & N. Poole. (Eds.). (2014). *Making It Better: Gender Transformative Health Promotion for Women*. Toronto: Canadian Scholars' Press Inc.

Greaves, L., N. Poole, & E. Boyle. (Eds.). (2015). *Transforming Addictions: Gender, Trauma, Transdisciplinarity*. New York: Routledge International.

Health Canada. (2000). *Health Canada's Gender-Based Analysis Policy*. Ottawa: Minister of Public Works and Government Services Canada.

Health Canada. (2003). *Exploring Concepts of Gender and Health*. Ottawa: Minister of Public Works and Government Services Canada.

Health Canada. (2004). *Canadian Handbook on Health Impact Assessment: Vol. 1. The Basics*. Ottawa: Author.

Health Canada. (2006). *An Overview of Women's Health*. Retrieved from http://www.hc-sc.gc.ca/hcs-sss/pubs/care-soins/1997-nfoh-fnss-v2/legacy_heritage8_e.html.

Health Canada. (2007). *Bureau of Women's Health and Gender Analysis*. Retrieved from http://www.hc-sc.gc.ca/ahc-asc/branch-dirgen/hpb-dgps/pppd-dppp/bwhga-bsfacs/index_e.html.

Hemsing, N., & L. Greaves. (2014). Igniting Global Tobacco Control. In L. Greaves, A. Pederson, & N. Poole (Eds.), *Making It Better: Gender-Transformative Health Promotion* (pp. 73–92). Toronto: Canadian Scholars' Press Inc.

Holdcroft, A. (2007). Gender Bias in Research: How Does It Affect Evidence Based Medicine? [Editorial]. *Journal of the Royal Society of Medicine* 100(1/2/3): 2–3.

Johnson, J. L., L. Greaves, & R. Repta. (2007). *Better Science with Sex and Gender: A Primer for Health Research*. Vancouver: Women's Health Research Network.

Keller, E. F. (1985). *Reflections on Gender and Science*. New Haven & London: Yale University Press.

Laurence, L., & B. Weinhouse. (1994). *Outrageous Practices: How Gender Bias Threatens Women's Health*. New York & Toronto: Random House.

Mehra, R., & G. R. Gupta. (2006). *Gender Mainstreaming: Making It Happen*. Washington, DC: International Center for Research on Women (ICRW).

NIH. (2014). New Supplemental Awards Apply Sex and Gender Lens to NIH-Funded Research. Bethesda, MD: Author.

Okojie, C. E. E. (1994). Gender Inequalities of Health in the Third World. *Social Sciences and Medicine* 3(9): 1237–1247.

Oliffe, J. L., & L. Greaves. (2011). *Designing and Conducting Gender, Sex, and Health Research*. Thousand Oaks, CA: SAGE.

Phillips, S. (2005). Defining and Measuring Gender: A Social Determinant of Health Whose Time Has Come. Commentary. *International Journal for Equity in Health* 4(11). doi10.1186/1475-9276-4-11.

Preves, S. E. (2000). Negotiating the Constraints of Gender Binarism: Intersexuals' Challenge to Gender Categorization. *Current Sociology* 48(3): 27–50.

Public Health Agency of Canada. (1999). *Towards a Healthy Future: Second Report on the Health of Canadians*. Retrieved from http://www.phac-aspc.gc.ca/ph-sp/phdd/report/toward/over.html.

Public Health Agency of Canada. (2004). *What Is the Population Health Approach?* Retrieved from http://www.phac-aspc.gc.ca/ph-sp/phdd/approach/approach.html#history.

Raphael, D., T., Bryant, & M. Rioux. (2006). *Staying Alive: Critical Perspectives on Health, Illness, and Health Care*. Toronto: Canadian Scholars' Press Inc.

Ratcliffe, K. S. (2002). *Women and Health: Power, Technology, Inequality, and Conflict in a Gendered World*. Boston: Allyn and Bacon.

Russell, W. (2000). Forging New Paths—Transdisciplinarity in Universities. *WISENET Journal* 53.

Sen, G., P. Östlin, & A. George. (2007). *Unequal Unfair Ineffective and Inefficient. Gender Inequity in Health: Why It Exists and How We Can Change It*. Final report to the WHO Commission on Social Determinants of Health. Retrieved from http://www.who.int/social_determinants/resources/csdh_media/wgekn_final_report_07.pdf.

United Nations. (1995). *Platform for Action: Report from the Main Committee of the Fourth World Conference on Women*. Beijing: United Nations.

Wizemann, T., & M. Pardue. (2001). *Exploring the Biological Contributions to Human Health: Does Sex Matter?* Washington, DC: Institute of Medicine.

Further Reading

Greaves L., et al. (1999). *CIHR 2000: Sex, Gender, and Women's Health.* Vancouver: BC Centre of Excellence for Women's Health: British Columbia Women's Hospital and Health Centre. Retrieved from www.bccewh.bc.ca/wp-content/uploads/2012/05/2000_CIHR_2000_report.pdf.

Johnson, J. L., L. Greaves, & R. Repta. (2007). *Better Science with Sex and Gender: A Primer for Health Research.* Vancouver: Women's Health Research Network. Retrieved from http://bccewh.bc.ca/wp-content/uploads/2012/05/2007_BetterSciencewithSexandGender PrimerforHealthResearch.pdf.

Oliffe, J., & L. Greaves. (Eds.). (2012). *Designing and Conducting Gender, Sex, and Health Research.* Thousand Oaks, CA: SAGE Publications.

Phillips, S. P. (2005). Defining and Measuring Gender: A Social Determinant of Health Whose Time Has Come. *International Journal for Equity in Health* 4(11). Retrieved from http://www.equityhealthj.com/content/4/1/11.

Wizemann, T., & M. Pardue. (2001). *Exploring the Biological Contributions to Human Health: Does Sex Matter?* Washington, DC: Institute of Medicine.

Relevant Websites

British Columbia Centre of Excellence for Women's Health: www.bccewh.bc.ca

Institute of Gender and Health, Canadian Institutes of Health Research: http://www.cihr-irsc.gc.ca/e/8673.htm

National Institutes of Health, Office of Research on Women's Health: http://orwh.od.nih.gov

The Source: www.womenshealthdata.ca

CHAPTER 2

Integrating Women's Health and Gender Analysis in a Government Context: Personal Reflections on a Work in Progress

Sari Tudiver[1]

Introduction

This chapter offers some personal reflections and lessons learned while working toward integrating an understanding of women's health and gender analysis into policies, programs, regulatory and other initiatives in a federal government department. It is directed to students and others interested in working with, and possibly within, government, particularly on issues pertaining to gender and women's health.

When I wrote the chapter for the first edition of this book in 2009, I had been employed as a senior policy analyst at the then Bureau of Women's Health and Gender Analysis at Health Canada for seven years. That position provided one particular vantage point from which to view a large and complex government organization.[2] I identified some key lessons learned from my work then: strategic ways to navigate government structures; the need to recognize and take advantage of opportunities for collaboration and mutual learning across traditional boundaries; and the importance of making the profound and sometimes emotionally charged concepts of "sex," "gender," and "diversity" relevant and meaningful to colleagues working within the paradigms and practices of the biomedical sciences, federal policy, and regulation. I noted that these and other lessons remained a work in progress, part of my ongoing attempt to keep the long-term goals of gender equality and better health for all in clear view while addressing the everyday business of government. The chapter included a standard disclaimer that "the views and opinions expressed herein are those of the author and do not necessarily reflect or represent the views of Health Canada or other federal departments or agencies." However, given the subject matter and that I was provided with work time to complete the paper, it was also standard practice for the contents to be vetted and approved by departmental communications staff and senior management. I wrote with that in mind.

This chapter revisits those reflections and learnings five years later when I am no longer working within government and at a time when the political landscape has changed dramatically. Indeed, many of the institutions and structures described in the original chapter no longer exist. In light of these changes, I have chosen to briefly highlight some key mechanisms and initiatives that had been established at the federal level since the 1970s to support research, policy, and program development in relation to women's health and gender analysis and then attempt to illustrate some of what is lost, as well as what remains in 2015. I emphasize the importance of preserving "corporate memory" about government initiatives and the need for critical reflection about the structural and policy changes that have occurred. There is much to learn from the past as we seek to transform social policies and governance structures to ensure gender equality and improved equitable health outcomes for all in the future.

Remembering Decades Past: Women's Health Advocacy and Government Responses

Since the early 1960s, a vibrant women's movement emerged among anglophone and francophone women across Canada advocating for gender equality, equity, and human rights (Adamson et al., 1988; Bégin, 1992; Black, 1993). Concerted pressure from many of these women's groups and organizations led to the establishment of the Royal Commission on the Status of Women (RCSW) in 1967. Its 1970 landmark report and recommendations were based on submissions and testimonies from women's groups across Canada and identified crucial social policy issues, including women's inequality in economic, legal, and social status; conditions of employment; and responsibilities for child care (*Report of the RCSW*, 1970). Follow-up to the report was coordinated by the Office of the Coordinator, Status of Women and an Inter-departmental Committee within the Privy Council Office (PCO) with direct access to the prime minister. Over 100 round tables, conferences, and informal discussions in church basements and shopping malls contributed to a vital discourse about gender roles and the changes needed to bring about gender equality in Canada. New federal and provincial structures were established, including a federal minister responsible for the status of women in 1971. However, the Royal Commission had important omissions: issues pertaining to violence against women and women's health did not feature in submissions to the Commission and were not addressed by Commissioners in the final report (Bégin, 1992).

What has come to be known as the women's health movement in Canada was in fact emerging by the late 1960s. Women's health groups and organizations, health and social service providers, and many individual patients and consumers had begun to identify inequities in how the health system responded to women's health needs and to document gaps and biases in policy, services, and research about women's health (Boscoe et al., 2005; Morrow, 2007; Chapter 1 in this volume). This activism took many forms: women came together in coalitions to advocate for reproductive rights and for legalization of birth control and abortion; to ensure the safety and efficacy of drugs and medical devices used by women; and to provide more comprehensive information about women's bodies, health, and wellness. New women-centred models of care provided services that addressed pregnancy, birthing, and menopause as natural stages of women's lives rather than medical conditions that necessarily required complex interventions (*Healthsharing Magazine*, 1979–1993).[3] As well, health researchers in Canada and internationally began to document sex and gender[4] differences between women and men in the prevalence, symptoms, and progression of many diseases; in the utilization of health services; and in the patterns of use of prescription drugs and other therapeutic interventions (Keitt, 2003; Doyal, 1995; Harding, 1986; Messing, 1998).

Concurrent campaigns organized by women in the global South demanding reproductive rights, safe medicines, and medical devices, and limitations on the marketing of infant formula were also taken up by Canadian women's health groups (Tudiver, 1986). Beginning in 1975, the UN Decade for Women helped strengthen information sharing between thousands of women of the global North and South who met in the pre-social media age at the NGO forums and the parallel Official UN Decade for women conferences in Mexico City, Nairobi, and later Beijing and at other international conferences on women's health. The "programs for action" that resulted from these meetings provided opportunities for women's health issues to be named, discussed, and placed on policy agendas as legitimate social issues to be addressed through health and social policies in Canada and other countries (*Nairobi Forward-Looking Strategies for the Advancement of Women*, 1985; United Nations, 1996; Morrow, 2007). Canada's subsequent ratification of the Convention on the Elimination of All Forms of Discrimination Against Women (CEDAW) in 1981 was a positive sign of federal government policy commitment to addressing "all forms of discrimination" against women, including "the discrimination against women in the field of health care in order to ensure, on a basis of equality of men and women, access to health care services, including those related to family planning" (Convention on the Elimination of All Forms of Discrimination Against Women, Article 12, p. 1).[5]

Health and Welfare Canada: Some Early Initiatives in Women's Health

In 1979, the federal department of health, then known as Health and Welfare Canada, established the position of Office of the Senior Adviser, Status of Women. Frieda Paltiel, the former PCO coordinator who had steered the follow-up to the Royal Commission Report, was appointed to the position. With her expert understanding of government and voluntary sector processes, perseverance, and ability to strategically leverage her position reporting directly to the minister of health, Paltiel began to take action on women's health issues, including family violence (Paltiel, 1997). Creative, substantive work was nurtured through this office. Among the earliest and enduring examples: in 1982, Health and Welfare Canada published *The Effects of Tranquillization: Benzodiazepine Use in Canada* by Ruth Cooperstock and Jessica Hill, complemented by *It's Just Your Nerves*, a training manual for facilitators (Cooperstock & Hill, 1982; Health and Welfare Canada, 1982). The substantive analyses presented in this work and the models of how to address issues of inappropriate prescribing, addictions, and other serious side effects of benzodiazepines remain highly relevant today (Women and Health Protection, 2006).

Throughout the 1980s, the Office of the Senior Adviser organized conferences and published reports on women, health and development, reproductive health, and health of adolescent girls, among many other issues. There was support for women's groups across Canada, such as DAWN, the Disabled Women's Network. The National Clearinghouse on Family Violence, and the Family Violence Initiative were also established and supported. In 1986, following the Nairobi UN End of Decade for Women conference, Health and Welfare Canada conducted a national survey of women's groups and organizations, women's health professionals, and researchers to identify key women's health issues. Subsequently, a National Symposium on Changing Patterns of Health and Disease in Canadian Women was held in Ottawa in April 1988 (Health and Welfare Canada, Status of Women, 1989). This was followed by the establishment of the Federal/Provincial/Territorial Working Group on Women's Health Issues to advise the Conference of Deputy Ministers of Health on women's health matters (Ford, 1990).

The FPT Working Group report, *Working Together for Women's Health: A Framework for the Development of Policies and Programs*, provided a conceptual framework to better understand women's health issues and prioritize appropriate actions for federal, provincial, and territorial jurisdictions (Ford, 1990). The report not only presented a list of key women's health issues,[6] but also addressed the social determinants of women's health, including their multiple roles as formal and informal caregivers for family and others. Of particular importance, it pointed to the diversity of women's situations and experiences in Canada and the impacts of discrimination on the health of women with disabilities, Aboriginal women, immigrant women, women of colour, adolescent girls, and senior women. The majority of issues identified remain pertinent 25 years after it was written.

The years following this report were characterized by policies of fiscal restraint, including cutbacks in funding to many women's organizations. However, the Office of the Senior Adviser at Health and Welfare Canada continued to convene round tables and conferences that encouraged cross-sector collaboration and research among policy-makers, academic researchers, community organizations, as well as public and private sector groups in areas affecting women, including HIV/AIDS, workplace health, mental health and addictions, and breast cancer (Paltiel, 1991; Neis, 1992; Ford, 1990; Harder, 1994).

The Women's Health Bureau and Its Mandate

In 1993, Health and Welfare Canada was restructured into two departments, Health Canada and Human Resources Development Canada. The Office of Senior Adviser, Status of Women was repositioned to become the Women's Health Bureau. Leadership passed to Abby Hoffman, a highly respected Olympic athlete and administrator, known for championing the rights of women in sport. The Bureau was to be the "focal point" for women's health within the federal government, with the mandate of "enhancing Health Canada's capacity to promote equitable health outcomes for women and men, boys and girls in Canada."[7] The Bureau's mandate was strengthened in 1995 when Canada adopted the Beijing *Platform for Action*, the concluding document from the Fourth UN World Conference on Women, and released the *Federal Plan for Gender Equality* in which Canada committed to the implementation of a women's health strategy (Status of Women Canada, 1995, Chapter 3).

The latter half of the 1990s continued to be a period of high-profile federal government initiatives focused on women's health. In 1996, the Women's Health Bureau organized and co-hosted the Canada–United States Women's Health Forum in Ottawa, bringing government officials, women's health researchers, health professionals, and activists together to share their cross-border perspectives on women's health issues. Papers were commissioned from each country to provide parallel overviews of a wide range of women's health issues. Participants discussed commonalities and differences, and identified possibilities for joint initiatives.

In that same year, Health Canada announced the establishment of five Centres of Excellence for Women's Health to be funded through the Women's Health Contribution Program (WHCP). The mandate of the regionally based Centres was "to generate and synthesize new knowledge about women's health, particularly in respect to the determinants of health, for the purposes of informing the policy process" (Health Canada, 1999, p. 23). The WHCP was to be a source of policy-relevant research for government, informed by community needs; to be considered, research projects had to demonstrate community/academic partnerships. The program also placed an emphasis on identifying health issues of concern to women whose voices were not commonly heard in policy circles due to geographic, economic, cultural, and other barriers of systemic discrimination. Many of the subsequent research studies employed participatory, community-based research models and qualitative methods to capture a contextual understanding of women's experiences. In addition, three working groups produced research relevant to the specific areas of women and health care reform; women and health protection, including issues of safety, efficacy, and regulation of therapeutic products; and research pertinent to Aboriginal women's health and healing.[8] The Canadian Women's Health Network, founded in 1993 at a meeting of over 70 independent women's groups, was also supported through the WHCP to provide a communications infrastructure for the Centres' work and a clearinghouse for popular, independent information about women's health issues (Health Canada, 1999, p. 23).

Health Canada's Women's Health Strategy (WHS) was released by then Minister of Health Alan Rock in 1999. It laid out Canada's international and federal commitments to women's health and the rationale for a strategy, including "the distinct nature of women's health issues." Four major objectives were identified, along with a total of 64 "key activities that will be undertaken to fulfil them." These addressed internal Health Canada policies and programs—such as planning, impact assessments, and advisory bodies—to ensure their responsiveness to sex and gender differences and women's health needs; making research more relevant to women's health concerns and accessible to wide audiences; supporting the provision of effective health services to women in the appropriate federal, provincial, and territorial jurisdictions that have direct responsibility for delivery of health services; and promoting good health through a wide range of preventive measures and reduction of risk factors, including occupational and environmental hazards that imperil women's health. It included a commitment to consult "women's organizations and health organizations interested in women's health on key policy files" (Health Canada, 1999, p. 22). Gender mainstreaming[9] was a primary pillar of the *Women's Health Strategy*. The WHS stated:

> In keeping with the commitment in the *Federal Plan for Gender Equality*, Health Canada will, as a matter of standard practice, apply gender-based analysis to programs and policies in the areas of health system modernization, population health, risk management, direct services, and research. (Health Canada, 1999, p. 21; archived)

Health Canada's Gender-Based Analysis (GBA) Policy was published the following year to support implementation of the stated GBA commitment. Drawing from resources developed by Status of Women Canada, the Organisation for Economic Co-operation and Development (OECD), Commonwealth Secretariat, and the work of Canadian and international women's health scholars, the document provided background about gender equality in the Canadian government context and definitions of key concepts. It emphasized the importance of integrating an understanding of how diversity within and among subgroups of women and men—in terms of age, race, ethnicity and culture, geographic location, sexual orientation, and abilities—may affect health over the life course, and how sex and gender interact with other health determinants, such as socio-economic status. The policy also noted the benefits of GBA's "challenge function" and the potential for identifying "more equitable, inclusive options" within government processes:

> GBA performs the challenge function that is essential to sound policies and programs. It challenges the assumption that everyone is affected in the same way by policies, programs and legislation, or that health issues such as causes, effects and service delivery are unaffected by gender. It probes concepts, arguments and language used, and makes the underlying assumptions and values transparent and

explicit. Where these are revealed to be biased or discriminatory, GBA points the way to more equitable, inclusive options. (Health Canada, 2000, p. 2; archived)

Back to Me . . .

When I began working at the Women's Health Bureau in the fall of 2000, there was a strong team spirit among the staff and a sense of working toward common goals of gender equality, equity, and improved health outcomes for all. In addition to the release of the *WHS* and GBA policy documents and the funding of the WHCP, Bureau staff had just helped organize the First International Conference on Women, Heart Disease, and Stroke held in Victoria, BC, co-sponsored by Health Canada, the U.S. Centres for Disease Control, the American Heart Association, the Heart and Stroke Foundation of Canada, and the Canadian Cardiovascular Society. There was considerable enthusiasm about the *2000 Victoria Declaration: Science and Policy in Action*, produced at this event, which called attention to the social determinants of women and heart health and laid out strategies for future action (Advisory Board, 2000). As well, the 1999 report of the Advisory Committee on Women's Health Surveillance, chaired by the Hon. Monique Bégin, had recommended that Health Canada's surveillance systems address deficiencies in the systematic collection, analysis, and dissemination of information pertaining to women's health, and expand its use of gender-based analysis (Advisory Committee on Women's Health Surveillance, 1999). There appeared to be a basis within the federal government from which to address gender gaps and inequities in key areas of health policy, surveillance, and research.

Daily Work: Building "The Business Case" for Women's Health and GBA

The work of the Bureau revolved around integrating considerations of women's health and gender-based analysis in the everyday business of Health Canada. The overall goals of this gender mainstreaming were articulated in the *Women's Health Strategy* and *GBA Policy* in terms of promoting health equity and gender equality. However, at a practical level, we knew that many senior managers and colleagues throughout the department considered these issues new, confusing, and often irrelevant to their work. We needed to provide a clear rationale and demonstrate *how* addressing women's health and conducting GBA were necessary and significant to the specific areas of the department's mandate and that any extra time, effort, and costs associated with implementing the policy would provide "added value." We could cite any of the 64 "key activities" identified in the *Women's Health Strategy* to justify our focus on an issue, but that was only the first step in a formidable process.

Bureau staff adopted several strategies for our work. First, to promote skills in gender-based analysis we developed, adapted, and promoted a variety of GBA resources and tools that could be applied to different areas of work/expertise. We were clearly told by colleagues that resources could not be overly academic in tone and that checklists and case studies were particularly useful. We designed and developed a core handbook, *Exploring Concepts in Gender and Health* (Health Canada, 2003) to provide easy-to-find background on the legislative and policy mandates for GBA, clarify key concepts, and present examples of questions that could be applied in the development and review of policies and programs. Four case studies offered examples of how GBA could be applied to prevention, treatment, and research on cardiovascular diseases; to performance indicators and measures for the mental health system; to research on violence; and to tobacco policy. We also conducted a baseline departmental survey to assess awareness about GBA—which was found to be low—and developed GBA training modules for in-person workshops and online. Bureau staff also encouraged the development of approaches to gender analysis that would be culturally appropriate to the diversity within and between First Nations, Inuit, and Métis communities.[10]

Second, we provided input on policy files specific to women's health (e.g., abortion, perinatal care, menopause) and worked with colleagues on gender-sensitive approaches to files such as tobacco, HIV/AIDS, mental health, and nutrition. Colleagues conducting regulatory reviews of the efficacy and safety of therapeutic products asked for our input about the social issues pertaining to the use of products such as emergency contraception and breast implants. There were occasional opportunities to contribute to the drafting of new legislation affecting women's health, for example, with the Assisted Human Reproduction Act, which acknowledges as one of its basic principles:

> while all persons are affected by these technologies, women more than men are directly and significantly affected by their application and the health and well-being of women must be protected in the application of these technologies. (An Act Respecting Assisted Human Reproduction, 2004, p. 1)

As part of everyday duties, Bureau staff dealt with ministerial correspondence pertinent to women's health, drafted or provided input to Question Period notes, and engaged in strategic planning. We contributed to the Government of Canada's positions and reporting on agreements and other instruments to advance domestic and international commitments for gender equality in health and, when appropriate, represented Canada at international meetings.

Since 2007, the Treasury Board of Canada Secretariat (TBS), the central agency responsible for management and expenditures of the federal government,[11] has required that gender-based analysis be applied to all its submissions. The Submission Guide states:

> Conducting a gender-based analysis should be considered. This type of analysis identifies how public policies differentially affect women and men. While gender implications may not be obvious in the first stage of analysis, they may emerge later. Therefore, gender questions should be raised throughout the analytical process. (Treasury Board of Canada Secretariat, 2007, p. 25)

Similarly, GBA must be referenced in Memoranda to Cabinet. These requirements made existing GBA policies more explicit at the highest levels of government. Increasingly, Bureau staff were called upon—often toward the final, rather than earlier, stages of preparation—to help colleagues in other areas of the department fulfil GBA requirements for these documents.

Third, we became involved in cross-branch and cross-sector initiatives where our participation could add particular value. For example, I served on the steering committee of Health Canada's *Health Policy Research Bulletin*, a publication focused on research about health policy (Health Canada, 2001–2011). Topics were diverse (e.g., health and environment, health promotion, health human resources, First Nations and Inuit health, regulation of natural health products, Canadian fertility trends) and involved the collaboration of a wide range of authors and editors with differing backgrounds and expertise. Bureau staff developed GBA guidelines for *Bulletin* authors and wrote articles, demonstrating how sex and gender analysis could contribute to a deeper understanding of the effects of particular health policies. We helped integrate considerations of women's health, gender, and diversity into the agendas of Health Canada science forums and worked with colleagues to develop the first Health Canada public consultations pertaining to regulatory approval of drugs and medical devices. In 2007, senior management asked us to chair the revision process for Health Canada's 1997 Guidance Document on inclusion of women in clinical trials. This initiative involved collaboration with clinical trial reviewers and researchers within Health Canada, representatives from the CIHR Institute of Gender and Health, and consultation with external stakeholders (Health Canada, 2013).

The Bureau also led a major initiative within Health Canada to encourage the development and validation of gender-sensitive health indicators with a specific focus on women's health indicators. The need for such indicators had been identified as one of the key activities in the *Women's Health Strategy*. On behalf of Health Canada, the Bureau developed a call for proposals from university-based researchers, supported the peer-review processes, and provided opportunities for the final research reports to be presented to staff at Health Canada, Statistics Canada, and other stakeholders (Tannenbaum, 2006; Bierman, 2007; Austin et al., 2007). The Bureau's focus on gender-sensitive indicators identified work being done in this area and served as a catalyst for a number of projects taken up by researchers at the Centres of Excellence for Women's Health and elsewhere (Colman, 2003; Chasey et al., 2010; Haworth-Brockman et al., 2011).

In the varied activities undertaken by Bureau staff, whenever possible, we drew upon the considerable research generated through the WHCP to leverage policy impact. There were many examples of policy engagement, as outlined in Box 2.1.

My involvement in various aspects of this work brought many personal satisfactions: rich collegiality with co-workers and daily opportunities to learn new things about the development and implementation of policy, the regulation of health products, health surveillance systems, and the discourse of government. My understanding of women's health and

Box 2.1

Examples of Policy Engagement

- *Including Gender in Health Planning: A Guide for Regional Health Authorities* was published by the Prairie Women's Health Centre of Excellence (Donner, 2003) and widely used by the Manitoba health care planners and managers to whom it was directed. Its clear explanations of concepts and case studies on mental health and diabetes using subpopulation health surveillance data inspired a more comprehensive guidebook of GBA case examples (Clow et al., 2009).
- A detailed economic and social analysis of the effects of breast implant surgeries on utilization of the public health care system (Tweed, 2003) contributed to Health Canada Advisory Committee policy recommendations for the establishment of a patient registry.
- The report by Women and Health Care Reform, *Gender-Based Analysis and Wait Times: New Questions, New Knowledge*, provided a gender analysis of wait times for hip- and knee-replacement surgeries (Jackson et al., 2006). It was appended to the *Final Report of the Federal Advisor on Wait Times* (Postl, 2006).
- Women and Health Protection, through representation from Health Canada, suggested that the International Conference on Harmonization (ICH)[12] develop a policy on inclusion of women in clinical trials. This led the ICH to undertake a pilot study of practices among its member regulatory authorities of Europe, Japan, and the United States. As a result, an ICH Considerations Paper, *Sex-Related Considerations in the Conduct of Clinical Trials* (ICH, 2004; revised 2009), was developed to which Health Canada provided input.
- Policy research concerning fetal alcohol spectrum disorder and women's health, supported by the BC Centre of Excellence for Women's Health, contributed to the development of gender-sensitive, low-risk drinking guidelines (lower for women than for men) that were endorsed by the federal/provincial and territorial governments in 2011 (Canadian Centre on Substance Abuse, 2011; Poole & Greaves, 2013).

gender analysis deepened as we applied the analysis to new issues, such as biotechnology and climate change. My colleagues and I were part of consultations and conferences that brought us in touch with researchers, clinicians, other policy analysts, senior bureaucrats, and representatives from the voluntary and private sectors in Canada and internationally. Of course, we recognized there were many complexities and obstacles to implementing the Bureau's mandate, but, as noted in the first edition of this book, we shared cautious optimism that "we are moving closer to more systematic application of gender-based analysis and attention to women's health needs in policies and programs, research, and regulatory work" (Tudiver, 2009, p. 23).

Changes

In her 2009 review of GBA implementation in a total of 10 federal departments and central agencies, including Health Canada, the auditor general documented that GBA was highly uneven in its application and called for more rigorous integration of gender-based analysis throughout the federal government (Auditor General of Canada, 2009).[13] Despite the auditor general's recommendations that GBA be integrated into all policies, programs, and legislative initiatives, Bureau staff were aware that our positioning within the bureaucracy was fragile. From 2006 on, departmental reorganizations resulted in many changes. The Bureau was shuffled from its position in the Health Policy Branch to a newly created Regions and Programs Branch, with no clear rationale beyond our administration of the WHCP. This marginalization was also reflected in our new designation as the Gender and Health Unit (GHU). While a name change in 2005 from the Women's Health Bureau to the Bureau of Women's Health and Gender Analysis acknowledged our GBA mandate, the change to the Gender and Health Unit signalled demotion within the department hierarchy and the demise of a focus on women's health within Health Canada.

When I decided to retire from Health Canada in January 2010, there was still a significant staff complement working on many of the women's health and GBA activities identified above, but the handwriting was on the wall. Government positions were being cut and long-time co-workers forced to compete for a single position. We knew the Bureau was under review. Morale plummeted as the flexibility associated with our work constricted. An announcement in 2012 confirmed that funding would not be renewed for the WHCP as of March 31, 2013. Currently (2015), the Gender and Health Unit is located within the Office of Grants and Contributions Services and Innovation, part of Health Programs and Strategic Initiatives, within the Strategic Policy Branch. The Unit is comprised of one full-time senior policy analyst.

Major cuts to government programs and staffing have occurred in past decades. Under the current government, cuts have been deep and wide across departments, affecting capacities for research and rigorous data collection and resulting in the loss of funding and demise of numerous voluntary/civil society organizations. In the following sections, I offer some personal thoughts on what I believe is lost and on what I believe remains within the bureaucracy that might provide a basis for federal support to advance gender equality and health equity in better times.

What Is Lost

As of 2015, there is no longer any position within the Health Portfolio with direct responsibility for women's health. The *Women's Health Strategy* document is archived, available for purposes of research and information only. While there is a mandate for what is now called sex- and gender-based analysis (SGBA), the lack of human resources means that only some requests for SGBA advice can be addressed in a limited way. There is no support to conduct internal research and writing or coordinate initiatives such as women's health indicators. The small but vibrant staff culture located in a Bureau of Women's Health and Gender Analysis that drew women and men of varying backgrounds, ages, and areas of expertise to promote women's health and gender equality within the department and beyond is gone.

The withdrawal of funding for the WHCP has seriously reduced the capacity for conducting and disseminating external, independent, policy-based research focused on social determinants of women's health. The Atlantic Centre of Excellence, the Prairie Women's Health Centre of Excellence, the Canadian Women's Health Network, Women and Health Care Reform, and Women and Health Protection, with their unique regional and topical issues, national and international projects, and diversity of voices, have all ceased formal operations. The BC Centre of Excellence and the National Network on Environments and Women's Health remain open for now, thanks to other sources of funding, but with reduced capacity.

Over the past several years, Health Canada has limited the opportunities for seeking the input and advice of researchers, clinicians, as well as women's health and community groups on health research and policy priorities. This is part of a much broader direction within the federal government. The demise of the WHCP reflects the loss of a collaborative model that provided regular opportunities for government policy-makers to engage with the women's health community and to hear from people traditionally marginalized from contributing to government processes because of poverty, geographic location, disability, language, sexual orientation, or other barriers to address gender inequities in health. Creative insights and practical solutions often come from the margins when the issues are demonstrated to be relevant to people's needs and when women and men are given the opportunity to participate equally. Authentic citizen consultation is integral to healthy public policy. Limiting mechanisms for such engagement with civil society is a serious loss of democratic process.

What Remains

In 2009, *Health Canada's GBA Policy* was revised as the *Health Portfolio Sex and Gender-Based Analysis Policy* (SGBA) and endorsed by Health Canada and the agencies that comprise the Health Portfolio (Health Canada, 2009).[14] The rationale for the policy is to "help ensure that the initiatives and activities of the Health Portfolio lead to sound science, advance gender-related health equality and are effective and efficient." The policy addresses accountability, including roles and responsibilities of senior management for implementation, reporting, and evaluation of the policy; seeks to incorporate "lessons learned and best practices in advancing gender equity and equality in health"; and asserts that SGBA remains "a natural part of doing the business of the Health Portfolio . . . fully integrated into organizational processes and practices." In contrast to the previous policy, there is no reference to historical inequities and disadvantages in health that affected women disproportionately to men. Canada's commitments to major international instruments concerning human rights and gender equality, such as CEDAW and the Canadian Charter of Rights and Freedoms are identified in an endnote. The policy emphasizes a principle of "balance": "SGBA will be used to evaluate the gender influences of research, policies and programs to ensure that the needs of one sex is [*sic*] not addressed more than another." The Gender and Health Unit, in collaboration with the Chief Financial Officer Branch, is to provide leadership and advice in policy implementation, evaluation, and reporting.

The new *Health Portfolio Sex and Gender-Based Analysis Policy* is aligned with the recommendations of the 2009 auditor general's report. That report called on Status of Women Canada (SWC) to develop a GBA implementation plan asking all departments and agencies to put in place elements of a GBA framework. These included: a GBA policy, mandatory training for senior departmental officials, identification of GBA frameworks in departmental plans and priorities and in performance reports, yearly reporting to SWC on departmental GBA practices, and a "responsibility centre" to monitor implementation (Auditor General of Canada, 2009).

Given the minimal staffing of the GHU, taking a leadership role in carrying out the SGBA policy mandate requires maximal sharing of tasks and resources across the Health Portfolio. The Health Portfolio SGBA Policy Implementation Working Group, chaired by the GHU, has developed a five-year plan. Current activities include a baseline survey to assess GBA knowledge and use, integrating questions about impacts of sex and gender into the funding of grants and contributions, and promoting collaborative pilot projects. Working Group members organize lunchtime learning sessions where colleagues present GBA-relevant work and encourage participation in SWC training workshops and "GBA boot camps." The Gender and Health Unit senior policy analyst responds to requests about how to best meet GBA requirements in Treasury Board submissions and Memoranda to Cabinet. She advises colleagues to identify early in the submission process SGBA questions and indicators that could make a significant difference to project outcomes and suggests resources they might use. In a few instances, departmental programs have developed GBA guides specific to their needs.

Overall, Health Canada's current SGBA work appears "thin" on the input that can be provided to health policy files; there is little capacity to dig deeply or take time to probe assumptions. As well, the pace of work and increasing restrictions across government on "number of characters" for comments can discourage analysts from identifying gender- and diversity-related implications of a policy or program. Health Canada's SGBA work is focused on "high level" corporate gender mainstreaming. It relies on engagement of colleagues and resources developed particularly by the CIHR Institute of Gender and Health (IGH), the Public Health Agency of Canada (PHAC), and Status of Women Canada (CIHR Institute of Gender and Health, 2012; Butler-Jones, 2012; Status of Women Canada, 2013).[15]

Today, many staff throughout the Health Portfolio have expertise in and commitment to addressing SGBA, women's health, and health equity in their work. Some were previously employed at the Bureau of Women's Health and Gender Analysis, worked on major collaborative projects addressing women's health and sex- and gender-based analysis, and/or gained expertise and interest through university-based research and curricula and other experiences. Even while opportunities for expression are limited, this expertise and commitment remain.

What also remain are the hundreds of WHCP research reports and other resources addressing a wide variety of issues relevant to the work of the Health Portfolio. These are available on the websites and databases of the Centres of Excellence and the Canadian Women's Health Network (CWHN) (see http://www.cwhn.ca for links to all sites). Policy-relevant research on topics such as synthetic chemical exposures among women workers, and prevention of fetal alcohol spectrum disorder are underway. Guidebooks that include SGBA case studies remain especially valuable to SGBA policy integration (e.g., Clow et al., 2009; CIHR IGH, 2012). Hopefully, the policy relevance of this work will be rediscovered, valued, and serve as a basis for progressive work.

Lessons Learned

In the following sections, I reflect on some of the lessons I learned over my nine years working within the federal government and in the five years since leaving the civil service. I consider a few of the challenges, including contradictions and tensions, faced trying to integrate women's health and gender-based analysis in a federal government context. I then offer a few practical strategies based on these lessons. These comments are not meant to be comprehensive, but to provide a starting point to explore what it means to work as a public servant trying to advance the goals of gender equality, health equity, and improved health outcomes.

Some Challenges

Demonstrating Added Value /Opportunity Costs

It was difficult to clearly and concisely demonstrate added value in terms of quality of care and improved health outcomes, or calculate the economic benefits to the health care system of gender and diversity-sensitive analyses in the short term, preferably in a four-year electoral cycle. Indeed, we often heard arguments that taking sex, gender, and diversity into account increased program or research costs; we countered with arguments about reduced health risks, health equity, and gender equality. We might have mobilized more effectively the talents of economists and other researchers interested in social costing to calculate the gendered impacts on health outcomes of *not* taking a particular course of action.

Crafting the "Right" Message

Our messages were often too nuanced and complex. We needed a variety of short, compelling, and user-friendly approaches to help deliver our rich conceptual content and case studies. For messages to be heard by senior management, they have to be crafted to the political environment, one increasingly focused on commercial innovation. This involves a very delicate balance demonstrating that SGBA can help identify new opportunities for innovation while promoting goals of equity, social justice, and gender equality (see, for example, Schiebinger et al., 2011–2013).

Implementing a Broad Mandate Dependent on Others

The Bureau's broad mandate of women's health and gender mainstreaming cut across work in other areas of the department and as a result presented particular challenges and tensions. It was difficult to establish priorities and identify indicators for progress with regard to the 64 areas identified in the WHS to improve the health status of women and girls. Each action was framed as a commitment: for example, "Health Canada initiatives in support of health system modernization and expansion will include a gender impact assessment." However, the mechanisms needed to achieve such broad commitments were unspecified. Having the support of others in the department, especially senior management who held primary responsibility for the particular areas covered by the WHS commitment, was critical to moving forward, but varied considerably. We were not directly integrated into the work and were conscious of not wanting to be considered "the gender police" who tried to influence and challenge how the file work of others was being conducted. We took a great deal of time to build trust and collaborative ways of working with colleagues across the department.

Integrating Qualitative and Critical Social Research into Policy

The institutions and organizations funded through the Women's Health Contribution Program were mandated to develop action-oriented and policy-relevant social research through academic-community partnerships, yet the very nature of this mandate had many contradictions in a government context. The emphasis on social and not biomedical determinants of health produced many detailed qualitative studies of women's and girls' experiences; however, it was challenging for policy analysts to transfer this knowledge, often perceived by government as "anecdotal" and less credible, into the types of evidence demanded for policy documents. Further, research reports that drew conclusions critical of government policy and recommended major changes were not well received by the funder. Independent critique, highly valued in academic and community settings, was seen very differently in the government context, where negative publicity is to be avoided (Majury, 1999; Austin & Hirschkorn, 2014). Over the course of the WHCP, the "challenge function" of asking critical questions and interrogating assumptions, originally conceived to be part of gender-based analysis and the WHCP mandate, became increasingly unwelcome.

Moving Gender-Sensitive Policies into Action

Many opportunities for significant change to improve the work of government and the health of Canadians have been passed over. For example, the plan of action and follow-up research pertaining to women's health surveillance in Canada (Advisory Committee on Women's Health Surveillance, 1999; Des Meules et al., 2003) identified key gaps in surveillance data-gathering and gender-sensitive strategies for improving the systems, but resulted in few major changes. The results of work to develop and validate gender-sensitive health indicators, an area of leadership for Health Canada in the early 2000s, have not received much uptake in government, despite widespread interest in such work internationally. Sex- and gender-based analysis, when applied to the key federal government policy issue of wait times, remained as an appendix, not fully integrated into further actions of the federal wait times response. These and other examples reflect failures in political will and leadership and a lack of coherent vision to take advantage of creative, gender-sensitive policy directions that would positively affect the health of Canadians.

Navigating the Complexities of Gender Mainstreaming

Gender mainstreaming is a complex and often contested set of practices, particularly, but not only, in a government context (Walby, 2005; Rankin & Wilcox, 2004; Sweetman, 2012). Policy requirements to apply SGBA to *all* the business of government provide important leverage for those working in and outside government to promote gender equality and equity (Auditor General of Canada, 2009; Standing Committee on the Status of Women, 2008). The scope of activities can be contained, bureaucratic, and tenuous at a point in time, but the critical conceptual framework and challenge functions provided by such analysis can have transformative potential.

Some Practical Strategies

In conclusion, here are a few practical strategies I have learned along this journey. I encourage anyone thinking about a career in the public service to seek out many people with diverse vantage points in this complex system in order to gain perspectives, stories, and insights different from my own.

Know the Government Structures

It is essential to know the formal structures of the various branches and agencies of government, and their particular mandates and responsibilities, including the appropriate channels for setting agendas and reporting. In large bureaucracies with a wide range of functions, and a military-style model of command, this can be a formidable task. Take courses on policy processes and how government works. Read the auditor general reports for their insights into how well government functions and the recommendations for change, particularly in areas related to your work. It is important to understand *how* policy decisions are made in the rapidly changing "real world" environment in order to identify possible points of leverage for sex- and gender-based analysis in health policy work.

Build Your Networks, Credibility, and Expertise

Build relationships within and beyond your immediate circle of colleagues. Identify who is knowledgeable about particular issues and who is holding the pen on a policy file relevant to your work. In order to respond rapidly to a request for information or seek other advice, it is crucial to know who to call. In turn, know your files and be someone who can offer people credible help. Rigour and due diligence involve careful attention to available evidence on a subject—including what is not known—and presenting the evidence and analysis in a clear, balanced way to inform policy options. Hone your skills in applying sex- and gender-based analysis to policy, research, and regulation to determine the implications and potential impacts of policy options for diverse populations of women and men, and boys and girls. Seek out mentors and engage with others as you build your expertise and credibility.

Words Matter

In government, words *always* matter. Legislation and regulation, international agreements, conventions, and declarations to which Canada is a signatory, departmental policies or guidance documents set out various types of commitments for which the government has assumed accountability. Many of these instruments explicitly enshrine values of women's rights and gender equality. The wording of most documents reflects processes of consultation, committee work, and negotiation. Policy analysts should understand the historical contexts within which the language of past documents was forged as well as the present context and rationales for change. The choice of words is carefully framed and reviewed to be aligned with current government policies. When reviewing proposals, be aware of nuances that may enhance or undermine the health of women and girls and affect gender equality. Changes to a phrase or a single word may alter or strengthen the overall meaning and intent of a recommendation or policy. Remember that words can also have very different implications in different languages, cultural contexts, and in translation.

Be aware of the forms of discourse that characterize government processes and how these differ from non-governmental sectors. Be clear about the intended audiences for your work, but always try to bring clarity and not obscure an issue.

Seek Creative Spaces and Opportunities for Learning

Creative spaces for critical discussion about gender equality, diversity, equity, and women's health have significantly narrowed. Take advantage of any learning opportunities that may be available across government, at universities, and in the women's health community. These opportunities can help you "stay ahead of the wave" on current research about sex, gender, and diversity in health and about the strengths and pitfalls of gender mainstreaming strategies to better situate your work.

Seek alternative ways of reducing isolation and keeping the issues of gender and women's health alive and well in a chilly environment. Organize a journal club or other regular meeting time and invite new people with diverse backgrounds and interests to talk about their work. Use creative approaches to encourage "aha" moments about the value of SGBA. Small spaces can yield transformative insights and results.

Be Politically Astute and Aware of Your Moral Compass

While it is understandable that governments wish to speak with a consistent voice regarding major policies, who is allowed to speak, on what topics, and with what specific messages varies considerably with the government in power. You may be asked to respond to an issue in a way that makes you uncomfortable. Seek out ethics courses or talk with an ethics ombudsman. Be astute about what issues you are working on that might place the public good in jeopardy. While there are some safeguards, there are serious repercussions for public servants who criticize government policies. Are there words you will not speak or write and moral lines you will not cross? It is wise to think about these issues in advance.

Remember the Past

Governments are elected on a four-year cycle and priorities and policies change. What comes to be institutionalized as the "new normal" reflects a mix of political and ideological positions, interpersonal power dynamics, campaign promises, and other circumstances affecting those elected to govern at a particular period in time. Current policies have significant and negative impacts on programs and policies designed to redress economic and other inequities and promote women's equality. To envision change in the future, it is important to remember in what ways things were different in the past and debate the lessons learned from policies and initiatives intended to advance gender equality and health equity. Particularly in these times, it is important to seek inspiration from others who have worked and continue to work boldly and with perseverance—within and outside government structures—toward the goals of gender equality and social justice for all.

Notes

1. The origin of this article was a presentation made to the Ontario Training Centre Summer Institute, York University, Toronto, May 15, 2006, at the invitation of Dr. Pat Armstrong. Updated versions of the talk were presented to summer courses on "Gender-Based Analysis: Engendering Change" for international interns at the McGill Centre for Research and Teaching on Women in August 2006 and in July 2007. This article is a major revision of this early work.

   I wish to thank Dr. Pat Armstrong and Ann Pederson for the opportunity to participate in this project. As my key contact in the current process, Ann was steadfast, generous with her time, and a constant source of wise insights. She sustained me through many trying moments. I extend special thanks to my former Bureau colleagues now working in many areas of government and beyond who have inspired me over the past 15 years. You have taught me so much more than I can capture here. You know who you are.

   The views and opinions expressed in this article about my work in the federal government are my own.
2. For information about Health Canada, including its mission and structure, go to www.hc-sc.gc.ca. Explore the links through the different branches of the department.

3. *Healthsharing Magazine* was published from 1979 to 1993 and was groundbreaking for its time, providing critical information on women's health from a non-medical perspective, with a Canadian focus. The issues addressed provide a survey of the Canadian women's health movement throughout those years.
4. In this chapter, the concepts of "sex," "gender," and "sex- and gender-based analysis" are used according to the definitions provided in the *Health Portfolio Sex and Gender-Based Analysis Policy* (2009) and in CIHR documents. See CIHR (2014a), CIHR (2014b), and CIHR IGH (2012).
5. In addition to CEDAW, Canada has ratified all the major international human rights treaties, including the Universal Declaration of Human Rights; the International Covenant on Economic, Social, and Cultural Rights; the International Covenant on Civil and Political Rights; and the Convention on the Rights of the Child. Canada is also committed to international agreements such as the United Nations Declaration on Violence against Women, and to the consensus reached at the various UN conferences such as the Cairo Conference on Population and Development, the Vienna World Conference on Human Rights, and the Fourth United Nations World Conference on Women, in Beijing.
6. The issues included: women's mental health, reproductive health, violence against women, chronic and degenerative health conditions, female cancers, occupational and environmental health, nutrition, and active living.
7. The Health Canada website link to the mandate of the then Women's Health Bureau provided in the 2009 edition of this chapter is no longer available.
8. The original five Centres of Excellence were the British Columbia Centre of Excellence for Women's Health, the Prairie Women's Health Centre of Excellence, the National Network on Environments and Women's Health, Centre d'excellence pour la santé des femmes (CESAF) and the Atlantic Centre of Excellence for Women's Health. After CESAF closed in 2001, Health Canada funded the Réseau québecois d'action pour la santé des femmes to do similar work.
9. The term "gender mainstreaming" came into widespread use through the United Nations Beijing Platform for Action. It has been adopted by many international organizations, including the World Bank and the European Union. The UN Economic and Social Council (United Nations, 1997, p. 28) definition is helpful for our purposes:

   > Mainstreaming a gender perspective is the process of assessing the implications for women and men of any planned action, including legislation, policies or programmes, in all areas and at all levels. It is a strategy for making women's as well as men's concerns and experiences an integral dimension of the design, implementation, monitoring and evaluation of policies and programmes in all political, economic and societal spheres so that women and men benefit equally and inequality is not perpetuated. The ultimate goal is to achieve gender equality.

   Other elements of gender mainstreaming include institutionalizing gender concerns into an organization "to transform attitudes, culture, goals and procedures" and promoting women's participation in decision-making processes (Moser & Moser, 2005, p. 12; Redden, 2013).
10. For example, *Our Voices* is a sex- and gender-based analysis tool kit designed to be culturally appropriate and reflective of women's health issues specific to First Nations, Métis, and Inuit in Canada. Health Canada provided funding to conduct the Aboriginal Women and Girls' Health Roundtable in April 2005, which led to developing this resource (First Nations, Métis, and Inuit GBA, 2009). (See *Our Voices: A First Nations, Métis, and Inuit Sex- and Gender-Based Analysis Toolkit*, http://www.aboriginalgba.ca/.)

    The Native Women's Association of Canada has also developed culturally relevant GBA resources, http://www.nwac.ca/programs/culturally-relevant-gender-analysis.
11. The Treasury Board is a Cabinet committee of the Queen's Privy Council of Canada. It is responsible for accountability and ethics; financial, personnel, and administrative management; comptrollership; approving regulations; and most orders-in-council.

    A Treasury Board submission is a document submitted by a department or agency seeking approval for a proposed initiative. Even after Cabinet approves a policy initiative, Treasury Board approval is still needed to carry out the initiative. A submission includes details of design and delivery, yearly cost of the initiative, and expected results and outcomes. It may include other information, such as impact on gender. A Memorandum to Cabinet is the key instrument for providing written policy advice to Cabinet or seeking Cabinet support for a proposed course of action. It plays a pivotal role in Cabinet decision-making.

12. The full name is The International Conference on Harmonization of Technical Requirements for Registration of Pharmaceuticals for Human Use (ICH). It is a unique body in that it brings together the regulatory authorities and pharmaceutical industry of Europe, Japan, and the United States to discuss scientific and technical aspects of drug registration. ICH documents guide drug regulatory processes in Canada and internationally. Canada sits as an observer to the ICH.
13. The federal organizations included in the 2009 audit were: the Treasury Board of Canada Secretariat, the Privy Council Office, the Department of Finance Canada, Status of Women Canada, the Department of Justice Canada, Health Canada, Human Resources and Skills Development Canada, Indian and Northern Affairs Canada, Transport Canada, and Veterans Affairs Canada.
14. As of 2015, the Health Portfolio includes: Health Canada, the Public Health Agency of Canada, the Canadian Institutes of Health Research, the Patented Medicines Prices Review Board, and the Canadian Food Inspection Agency.
15. Status of Women Canada has introduced "the modernization of GBA" to GBA+. This approach emphasizes the consideration of other "intersecting identity factors" in addition to gender, such as age, education, language, geography, culture, and income.

References

An Act Respecting Assisted Human Reproduction and Related Research, also known as Assisted Human Reproduction Act (S.C. 2004, c. 2). Ottawa: Government of Canada. Retrieved from http://laws-lois.justice.gc.ca/eng/acts/A-13.4/page-1.html.

Adamson, N., L. Briskin, & M. McPhail. (1988). *Feminist Organizing for Change: The Contemporary Women's Movement in Canada*. Toronto: Oxford University Press.

Advisory Board, First International Conference on Women, Heart Disease, and Stroke. (2000). *The 2000 Victoria Declaration on Women, Heart Diseases, and Stroke*. Victoria, Canada. May 10. Retrieved from http://www.cwhn.ca/sites/default/files/resources/victoria_declaration/victoria.pdf.

Advisory Committee on Women's Health Surveillance. (1999). *Women's Health Surveillance: A Plan of Action for Health Canada*. Ottawa: Health Canada.

Auditor General of Canada. (2009). *The Spring 2009 Report of the Auditor General of Canada to the House of Commons*. Chapter 1: Gender-Based Analysis. Ottawa: Office of the Auditor General of Canada.

Austin, S., & K. Hirschkorn. (2014). Policy, Overview. In T. Teo (Ed.), *Encyclopedia of Critical Psychology* (pp. 1412–1419). New York: Springer.

Austin, S., S. Tudiver, M. Chultem, & M. Kantiebo. (2007). Gender-Based Analysis, Women's Health Surveillance, and Women's Health Indicators: Working Together to Promote Equity in Health in Canada. *International Journal Public Health* 52(1, Suppl. 1): S41–S48.

Bégin, M. (1992). The Royal Commission on the Status of Women in Canada: Twenty Years Later. In C. Backhouse & D. Flaherty (Eds.), *Challenging Times: The Women's Movement in Canada and the United States* (pp. 21–38). Montreal & Kingston: McGill-Queen's University Press.

Bierman, A. (2007). *Measuring Health Inequalities among Canadian Women: Developing a Basket of Indicators*. Ottawa: Health Canada's Health Policy Research Program.

Black, N. (1993). The Canadian Women's Movement: The Second Wave. In S. Burt, L. Code, & L. Dorney (Eds.), *Changing Patterns: Women in Canada* (2nd ed., pp. 70–85). Toronto: McClelland & Stewart.

Boscoe, M., G. Basen, G. Alleyne, B. Bourrier-Lacroix, & S. White. (2005). The Women's Health Movement in Canada: Looking Back and Moving Forward. *Canadian Woman Studies* 24(1): 7–13.

Butler-Jones, D. (2012). *The Chief Public Health Officer's Report on the State of Public Health in Canada, 2012: Influencing Health—The Importance of Sex and Gender.* Ottawa: Public Health Agency of Canada.

Canadian Centre on Substance Abuse. (2011). *Canada's Low-Risk Alcohol Drinking Guidelines.* Retrieved from http://www.ccsa.ca/Eng/topics/alcohol/drinking-guidelines/Pages/default.aspx.

Chasey, S., A. Pederson, & P. Duff. (2010). *Canadian Women's Health Indicators: An Introduction, Environmental Scan, and Framework Examination.* Vancouver: British Columbia Centre of Excellence for Women's Health.

CIHR. (2014a). Definitions of Sex and Gender. Ottawa: Author. Retrieved from http://www.cihr-irsc.gc.ca/e/47830.html.

CIHR. (2014b). *Gender, Sex, and Health Research Guide: A Tool for CIHR Applicants.* Ottawa: Author.

CIHR IGH. (2012). *What a Difference Sex and Gender Make: A Gender, Sex, and Health Research Casebook.* Vancouver: Author.

Clow, B. N., A. Pederson, M. Haworth-Brockman, & J. Bernier. (2009). *Rising to the Challenge: Sex- and Gender-Based Analysis for Health Planning, Policy, and Research in Canada.* Halifax: Atlantic Centre of Excellence for Women's Health.

Colman, R. (2003) *A Profile of Women's Health Indicators in Canada.* A report prepared for the Bureau of Women's Health and Gender Analysis by Dr. Ron Colman, GPI Atlantic. Ottawa: Health Canada.

Convention on the Elimination of All Forms of Discrimination against Women, G.A. res. 34/180, 34 UN GAOR Supp. (No. 46) at 193, UN Doc. A/34/46, entered into force September 3, 1981. Article 12. Retrieved from http://www.un.org/documents/ga/res/34/a34res180.pdf.

Cooperstock, R., & J. Hill. (1982). *The Effects of Tranquillization: Benzodiazepine Use in Canada.* Ottawa: Minister of National Health and Welfare.

Des Meules, M., A. Kazanjian, H. Maclean, J. Payne, D. E. Stewart, & B. Vissandjée. (2003). *Women's Health Surveillance Report: A Multi-Dimensional Look at the Health of Canadian Women.* Ottawa: Canadian Institute for Health Information.

Donner, L. (2003). *Including Gender in Health Planning: A Guide for Regional Health Authorities.* Winnipeg: Prairie Women's Health Centre of Excellence. Retrieved from www.pwhce.ca/pdf/gba.pdf.

Doyal, L. (1995). *What Makes Women Sick: Gender and the Political Economy of Health.* London: Macmillan Press Ltd.

First Nations, Métis, and Inuit GBA. (2009). *Our Voices: A First Nations, Métis, and Inuit Sex- and Gender-Based Analysis—About the Toolkit.* Retrieved from http://www.aboriginalgba.ca/about/.

Ford, A. R. (1990). *Working Together for Women's Mental Health: A Framework for the Development of Policies and Programs.* Prepared by the Federal, Provincial, and Territorial Working Group on Women's Health.

Harder, S. (1994). *Report on the National Forum on Breast Cancer*, Montreal, November 14–16, 1993. Ottawa: Parliamentary Research Branch. Retrieved from http://publications.gc.ca/Collection-R/LoPBdP/MR/mr117-e.htm.

Harding, J. (1986). Mood-Modifiers and Elderly Women in Canada: The Medicalization of Poverty. In K. McDonnell (Ed.), *Adverse Effects: Women and the Pharmaceutical Industry* (pp. 51–86). Toronto: Women's Press.

Haworth-Brockman, M. J., H. Isfeld, A. Pederson, B. Clow, A. Liwander, & B. A. Kinniburgh (Eds.). (2011). *Careful Measures: An Exploration of the Sex and Gender Dimensions of a Deprivation Index.* Vancouver: British Columbia Centre of Excellence for Women's Health.

Health Canada. (1999). *Health Canada's Women's Health Strategy.* Ottawa: Minister of Public Works and Government Services Canada (archived). Retrieved from http://www.hc-sc.gc.ca/ahc-asc/pubs/_women-femmes/1999-strateg/index-eng.php.

Health Canada. (2000). *Health Canada's Gender-Based Analysis Policy.* Ottawa: Minister of Public Works and Government Services Canada (archived). Retrieved from www.hc-sc.gc.ca/hl-vs/women-femmes/gender-sexe/policy-politique_e.html.

Health Canada. (2003). *Exploring Concepts of Gender and Health* (archived on June 24, 2013). Ottawa: Minister of Supply and Services Canada.

Health Canada. (2009). *Health Portfolio Sex- and Gender-Based Analysis Policy.* Retrieved from http://www.hc-sc.gc.ca/hl-vs/gender-genre/analys/policy-politique-eng.php.

Health Canada. (2013). *Guidance Document: Considerations for Inclusion of Women in Clinical Trials and Analysis of Sex Differences.* Retrieved from http://www.hc-sc.gc.ca/dhp-mps/prodpharma/applic-demande/guide-ld/clini/womct_femec-eng.php.

Health Canada Health Policy Research Bulletins. (2001–2011). Ottawa: Minister of Public Works and Government Services (archived on June 24, 2013). Retrieved from http://www.hc-sc.gc.ca/sr-sr/pubs/hpr-rpms/index-eng.php.

Health and Welfare Canada, Health Promotion Directorate. (1982). *It's Just Your Nerves: A Resource on Women's Use of Minor Tranquillizers and Alcohol.* Ottawa: Minister of National Health and Welfare.

Health and Welfare Canada, Status of Women. (1989). *Proceedings of the National Symposium on Changing Patterns of Health and Disease in Canadian Women: April 18–20, 1988, Ottawa, Canada.* Ottawa: Minister of Supply and Services Canada.

Healthsharing Magazine. (1979–1993). Toronto: Women Healthsharing Inc. Retrieved from http://www.cwhn.ca/en/node/46457.

International Conference on Harmonization of Technical Requirements for Registration of Pharmaceuticals for Human Use (ICH). (2004; revised 2009). ICH Considerations Paper, *Sex-Related Considerations in the Conduct of Clinical Trials.* Retrieved from http://www.ich.org/fileadmin/Public_Web_Site/ICH_Products/Consideration_documents/ICH_Women_Revised_2009.pdf.

Jackson, B., A. Pederson, & M. Boscoe (on behalf of the Women and Health Care Reform Group). (2006). *Gender-Based Analysis and Wait Times: New Questions, New Knowledge.* Retrieved from http://www.hc-sc.gc.ca/hcs-sss/pubs/system-regime/2006-wait-attente/gender-sex/index-eng.php.

Keitt, Sarah K. (2003). Sex and Gender: The Politics, Policy, and Practice of Medical Research. *Yale Journal of Health Policy, Law, and Ethics* 3(2): Article 2. Retrieved from http://digitalcommons.law.yale.edu/yjhple/vol3/iss2/2.

Majury, D. (1999). *Promoting Women's Health: Making Inroads into Canadian Health Policy. A Policy Advice Framework Report to the Centres of Excellence for Women's Health Program.* Synopsis. Ottawa: Health Canada, Women's Health Bureau.

Messing, K. (1998). *One-Eyed Science: Occupational Health and Women Workers.* Philadelphia: Temple University Press.

Morrow, M. (2007). Our Bodies Our Selves in Context: Reflections on the Women's Health Movement in Canada. In M. Morrow, O. Hankivsky, & C. Varcoe (Eds.), *Women's Health in Canada: Critical Perspectives on Theory and Policy* (pp. 33–63). Toronto: University of Toronto Press.

Moser, C., & A. Moser. (2005). Gender Mainstreaming since Beijing: A Review of Success and Limitations in International Institutions. *Gender and Development* 13(2): 11–22.

Nairobi Forward-Looking Strategies for the Advancement of Women. (1985). Adopted by the World Conference to review and appraise the achievements of the United Nations Decade for Women: Equality, Development, and Peace, held in Nairobi, Kenya, July 15–26, 1985. Retrieved from http://www.un-documents.net/nflsaw.htm.

Neis, B. (1992). *Proceedings of the Research Round Table on Gender and Workplace Health: June 22-23, 1992, Ottawa, Canada.* Ottawa: Office of the Senior Adviser, Status of Women, Health and Welfare Canada.

Paltiel, F. (1991). *Understanding Women and AIDS: What We Know, What We Need to Know, What We Can Do: Proceedings of the Health and Welfare Canada Seminar for World AIDS Day 1990, December 3, 1990.* Ottawa: Office of the Senior Adviser, Status of Women, Health and Welfare Canada.

Paltiel, F. (1997). State Initiatives: Impetus and Effects. In C. Andrew & S. Rogers (Eds.), *Women and the Canadian State* (pp. 27–51). Montreal and Kingston: McGill-Queen's University Press.

Poole, N., & L. Greaves. (2013). Alcohol Use during Pregnancy in Canada: How Policy Moments Can Create Opportunities for Promoting Women's Health. *Canadian Journal of Public Health* 104(2): e170–e172.

Postl, B. D. (2006). *Final Report of the Federal Advisor on Wait Times.* Ottawa: Health Canada. Retrieved from http://www.hc-sc.gc.ca/hcs-sss/pubs/system-regime/2006-wait-attente/index-eng.php.

Rankin, L. P., & K. D. Wilcox. (2004). De-Gendering Engagement? Gender Mainstreaming, Women's Movements, and the Canadian Federal State. *Atlantis* 29(1): 52–60.

Redden, S. (2013). Gender Mainstreaming: A Review Paper. Gender Equality Measurement Project (GEM). Unpublished manuscript, Carleton University, Ottawa.

Report of the Royal Commission on the Status of Women in Canada (RCSW). (1970). Ottawa. Retrieved from http://epe.lac-bac.gc.ca/100/200/301/pco-bcp/commissions-ef/bird1970-eng/bird1970-eng.htm.

Schiebinger, L., I. Klinge, I. Sánchez de Madariaga, M. Schraudner, & M. Stefanick. (Eds.). (2011–2013). *Gendered Innovations in Science, Health & Medicine, Engineering and Environment.* Stanford University. Retrieved from genderedinnovations.stanford.edu.

Standing Committee on the Status of Women. (2008). Eleventh Report. 39th Parliament, 2nd Session. *Towards Gender Responsive Budgeting: Rising to the Challenge of Achieving Gender Equality.* Ottawa: Government of Canada.

Status of Women Canada. (1995). *Setting the Stage for the Next Century: The Federal Plan for Gender Equality.* Ottawa: Status of Women Canada.

Status of Women Canada (2013). *GBA+ Resources.* Retrieved from http://www.swc-cfc.gc.ca/gba-acs/resources-ressources-eng.html.

Sweetman, C. (2012). Introduction. *Gender and Development: Beyond Gender Mainstreaming* (Special issue) 20(3): 389–403.

Tannenbaum, C. (2006). *Towards a Better Understanding of Women's Mental Health and Its Indicators.* A report funded through Health Canada's Health Policy Research Program. Ottawa: Health Canada.

Treasury Board of Canada Secretariat. (2007). *Treasury Board of Canada Secretariat: A Guide to Preparing Treasury Board Submissions.* Ottawa: Author.

Tudiver, S. (1986). The Strength of Links: International Women's Health Networks in the Eighties. In K. McDonnell (Ed.), *Adverse Effects: Women and the Pharmaceutical Industry* (pp. 187–214). Toronto: Women's Press.

Tudiver, S. (2009). Integrating Women's Health and Gender Analysis in a Government Context: Reflections on a Work in Progress. In P. Armstrong & J. Deadman (Eds.), *Women's Health: Intersections of Policy, Research, and Practice* (pp. 21–34). Toronto: Women's Press.

Tweed, A. (2003). *Health Care Utilization among Women Who Have Undergone Breast Implant Surgery.* Vancouver: British Columbia Centre of Excellence for Women's Health.

United Nations. Department of Public Information. (1996). *Platform for Action and the Beijing Declaration: Fourth World Conference on Women, Beijing, China, 4–15 September, 1995.* New York. Retrieved from http://www.un.org/womenwatch/daw/beijing/platform/plat1.htm.

United Nations. Economic and Social Council. (1997). *Mainstreaming the Gender Perspective into All Polities and Programmes in the United Nations System.* Retrieved from http://www.un.org/en/ecosoc/docs/2009/resolution%202009-12.pdf.

Walby, S. (2005). Introduction: Comparative Gender Mainstreaming in a Global Era. *International Feminist Journal of Politics* 7(4): 453–470.

Women and Health Protection. (2006). *Remembering Ruth Cooperstock: Women and Pharmaceuticals Twenty Years Later. A Symposium held at the University of Toronto, November 1, 2005.* Retrieved from http://www.whp-apsf.ca/pdf/coopProceedingsEN.pdf.

Further Reading

Auditor General of Canada. (2009). *The Spring 2009 Report of the Auditor General of Canada to the House of Commons: Chapter 1 Gender-Based Analysis.* Ottawa: Office of the Auditor General of Canada.

Bégin, M. (1992). The Royal Commission on the Status of Women in Canada: Twenty Years Later. In C. Backhouse & D. Flaherty (Eds.), *Challenging Times: The Women's Movement in Canada and the United States* (pp. 21–46). Montreal & Kingston: McGill-Queen's University Press.

CIHR IGH. (2012). *What a Difference Sex and Gender Make: A Gender, Sex, and Health Research Casebook.* Vancouver: Author. Retrieved from http://www.cihr-irsc.gc.ca/e/44734.html.

Health Canada. (2003). *Exploring Concepts in Gender and Health.* Ottawa: Minister of Supply and Services Canada. Retrieved from http://www.hc-sc.gc.ca/hl-vs/pubs/women-femmes/explor-eng.php.

Health Canada. (2009). *Health Portfolio Sex and Gender-Based Analysis Policy.* Retrieved from http://www.hc-sc.gc.ca/hl-vs/pubs/women-femmes/sgba-policy-politique-ags-eng.php.

Health Canada. (2013). *Guidance Document: Considerations for Inclusion of Women in Clinical Trials and Analysis of Sex Differences.* Retrieved from http://www.hc-sc.gc.ca/dhp–mps/prodpharma/applic-demande/guide-ld/clini/womct_femec-eng.php.

Paltiel, F. (1997). State Initiatives: Impetus and Effects. In C. Andrew & S. Rogers (Eds.), *Women and the Canadian State* (pp. 27–51). Montreal and Kingston: McGill-Queen's University Press.

Relevant Websites

Canadian Women's Health Network: www.cwhn.ca

Status of Women Canada. GBA+ Resources: http://www.swc-cfc.gc.ca/gba-acs/resources-ressources-eng.html

Schiebinger, L., I. Klinge, I. Sánchez de Madariaga, M. Schraudner, & M. Stefanick. (Eds.). (2011-2013). *Gendered Innovations in Science, Health & Medicine, Engineering and Environment*: genderedinnovations@stanford.edu

CHAPTER 3

Sex, Gender, and Systematic Reviews: The Example of Wait Times for Hip and Knee Replacements

Ann Pederson and Pat Armstrong[1]

Introduction

Health care, health policy, and health services reforms depend to varying degrees upon evidence drawn from research. Increasingly, research is identifying sex and gender differences in the underlying determinants of health and illness, the experiences men and women have of disease and care within the health care system, and the roles that they play within health care as paid and unpaid health care providers. Yet this research base remains small and its impact on health policy even smaller. This chapter reflects upon the use of one form of research evidence synthesis—systematic reviews—to understand the influences of sex and gender on one specific aspect of health care delivery as measured by wait times for total joint arthroplasty (TJA), more commonly known as hip- and knee-replacement surgery.

This study extends a previous narrative review prepared by members of Women and Health Care Reform and published as part of the federal wait times advisor's report in 2006 (Postl, 2006).[2] Based on a review of the published peer-reviewed literature, discussions with key informants familiar with that research, and an analysis of the available grey literature on the issue of wait times in Canada, it suggested that there was evidence of potential bias in the referral of women for hip- and knee-replacement surgery (see Jackson, Pederson, & Boscoe, 2009).

This study revisits the issue of wait times for TJA and gender through the methods of systematic review. Such reviews have become central in health services as a means of informing practices so we thought it was important to see the extent to which sex and gender are integrated in the methods of these reviews. Inspired by the work of the Cochrane and Campbell Collaborations, as well as by the tools described by the National Institute for Health and Care Excellence in the United Kingdom, we identified a research question, established inclusion and exclusion criteria for studies, conducted a systematic library search to identify relevant literature, critically reviewed that literature in a standardized approach, and summarized our findings across the set of included studies. Then we synthesized what that literature could tell us about how sex and gender influenced wait times for TJA.

The available literature on TJA provided only a limited view of sex as an independent variable and even less on the contribution of gender. Equally important, most of the literature sought to ignore context, while gender can be understood only in context. Our findings suggest that an approach to evidence synthesis that explicitly aims to take context into account, such as realist review (Pawson et al., 2005) or other methods of synthesis that are designed to bring multiple forms of evidence together to develop insight on a topic (see Dixon-Woods et al., 2005; Mays, Pope, & Popay, 2005), may be more suitable to the complex challenge of incorporating sex- and gender-based analysis into evidence synthesis.

Sex- and Gender-Based Analysis

Sex- and gender-based analysis (SGBA) involves asking questions about implications of the research, policy, or program for men and women and/or boys and girls (Clow, Pederson, & Haworth-Brockman, 2009). It is not a technique so much as a process of inquiry; it relies in part upon the reporting of information about a topic by sex—that is, by male and female—but such sex-disaggregated data are a minimum prerequisite to an SGBA.

In SGBA, "sex" is defined as the biological categorization of all species into male and female according to their reproductive characteristics whereas "gender" is understood to refer to "the array of socially constructed roles and relationships, personality traits, attitudes, behaviours, values, relative power and influences that society ascribes to the two sexes on a differential basis" (Health Canada, 2003, p. 8). Thus gender needs to be understood as a multi-dimensional phenomenon inclusive of processes that organize social relations, generate identities, establish and sustain social practices, and structure social institutions in specific contexts (see Johnson, Greaves, & Repta, 2007, 2009). However, while the distinctions between sex and gender have been prominent in health research circles in recent years, and have helped to spur research in important directions, they are intertwined and difficult to disentangle both in research and in their effects. Moreover, "Our common binary understanding of sex (male/female) is limiting and unrepresentative of the breadth and variety that exists with respect to human sexual characteristics" (Johnson, Greaves, & Repta, 2009, p. 5). Context shapes bodies and minds. Thus, ensuring sex and gender are taken into account requires understanding the context in which this shaping takes place.

Both sex and gender matter in health. Research has begun to demonstrate myriad ways that the human body is affected by biological variation, including those physiological and anatomical differences arising from the sex chromosomes, and from social practices that constrain and shape the body throughout the life course. From influencing prenatal exposures to regulating patterns of work, education, recreation, and reproduction, gender affects what we eat, how we are treated, our access to resources and opportunities, our self-concept, our safety, and our relationships. Because gender is a "complex, and powerfully effective, domain of social practice" (Connell, 2000, p. 18), it has the potential to have a profound impact on the nature of human health and illness as well as on how we respond to them through the social institutions of medicine, the family, and policy. To complicate matters further, sex and gender also affect health through their interaction with other key determinants of health, including income, paid and unpaid work, age, disability, racialization, geography, and language. In the analysis reported here, we ask whether systematic reviews are useful for understanding this complex array of factors and, in particular, for understanding gender as fundamentally tied to social context.

Gender and Wait Times for TJA as a Policy Issue

For individuals with advanced osteoarthritis of the hip or knee, total joint arthroplasty is the definitive treatment (Blackstein-Hirsch et al., 2000; Hawker, 2004). National statistics show that demand for hip- and knee-replacement surgery continued to grow in Canada over the past decade. For example, data from 2006–2007 indicate a 10-year increase of 101 percent and a 6 percent annual increase (Canadian Institute for Health Information, 2009a). Delayed procedures can result in poorer health outcomes and there are cost savings associated with hip/knee replacement performed earlier in the course of disease (Fortin et al., 1999; Ferrata et al., 2011), so timely access to care is important for patients in both the short and long term.

In the early 2000s, Canadian officials recognized that wait lists had developed in response to high levels of demand for numerous medical procedures, including TJA. In Canada, access to care is supposed to be related to medical need rather than other factors such as the ability to afford to pay for care. However, like many advanced capitalist countries with universal health insurance, Canada began to experience an increase in demand for surgical and diagnostic procedures that led to wait lists for the procedure. These wait lists raised concern about the erosion of public confidence in medicare in the 1990s. According to Roy Romanow's Royal Commission Report, "long waiting times are the main, and in many cases only reason Canadians say they would be willing to pay for treatments outside of the public health system" (Romanow, 2002, p. 138).

In the 2004 Health Accord, federal, provincial, and territorial first ministers agreed to establish clinically acceptable wait times in five priority areas and to make significant reductions in wait times by March 2007. In 2005 Canada's federal, provincial, and territorial ministers responded to public demand to reduce wait times by identifying priority areas for wait times interventions through dedicated funding. A $4.5 billion Wait Times Reduction Fund was thus established and a federal wait times advisor, Dr. Brian Postl, was appointed.

Dr. Postl invited members of Women and Health Care Reform (WHCR), a research group drawn from the Centres of Excellence for Women's Health and the Canadian Women's Health Network, to comment upon how gender might be a factor in wait times. Entitled *Gender-Based Analysis and Wait Times: New Questions, New Knowledge*, our report reviewed the findings of a gender-based analysis on total hip-/knee-replacement surgery wait times. As noted above, that initial analysis suggested that disparities exist between and among women and men with regard to the need for and use of TJA: while both men and women appeared to need more access to TJA than they were able to get, women were underusing TJA more than men. These findings were appended to the federal wait times advisor's report released later that year (Postl, 2006) and were referenced in the main text.

One explanation for the greater underuse of TJA among women than men put forward in the literature we reviewed was that so-called "gender-blind" or "objective" diagnostic tools, such as radiography, cannot distinguish how arthritis disease appears differently in women and men. A study examining function in patients awaiting knee replacement revealed that despite similar radiographically determined knee damage, women reported greater disability, impairment, and pain than men (Pagura et al., 2003). Other studies suggested that women were less likely to be referred, or were referred after a longer interval, to orthopedic surgeons for consideration for arthroplasty (e.g., Hawker et al., 2000). These findings are consistent with evidence of gender bias in diagnosis and treatment, and gender differences in clinical communication (Hawker et al., 2000, p. 1021). Diagnostic tools and referral practices must therefore be informed by gender and diversity analyses to ensure that they are valid for women and men across social locations. Simply counting the number of women and men is not enough.

Through our analysis, we determined that there was very little information about how women and men are affected by waiting, especially about how waiting for TJA is affected by factors known to be influenced by sex and gender. We wondered how wait times are affected by the kinds of paid and unpaid work men and women do, the supports they have, or when their responsibilities as wage earners and/or caregivers for family members and others are taken into account (see Jackson, Pederson, & Boscoe, 2008; Badley & Kasman, 2004). Instead, studies, to the extent that they address waiting at all, focus on the clinical impact of waiting, including the impact of waiting on patient-reported pain, functional limitations, and overall quality of life. Moreover, the literature provided little explicit evidence on how sex and gender were implicated in wait times for hip- and knee-replacement surgery.

To further examine the relationship between sex, gender, and wait times for TJA, we decided to approach the topic using a different methodological approach to complement our initial narrative review. What would we learn about the use of wait times for TJA using a systematic review? Could a systematic review approach incorporate SGBA? What follows is a step-by-step description of our process, something that is required in these forms of systematic reviews.

Knowledge Synthesis

The synthesis of evidence to inform health care decision-making has grown substantially over the past two decades. In general, systematic reviews are informed by an evidence hierarchy in which randomized clinical trials are the most valued and findings are compiled and compared statistically. Evidence is collected systematically following a predetermined protocol. The overall goal is to identify, evaluate, and summarize the findings of all relevant studies of a given treatment or procedure, and analysts rely on librarians and extensive research networks to identify all potentially relevant materials from a wide range of electronic sources and key informants. The main purpose of such reviews is to establish the effectiveness of interventions, whether these be health, medical, or social, and to generate generalizable findings across interventions to determine what works.

Conventional systematic reviews are designed to be replicable and multiple steps are undertaken to reduce potential bias in the acquisition, interrogation, or synthesis of findings. The process is intended to be rigorous, replicable, and transparent, as well as update-able should new studies be identified. Through the use of standardized quality-appraisal techniques and the application of tools for extracting and synthesizing findings, such reviews are intended to identify the best studies and to rigorously scrutinize all existing research.

It has been suggested, however, that the methods of conventional systematic reviews may not be applicable to some topic areas. The linear protocol and narrow hierarchy of evidence limit the flexibility of the process and do not permit the straightforward integration of multiple forms of evidence, including qualitative evidence (see Dixon-Woods et al., 2005). In particular, conventional reviews give little attention to context and/or the constraints on decision-makers in trying to interpret research or apply it in practice—a large problem given that gender is understood as context specific. "Decision-makers must address complicated questions about the nature and significance of the problem to be addressed; the nature of proposed interventions; their differential impact; cost-effectiveness; acceptability and so on" (Mays, Pope, & Popay, 2005, p. 6). Thus, researchers are beginning to suggest the need to develop and use a wider array of approaches to knowledge synthesis to address complex policy questions. Nevertheless, such systematic reviews remain the gold standard in evidence assessment.

In their work on cardiovascular disease, Doull et al. (2010) suggested that sex and gender are seldom considered in conducting systematic reviews and that this omission has important implications for assuring the quality of research and for achieving equitable health outcomes for women and men. However, Doull et al. applied their analysis of sex and gender to the set of systematic reviews themselves. In our study, we attempted to apply a sex- and gender-based analysis within the conduct of a systematic review and to look at the primary studies and see what we could learn about potential sex differences and gender influences on who had access to TJA, who chose to undergo TJA, and their experience of the process of TJA.

Methods

Three research questions animated this study: (1) What are the factors associated with wait times for total joint arthroplasty? (2) Are sex and gender considered in this literature? (3) If so, what does this literature say about the influence of sex and gender on wait times for TJA? Our purpose in framing the research questions this way was to see how the literature represented the issue of wait times for TJA and specifically whether sex and gender would be identified, alone or in association with other dimensions or aspects of social location such as age, socio-economic status, and race as factors influencing wait times for TJA.

Two sets of searches were conducted by a medical librarian and then combined to generate the final set of articles for review. Both medical and social science databases were searched because of the research question's breadth and the potentially wide list of factors that might be associated with wait times for TJA. Where databases allowed for language and date limits, records were restricted to articles written in English with a date range of 1985 to September 30, 2009. The first search produced a set of 1,447 references and the second 8,465 for a total of 9,912 references for further examination by members of the review team. Table 3.1 illustrates the distribution of articles in the second search by the various databases; most of the articles were obtained from medical sources, but there was clearly some literature from the social sciences as well included in the set of references.

To select relevant studies for detailed review, titles were initially scanned by two reviewers to remove studies that were clearly irrelevant and to identify duplicate articles. Next, references were screened for relevancy based on the titles. Then three reviewers examined the abstracts against formal inclusion and exclusion criteria to eliminate further ineligible references. Articles were included if they were English language and reported on research or provided a comment on wait times for TJA for hips and/or knees.

Articles were formally excluded if they dealt with:

a. other orthopedic procedures, including those for acute hip fracture and TJA for other joints, such as shoulders, ankles, etc.;
b. outcomes of pharmacological interventions or surgical techniques;
c. hospital report cards when they did not discuss wait times or TJA;
d. effectiveness of post-operative rehabilitation techniques (except if they explicitly relate to reducing wait times);
e. patient education materials, procedures, and approaches unrelated to wait times (e.g., discussions of resources designed to simply explain TJA to patients);
f. referrals to rehabilitation if unrelated to decision-making regarding the surgery; or
g. patient experiences of rehabilitation processes or techniques.

Database	Number of Titles Retrieved
Medline (OvidSP)	2,724
Medline in process	188
Embase	3,511
All EBM	940
CINAHL	940
PsycInfo	152
Sociological abstracts	10
Total	**8,465**

TABLE 3.1: Number of Articles Retrieved from Various Databases in Second Search

The first process yielded 188 articles for full-article review and the second produced 60. Once this sifting process was complete, electronic full-text articles were retrieved for a total of 248 studies, reports, and reviews for full assessment.

Based on the criteria, a further 21 were subsequently excluded based upon examination of the full article. Thus, the final total of articles for full review by three team members was 227. All 227 articles were subsequently reviewed and summarized by a team from the BC Centre of Excellence for Women's Health familiar with systematic reviews.

Three reviewers each reviewed approximately 76 full articles based on eight questions, namely, the type of article, country of context, research question, outcome of interest, whether "sex" and/or "gender" was defined, whether the outcome of interest was associated with sex and/or gender, whether the data were disaggregated in terms of sex, and whether other social location variables were considered. A subset of the articles was subsequently selected for further analysis on the basis that the article had explicitly associated an outcome of interest with sex and/or gender. These articles were used to explore how quantitative research approached sex- and gender-based analysis.

A conventional systematic review identifies a specific outcome of interest for assessment and documents an explicit quality-appraisal mechanism. Typically, the quality of evidence is established using a hierarchy of evidence that ranks randomized, controlled studies at the highest level, followed by meta-analyses or systematic reviews of randomized controlled trials (RCTs), then systematic reviews of other types of studies such as non-randomized clinical trials, case-control studies, cohort studies, and correlational studies. The lowest ranked evidence will usually include non-analytic studies such as case reports followed by expert opinion and formal consensus processes. It was impossible to apply this type of appraisal process to the literature on the factors associated with wait times for total joint arthroplasty. We therefore limit the discussion below to the nature of the studies and the approach they take to incorporating sex and gender into the analyses, rather than imposing an inappropriate evidence hierarchy on the body of literature available.

Main Findings

A total of 246 studies formed the core set of articles for this review. The final set of literature included material that ranged from editorial commentaries to reports of empirical research. A small subset of the material consisted of research on clinical assessment tools to document the patient experience of waiting for total joint-replacement surgery, including statistical analyses of the properties of the instruments themselves. A very small number of articles reported on the results of medical chart reviews of patients to provide a profile of the surgical load at a particular hospital or service or their efforts at improving patient flow through the service. Finally, nine articles were either narrative or systematic reviews.

Type of Article	Number of Articles
Editorial/commentary/essay (not a research study)	51
Empirical study	136
Instrument statistical assessment	22
Medical record analysis (audit)	9
Other (foreign language, missing, repetition, irrelevant)	19
Review (systematic or narrative)	9
Total	**246***

* The sample size is larger than 227 because the categories are not mutually exclusive.

TABLE 3.2: Breakdown of Articles by Type

As the review was limited to English literature, the distribution of articles reflects that limitation with the largest number of articles describing wait times and TJA issues about Canada, followed closely by the United Kingdom and the United States. A few were retrieved from the Nordic countries, Australia, and New Zealand. All these countries share similar concerns regarding access to surgical services, aging populations, and costs.

Given the complexity of the wait times issue, the articles addressed a number of approaches and strategies to monitor, reduce, or evaluate total joint-replacement procedures or wait times for surgery. From most frequent to least frequent, the articles were concerned with:

a. tools for setting priorities among patients based upon clinical need;
b. impact of waiting on patients, including quality of life, pain, and functional impairment;
c. organization of hip- and knee-replacement services;
d. economic cost evaluations;

e. the effectiveness of pre-surgical interventions (pre-habilitation initiatives designed to improve the patient's fitness for surgery and possibly improve post-operative outcomes such as these may include weight loss to reduce BMI, strength training to improve overall muscle strength, medical management of co-morbid conditions such as hypertension that may affect surgery, and so on);
f. reports on clinical outcomes of TJA;
g. population studies of the need for TJA and access to care;
h. reports on rehabilitation processes and outcomes;
i. decision-making aspects of the TJA process;
j. studies of patient quality of life during the wait period;
k. patients' reports of the acceptability of wait times;
l. the model of care;
m. profile of patients on a wait list;
n. revision outcome reports;
o. efforts to measure wait times;
p. benchmarks for wait times for TJA;
q. pre-surgery screening;
r. alternative management processes;
s. social support; and
t. provider training.

Approximately 30 percent of the articles actually examined sex or gender in relation to outcomes such as patient reports of pain, length of wait time, and choice of care provider. The majority, however, did not address either sex or gender in relation to the outcome of interest.

The most common way that "sex" was reported in the literature was simply as a feature of the study sample. That is, authors reported the sample as percentage female or offered a female/male ratio. No further analysis of sex was provided. Using keyword searching, 27 articles were identified as reporting sex-disaggregated data. Subsequent detailed examination of the articles suggested that not all of these articles actually reported clear sex-disaggregated findings, reducing the sample to 20. Thirteen articles reported findings in which sex was controlled hence the findings eliminate the effects of sex and render its effects invisible. Thirteen articles (discussed in detail below) performed multivariate analyses (typically multiple regression) in which sex was included as an independent (predictor) variable. Four articles described a study focused on the outcomes specifically in relation to women. Two of these provided sex-disaggregated data as part of the results, but the focus of the study was actually upon women. No articles said they were only about men.

The articles were also examined for whether they provided information about other aspects of identity, demographic characteristics, or social location. Slightly fewer than half the articles included some additional information about the study population (n = 96), most

Nature of Analysis	Number of Articles
Sex only as a demographic characteristic of sample	36
Analyzed sex differences	27
Controlled sex as a variable	13
Analyzed sex as a predictor of study outcome	13
Focus on "women"	4
Ethnicity/race	20
Age	72

TABLE 3.3: Nature of Analysis with Respect to "Sex", Ethnicity/Race and Age

commonly their age, followed by income and ethnicity or race. Other aspects of diversity noted included geographic location of the study population, disability, obesity, and the existence of social support networks.

The second aspect of this review was to characterize the content of the articles with respect to what the articles suggested regarding the influence of sex and gender on the issue of wait times for TJA. This analysis was performed by three reviewers who each read a third of the articles and then met to generate a thematic summary of their respective set of articles. A second reading was done to confirm details of particular studies. Three main questions animate this literature: (1) Who is waiting for total joint arthroplasty? (2) What is the effect of waiting? (3) Is this fair?

Overall, we found that the literature is concerned with access to care (with wait times for TJA as the example) and fairness (who gets care). More specifically, the literature describes the need for and impact of wait lists to manage demand for TJA in Canada, the United States, the United Kingdom, Ireland, Denmark, Norway, Finland, Sweden, Australia, New Zealand—all but the United States with a large public component to their health care. Some documentation considers the history of concern with access to TJA, beginning in the early 1990s with New Zealand and Britain struggling to meet demand and with explicit efforts to address wait lists for care.

Wait lists are understood in this literature as an explicit rationing system. The basic principle is that there is a queue for surgery based upon first come, first served. With demand exceeding supply, issues of determining how many people are waiting for care, the impact of waiting, and who gets care and when become more prominent. Discussions emerge about how to fairly distribute the scarce resource and with that, technical tools for assessing relative need for care. Procedures are identified to streamline the actual surgical procedures, reduce inefficiencies such as last-minute cancellations of surgery, and enhance communication of who is waiting for care. Studies often measure both medical/clinical and psychosocial outcomes, most commonly through various tools.

Some studies examined the perspective of patients on waiting and the "acceptability" of the wait. This literature documents patients' anxiety and concerns associated with waiting. Although sometimes captured qualitatively, more often formal Quality of Life assessments before and after surgery are used. Some of the literature explores patient decision-making about surgery regarding the location, surgeon, and timing of surgery. Much of this is concerned with identifying how patient decisions influence patient compliance with medical advice and the acceptability of waiting. A few articles address issues that might interfere with a patient's decision to accept surgery, such as the availability of social support and employment issues.

Those studies that examined the impact of waiting on patients focused largely on clinical aspects of the patients' experiences. For example, does waiting increase pain? Can this pain be effectively managed? How does this relate to patient reports of quality of life? A complex set of procedures has been introduced into the clinical pathway to TJA that is now known as "pre-hab." They include education and information about the procedure, preparation for surgery, and rehabilitation; exercise programs to promote strength and weight loss; weight management programs; and management of other medical conditions that might influence the outcome of surgery, including hypertension. Sometimes the waiting period is simply treated as the time frame pre- and post-test examinations, but not actually noted; other times, the waiting period is actually measured and assessed.

A few articles were clinical case summaries by surgeons who described TJA patient demographics and medical profile, including the reasons for surgery as well as other clinical information such as other illnesses and surgical outcomes. Other articles identified patients by medical status, where they were from, who provided care, and where the care was provided. Some of these considered the effectiveness of the surgery, documenting the impact of TJA on pain, quality of life, mobility, and functionality.

The published literature is also concerned with generating discussion of ways to improve the system of care. A major theme was how to identify those people needing care and ensure that they were receiving it in a timely manner. Some were concerned with the development, use, statistical validation, and evaluation of clinical priority-setting tools at both the individual and system level. These discussions often touched on issues of fairness, framing "fairness" in this case as ensuring that those with greatest medical need receive care first. There was little discussion of alternative ways of conceptualizing fairness.

With examples from Toronto, Vancouver, and Winnipeg, some articles exposed the complexity of responses to wait times for TJA. Some of these discussions are accompanied by cost analyses, suggesting that upfront investments enhance the flow of patients through the system and increase the likelihood that once in the queue, a patient will follow through to surgery and come through surgery well. Some articles also considered how alternative health care providers such as advanced practice physiotherapists, acupuncturists, or case managers could be used to promote a comprehensive approach to care.

The final aspect of the review focused on sex and gender within the articles, asking what we can learn about sex and gender through the systematic review process. Some articles examined sex as a demographic variable and some performed a statistical analysis using sex as an independent variable. These analyses raise questions about how to conceptualize and measure sex and gender as well as about the limits of approaching SGBA in the manner that was possible using the techniques of conventional systematic review.

Sex Differences

Seventeen studies reported data by sex. The majority of studies reported sex differences in relation to patient health status pre- or post-operatively and with respect to the impact of waiting on health outcomes. The studies all conducted statistical analysis to investigate sex as one of the potential predictors for their outcome among others. Such an analysis eliminates the possibility of attributing the outcomes to sex when it is a function of another variable.

Fourteen of these studies reported the results of multivariate analyses in which sex was included. The majority found some association. Of these, the largest number examined post-operative outcomes such as pain, co-morbidities, complications, length of rehabilitation, and level of recovery of function. Only a small body of literature examined other aspects of social location in relation to TJA and while some of the studies examined utilization of TJA by different age, racial, or income groups, none measured wait times per se. Research from the United States did suggest that individuals with lower incomes, who were black or who were women were less likely to receive TJA than those with higher incomes, who were white, or men. Given the association of the need for TJA with overweight and obesity, some studies also examined use of TJA in relation to these factors.

Discussion

This chapter analyzes not only wait times for hip and knee surgery but also the systematic review process. To some extent, our findings on TJA were confirmed. At the time of the initial study, publicly available wait times data for TJA were rarely disaggregated by sex (male and female) and there was a glaring absence of awareness of gender in the scientific literature. Since the publication of the federal wait times advisor's report, some wait times reporting provides sex disaggregation of data for who receives surgery. For example, the *Canadian Joint Replacement Registry 2008–2009 Annual Report* (Canadian Institute for Health Information, 2009b) included age- and sex-specific rates for joint replacements, documenting notable increases in knee replacement for both males and females in the 45 to 54 age group. Increases in the number of procedures performed were noted for both males and females, with different patterns by age group. Data from the Canadian Joint Replacement Registry (CJRR) and from the Hospital Morbidity Database (HMDB) suggested that females received more joint-replacement surgeries than males in 2006–2007, though it remains unclear whether these rates reflect changes in surgery rates by sex or whether they reflect the burden of illness by sex and hence the need for surgery. Osteoarthritis was the most prevalent diagnosis for hip/knee replacements for both males and females.

Yet all these data still provide only a partial view of the relationship between the need for TJA and access to services in relation to sex. Moreover, virtually no information is provided that would enable decision-makers to determine whether the rates of TJA were appropriate given gender influences on the need for surgery, referral rates for surgery, and actual procedures performed. While official statistics may now report some breakdown by sex, the scientific literature has little to say about the factors influencing wait times for hip- and knee-replacement surgery and even less to say about how sex and gender influence those wait times. Instead, a thematic assessment of the literature suggests that researchers are concerned with examining the clinical effects of waiting, efforts to reduce waiting through changes in clinical and organizational practices, and the use of clinical assessment procedures to ensure that those who are referred for surgery are appropriate candidates for the procedure. There is some discussion about access to surgery, but it is framed in terms of ensuring that those who are in greatest medical need receive care ahead of less clinically urgent cases. Hence the discussion of access to and use of TJA is largely framed as one of being able to accurately identify and assess medical need.

For this review, three related research questions were posed: (1) What are the factors associated with wait times for total joint arthroplasty? (2) Are sex and gender considered in this literature? (3) If they were, what does the literature say about the influence of sex and gender on wait times for TJA? These questions were designed to construct a method for conducting a systematic review of a complex health policy topic from the perspective of sex and gender. While we identified a vast literature related to the topic of TJA, only a small portion of it dealt explicitly with the issue of waiting for TJA, and very little of it considered factors associated with waiting that were not strictly medical in nature, apart from a small number of epidemiological studies concerned with capturing the relationship between potential need for TJA and use of TJA in the United States.

The response to our first question is rather limited. While the literature identifies a number of factors as associated with hip- and knee-replacement surgery, it says relatively little about waiting for TJA and even less about the influence of sex and gender. In this literature, "wait time" for TJA is more often the context or setting for the research than the focus of the research. Few studies examined wait times per se or factors associated with wait times. Rather, there was an assumption that wait times could be reduced by improved care practices and therefore the emphasis was on better measures of clinical need and various practices to enhance patient fitness for surgery. "Wait time" was often only mentioned as the period of time during which a study was conducted, but the focus was on whether patients might experience clinical deterioration in a joint or change their minds about surgery or become unfit for surgery during that period, not whether wait times could be reduced per se. Most wait times were not measured and few of the articles we reviewed provided any discussion of changes in wait times as such. When wait times were the issue, the articles focused on systemic, clinical, and programmatic factors that might reduce them, but did not necessarily measure wait times per se. This literature, despite the systematic nature of the library search, did not focus on measuring or changing wait times. Rather, the literature addressed the effects of waiting on patient health, clinical outcomes such as pain and mobility, and patient quality of life. A large body of material was concerned with identifying clinical need through patient- or physician-administered questionnaires or procedures.

Sex and gender, however, were minor notes in this literature. Most often, sex was only mentioned as a patient characteristic and we seldom learned whether the outcome—wait time, pain, and satisfaction with surgery—was associated with sex or not. More importantly, this limited attention to sex as an independent variable did little to address the concept of gender and its potential contribution to wait times for TJA.

Indeed, discussions about gender were essentially non-existent. In part, this reflects the complexity of the concept of gender and the fact that gender is fundamentally about context—that is, historic, social, and economic practices—which systematic reviews and most primary research strip away as part of the research process. It may also reflect the assumption that researchers have made that neither sex nor gender is a relevant factor in understanding medical care. Yet research is beginning to challenge this view. As Hawker et al. (2002) have begun to document, there may be gender biases in the process of referral to TJA surgery and we may see gender norms enacted in patient decision-making about the timing and use of TJA. "Women, compared with men, have disproportionately greater potential unmet need for hip/knee arthoplasty after taking into consideration age, disease severity, and willingness to consider arthroplasty" (Hawker et al., 2002, p. 3337).

Conclusions

The challenges of examining sex and gender within this review process raise questions about the suitability of this approach to systematic reviews for analyzing sex and gender. Given that a previous narrative review was able to locate, identify, and summarize aspects of wait times for TJA that are associated with sex and gender, the fact that this systematic literature search and careful review process was not able to replicate those findings suggests that an alternative approach to the review process might be more appropriate for the assessment of sex and gender. It may be appropriate to consider approaches such as "realist review" as described by Pawson et al. (2005), for example. Realist reviews, which examine not simply what works but under what conditions, may be useful for articulating theories that suggest how sex and gender might shape the conditions and practices of patient decision-making, patient-practitioner interaction, and overall patient access to care. Realist review methods might also be better able to help reviewers identify under what conditions, in what contexts, and with what effects women and men, and subgroups of women and men, are able to access various health care services. Such an approach may help in developing responses not simply to clinical needs but to addressing health inequities that arise from fundamental differences in access to the determinants of health among some populations as well as to health care procedures. Evidence for equity, particularly gender equity, may require the use of review methods that can combine multiple forms of evidence and generate new theories about how health care decisions are undertaken, how procedures are allocated, how funds are distributed, and how care is accessed—or not.

Notes

1. This chapter is based upon a report prepared by a team of researchers from Women and Health Care Reform and the BC Centre of Excellence for Women's Health in 2010 with the support of the Women's Health Contribution Program of Health Canada. The views expressed are not necessarily those of Health Canada. The members of the project team were Patrice Allen, Pat Armstrong, Lorraine Greaves, Beth Jackson, Teresa Lee, Ann Pederson, Morgan Seeley, and Annie Qu. We are grateful for the intellectual, practical, and analytic contributions of all team members.
2. The full report is available upon request from Ann Pederson at apederson@cw.bc.ca.

References

Badley, E. M., & N. M. Kasman. (2004). The Impact of Arthritis on Canadian Women. *BMC Women's Health* 4(Supp. 1): S18–S27.

Blackstein-Hirsch, P., J. D. Gollish, G. Hawker, H. J. Kreder, N. N. Mahomed, & J. I. Williams. (2000). *Information Strategy: Urgency Rating, Waiting List Management, and Patient Outcomes Monitoring for Primary Hip/Knee Joint Replacement.* Toronto: Institute for Clinical Evaluative Sciences.

Canadian Institute for Health Information. (2009a). *Wait Times Tables—A Comparison by Province, 2009.* Retrieved from http://secure.cihi.ca/cihiweb/dispPage.jsp?cw_page=PG_2010_E&cw_topic=2010&cw_rel=AR_1909_E.

Canadian Institute for Health Information. (2009b). *Hip and Knee Replacements in Canada—Canadian Joint Replacement Registry (CJRR) 2008-2009 Annual Report.* Ottawa: Author.

Clow, B., A. Pederson, & M. Haworth-Brockman. (2009). *Rising to the Challenge: Sex- and Gender-Based Analysis for Health Planning, Policy, and Research in Canada.* Halifax: Atlantic Centre of Excellence for Women's Health.

Connell, R. W. (2000). *The Men and the Boys.* Berkeley: University of California Press.

Dixon-Woods, M., S. Agarwal, D. Jones, B. Young, & A. Sutton. (2005). Synthesising Qualitative and Quantitative Evidence: A Review of Possible Methods. *Journal of Health Services and Research Policy* 10(1): 45–53.

Doull, M., V. E. Runnels, S. Tudiver, & M. Boscoe. (2010). Appraising the Evidence: Applying Sex- and Gender-Based Analysis (SGBA) to Cochrane Systematic Reviews on Cardiovascular Diseases. *Journal of Women's Health (15409996)* 19(5): 997–1003.

Ferrata, P., S. Carta, M. Fortina, D. Scipio, A. Riva, & S. Di Giacinto. (2011). Painful Hip Arthroplasty: Definition. *Clinical Cases in Mineral Bone Metabolism* 8(2): 19–22.

Fortin, P. R., et al. (1999). Outcomes of Total Hip and Knee Replacement: Preoperative Functional Status Predicts Outcomes at Six Months after Surgery. *Arthritis and Rheumatism* 42(8): 1722–1728.

Hawker, G. A. (2004). The Quest for Explanations for Race/Ethnic Disparity in Rates of Use of Total Joint Arthroplasty. *The Journal of Rheumatology* 31(9): 1683–1685.

Hawker, G. A., et al. (2002). The Effect of Education and Income on Need and Willingness to Undergo Total Joint Arthroplasty. *Arthritis and Rheumatism* 46(12): 3331–3339.

Hawker, G. A., et al. (2000). Differences between Men and Women in the Rate of Use of Hip and Knee Arthroplasty. *New England Journal of Medicine* 342(14): 1016–1021.

Health Canada. (2003). *Exploring Concepts of Gender and Health.* Ottawa: Women's Health Bureau, Health Canada.

Jackson, B. E., A. Pederson, & M. Boscoe. (2009). Waiting to Wait: Improving Wait Times Evidence through Gender-Based Analysis. In P. Armstrong & J. Deadman (Eds.), *Women's Health: Intersections of Policy, Research, and Practice* (pp. 35–52). Toronto: Women's Press.

Johnson, J. L., L. Greaves, & R. Repta. (2007). *Better Science with Sex and Gender: A Primer for Health Research.* Vancouver: Women's Health Research Network.

Johnson, J. L., L. Greaves, & R. Repta. (2009). Better Science with Sex and Gender: Facilitating the Use of a Sex- and Gender-Based Analysis in Health Research. *International Journal for Equity in Health* 8(14): 1–11.

Mays, N., C. Pope, & J. Popay. (2005). Systematically Reviewing Qualitative and Quantitative Evidence to Inform Management and Policy-Making in the Health Field. *Journal of Health Services Research and Policy* 10(Supp. 1): 6–20.

Pagura, S. M.C., S. G. Thomas, L. J. Woodhouse, & S. Ezzat. (2003). Women Awaiting Knee Replacement Have Reduced Function and Growth Hormone. *Clinical Orthopaedics and Related Research* 415(October): 202–213.

Pawson, R., T. Greenhalgh, G. Harvey, & K. Walshe. (2005). Realist Review—A New Method of Systematic Review Designed for Complex Policy Interventions. *Journal of Health Services Research and Policy* 10(Supp. 1): 21–34.

Postl, B. D. (2006). *Final Report of the Federal Advisor on Wait Times.* Ottawa: Health Canada.

Romanow, R. J. (2002). *Building on Values: The Future of Health Care in Canada—Final Report.* Ottawa: Commission on the Future of Health Care in Canada.

Further Reading

Clow, B., A. Pederson, & M. Haworth-Brockman. (2009). *Rising to the Challenge: Sex- and Gender-Based Analysis for Health Planning, Policy, and Research in Canada.* Halifax: Atlantic Centre of Excellence for Women's Health.

Doull, M., V. E. Runnels, S. Tudiver, & M. Boscoe. (2010). Appraising the Evidence: Applying Sex- and Gender-Based Analysis (SGBA) to Cochrane Systematic Reviews on Cardiovascular Diseases. *Journal of Women's Health* (15409996), 19(5), 997–1003.

Hawker, G. A. (2004). The Quest for Explanations for Race/Ethnic Disparity in Rates of Use of Total Joint Arthroplasty. *The Journal of Rheumatology* 31(9): 1683–1685.

Hawker, G. A., et al. (2002). The Effect of Education and Income on Need and Willingness to Undergo Total Joint Arthroplasty. *Arthritis and Rheumatism* 46(12): 3331–3339.

Relevant Websites

Canadian Institute for Health Information: www.cihi.ca
Ontario Women's Health Network (OWHN): www.owhn.on.ca
Women and Health Care Reform: http://www.cwhn.ca/en/taxonomy/term/4335

CHAPTER 4

Women and Heart Disease—Getting to the Heart of the Matter

Karin Humphries

Introduction

Most of what we know about heart disease comes from studying men. This is despite the fact that every year heart disease claims the lives of women and men in almost equal numbers. Only in the past few decades have we begun to appreciate that heart disease is an important cause of death in women, and that sex matters with respect to risk factors and the likelihood of dying from heart disease. Heart disease is highly preventable, so understanding the risk factors and modifying them accordingly can significantly reduce the risk of death.

Myth #1: **Heart disease is a man's disease.** Truth: Heart disease is a major cause of death in women in North America and Europe.
Myth #2: **Women are not at risk for a heart attack until after menopause.** Truth: While risk increases with age, even among women 25 to 44 years of age, heart disease is the third most common cause of death.
Myth #3: **Current research on heart disease applies equally to women and men.** Truth: Women comprise only 20–25 percent of clinical trial participants, but emerging evidence suggests the effectiveness of treatments varies by sex.
Myth #4: **Women and men receive the same level of treatment.** Truth: Women are less likely to be cared for by a cardiologist when admitted to hospital and less likely to be treated with evidence-based medications.
Myth #5: **Women and men present with completely different heart attack symptoms.** Truth: Women and men are more alike than different with respect to symptoms of a heart attack. In both sexes, chest pain is the most common symptom.

TABLE 4.1: Common Heart Disease Myths

Risk Is Still Underestimated

Surveys in the United States and Canada have revealed that women fail to appreciate that they are more likely to die of heart disease and stroke than any other single condition. Breast cancer emerges as the health risk that most women fear, even though they are six to seven times more likely to die of heart disease. Awareness campaigns from the American Heart Association and the Heart and Stroke Foundation of Canada have almost doubled awareness in the past 15 years, but even so, only 50 percent of women can identify heart disease and stroke as the leading cause of death in women.

Sex Differences in Risk Factors

Research is starting to identify biological, clinical, and social differences in women and men with respect to their risks and their responses to heart disease. As knowledge increases, better and more tailored diagnostic strategies and interventions can be designed to meet the needs of both women and men.

Blood Lipids

In both women and men, elevated levels of cholesterol, specifically low-density lipoprotein (LDL) cholesterol (bad) are associated with an increased risk of heart disease. Prior to menopause, the higher level of estrogen helps keep LDL cholesterol low and high-density lipoprotein (HDL) cholesterol (good) high. High levels of triglycerides, another form of blood lipids, are more strongly associated with heart disease risk in women than men. High levels of triglycerides combined with declines in HDL cholesterol after menopause have been shown to increase the risk of death from heart disease in women over the age of 65.

Diabetes

This is a risk factor in both women and men, but the impact is greater in women. Diabetic women are three times more likely to develop heart disease than non-diabetic women; diabetic men are 1.7 times more likely to develop heart disease than non-diabetic men. It is not clear if this increased risk is due to the higher rate of concomitant obesity, hypertension, and high cholesterol in women, or whether diabetes in and of itself increases the risk of heart disease more in women than men.

Smoking

Again, smoking is a risk factor in both women and men, but women who smoke are twice as likely to experience a heart attack as their male counterparts. It is also important to note that women find quitting more challenging than men, perhaps because the menstrual cycle affects tobacco withdrawal symptoms. There is evidence to suggest that nicotine replacement therapy is not as effective in women.

Metabolic Syndrome

This is a constellation of risk factors—high blood pressure, glucose intolerance, low HDL cholesterol, high triglycerides, and a waist circumference greater than 88 cm (35 inches). The metabolic syndrome increases the risk of heart disease in both women and men, but among young women it may be the most important risk factor associated with the risk of a heart attack. Women with metabolic syndrome are also more likely to die within eight years of their bypass surgery than men.

Gestational Diabetes

Gestational diabetes, or glucose intolerance that is first identified during pregnancy, has been shown to be associated with cardiovascular disease two to three decades later. Gestational diabetes affects between 4 percent and 14 percent of pregnancies every year. Older age at pregnancy, obesity before pregnancy, and excessive weight gain during pregnancy are associated with a greater risk of gestational diabetes. It is unclear if this greater risk of cardiovascular disease is directly due to gestational diabetes or if the elevated risk is because women with gestational diabetes are at increased risk of developing Type 2 diabetes later in life; 93 percent of women with gestational diabetes develop Type 2 diabetes later in life.

Pre-eclampsia

Pre-eclampsia, or elevated blood pressure during or immediately after pregnancy, can double the risk of heart attack, stroke, and blood clots within two decades after pregnancy. Pre-eclampsia affects between 5 percent and 8 percent of pregnancies. Exactly how pre-eclampsia increases the risk of future cardiovascular disease is unknown at this time, but researchers theorize that the additional strain that pregnancy places on the cardiovascular system may unmask early underlying cardiovascular disease, in much the same way that a stress test is used to identify heart disease in a clinical setting.

Multiple Risk Factors

A recent Canadian study examined sex differences in the impact of traditional risk factors—diabetes, high blood pressure, elevated lipids, and smoking—and the risk of having blockages in the coronary arteries (Ko et al., 2014). For each of the four risk factors the impact was greater in women than in men, and in the presence of all four risk factors the risk of coronary artery blockages was almost two times greater in women than in men. Similarly, in a large international study of risk factors for heart attacks, the presence of high blood pressure and diabetes, as well as low physical activity, increased the risk of a heart attack more in women than men. Interestingly, the associations of risk factors were stronger among younger than older women and men (Anand et al., 2008).

In another Canadian study of heart attacks in young adults (under 55 years of age), the risk factor burden was greater in women than men; 24 percent of women and 15 percent

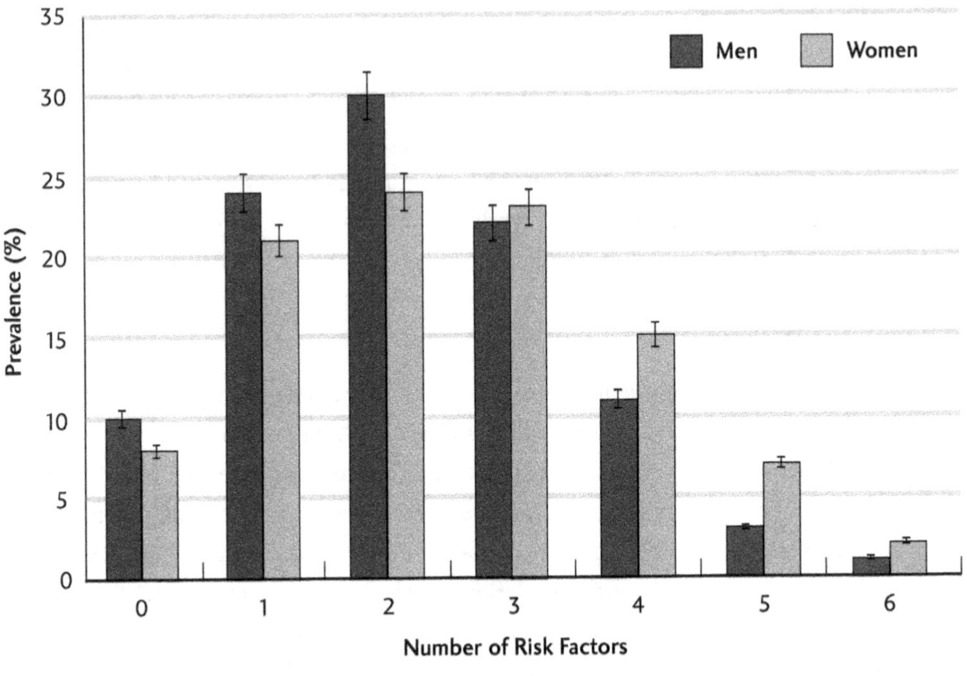

FIGURE 4.1: Proportion of patients with 0-6 traditional risk factors, according to sex

Source: J. Choi et al., 2014, Sex- and Gender-Related Risk Factor Burden in Patients with Premature Acute Coronary Syndrome. *Canadian Journal of Cardiology 30*(1): 113. Copyright 2014 by the Canadian Cardiovascular Society.

of men had four or more traditional risk factors. Among these young adults, 80 percent were current or former smokers, 55 percent had elevated lipids, and 48 percent had high blood pressure. Women were significantly more likely than men to have diabetes and a family history of heart disease.

Sex Differences in Presentation

There is considerable controversy about whether women and men present differently when they have a heart attack. In 2003, a key paper examining symptoms of a heart attack in women, both before and at the time of the event, was published. While this did not answer the question as to whether women presented differently from men, it provided important insights into the types of symptoms women experience before a heart attack (McSweeney et al., 2003). In particular, 71 percent of women experienced extreme fatigue in the week prior to their heart attack and almost half reported sleep disturbance. The most comprehensive description of symptoms in patients presenting with a heart attack is derived from a Canadian study among young adults under 55 years of age (Khan et al., 2013) and from a review of U.S. data (Canto et al., 2012).

A key finding is that women and men are more alike than different with respect to the signs of a heart attack. Most heart attacks involve chest discomfort that lasts several minutes or goes away and then comes back. This discomfort includes uncomfortable pressure, squeezing, a sense of fullness, or a stabbing pain. Chest discomfort is more likely in younger adults, with over 80 percent experiencing some type of chest discomfort, but among older adults chest discomfort may occur in only 50 percent of subjects experiencing a heart attack. Importantly, not all heart attacks involve chest pain, and in women in particular, other symptoms are quite common. These include:

- pain radiating to the neck, shoulder, back, arm, or jaw
- a rapid heartbeat that changes rhythm
- difficulty breathing
- heartburn, nausea, vomiting, or abdominal pain
- cold sweats or clammy skin
- dizziness

Microvascular Coronary Dysfunction

We classically associate a heart attack with a blockage in one or more coronary arteries. The buildup of cholesterol, other lipids, inflammatory cells, and fibrous tissue creates these blockages, or plaques. If the plaques build up to the point where they restrict blood flow, this can cause chest pain. If the plaque ruptures, the resulting blood clot will cause a heart attack. Blockages are visualized using a diagnostic test called a coronary angiogram, which provides a detailed X-ray picture of your heart and blood vessels. In women presenting for a coronary angiogram because of symptoms suggestive of a heart attack, a diagnosis of "normal" coronary arteries is five times more common than in men. While the term "normal" is somewhat subjective, it generally means there are no visible blockages, or the blockages are not significant enough to reduce blood flow through the coronary arteries.

Microvascular coronary dysfunction is associated with problems in the smaller blood vessels of the heart rather than the large coronary arteries that are visualized during a coronary angiogram. In patients with microvascular coronary dysfunction these small vessels do not function properly and as a result blood flow to the heart muscle is either reduced or completely absent. While men can present with microvascular coronary dysfunction, it is much more common in women. Because microvascular disease is an emerging area, the diagnosis of this condition remains a challenge and evidence for treatment is also lacking. It is also important to recognize that patients who present with chest pain, but without evidence of blockages in the major coronary arteries, are still at risk of cardiovascular events like a heart attack. They are also at a higher risk for depression and have a lower quality of life.

Sex Differences in Treatment and Outcomes

The overall consensus from research is that women are more likely than men to die within the first year of their heart attack. The reasons for this are not entirely clear, but there is evidence that women are diagnosed later than men; even when they are diagnosed, they are treated less aggressively; they are less likely to be prescribed medications; and they are less likely to be referred to cardiac rehabilitation programs. The reasons for these differences are also multi-fold. Women themselves tend to underestimate their risk of heart disease and thus may delay seeking treatment. Diagnosis can be more challenging in women than men, especially given that women are more likely than men to present with atypical symptoms like nausea, fatigue, or back pain, which are common to many other conditions, making the diagnosis of a heart attack more difficult in women.

In addition, women develop heart disease on average 10 years later than men. With increased age come more coexisting health conditions like high blood pressure, diabetes, and high cholesterol. These coexisting conditions increase the risk of complications and death.

In order to improve the outcomes of women with heart disease, more research is required. Importantly, the medical and research community needs to ensure that women are adequately represented in clinical trials and other research studies, and that the results of those studies are reported by sex, not just as an overall result.

How Women Can Reduce Their Risk of Heart Disease

There are several things women can do to reduce their risk of heart disease:

- *Don't smoke.* Your risk of a heart attack doubles if you smoke, even if you smoke as few as one to four cigarettes a day. Ongoing exposure to second-hand smoke can also increase your risk.
- *Increase your level of physical activity.* Aim for at least 30 minutes per day of moderate-intensity exercise five days a week. Brisk walking is considered moderate-intensity exercise. In addition, you can increase your level of activity by taking the stairs instead of the elevator or parking farther from your destination and walking.
- *Make healthier food choices.* A heart-healthy diet includes whole grains, a variety of fruits and vegetables, nuts, poly- or unsaturated fats instead of saturated fats, and fatty fish like salmon. Reduce or eliminate your intake of trans fats. Limit your salt intake—there is hidden salt in many processed foods.
- *Maintain a healthy BMI.* BMI stands for body mass index. It is calculated as your weight in kilograms divided by the square of your height in metres. Maintain your BMI between 18.5 and 24.9.
- *Decrease your waist circumference.* This measurement is taken at the level of your navel. For women the measurement should be no more than 88 cm or 35 in. For

Asian and South Asian women the waist circumference should be no more than 80 cm or 32 in.

- *Keep blood lipids in healthy range.* Know your cholesterol and lipid levels and keep them in the healthy range. For women the numbers you should aim for are outlined in Table 4.2.
- *Maintain a healthy blood pressure.* Ideally, your blood pressure should be less than 120/80 mm Hg. Regular exercise and achieving a healthy body weight can help you achieve this goal.

Cholesterol Targets	
Total cholesterol	< 5.2 mmol/L
HDL cholesterol	> 1.3 mmol/L
LDL cholesterol	< 3.4 mmol/L
Triglycerides	< 1.7 mmol/L

TABLE 4.2: Healthy Cholesterol and Triglyceride Values

Sex and Gender—Why Both Matter When It Comes to Heart Disease

In many articles the terms "sex" and "gender" are used interchangeably. While they are clearly related, these are distinct concepts. The Canadian Institutes of Health Research (2014) provides perhaps the most comprehensive definition of these two terms:

- Sex refers to a set of biological attributes such as physical and physiological features, including chromosomes, gene expression, hormone levels and function, and reproductive/sexual anatomy. Sex is usually categorized as female or male.
- Gender refers to the socially constructed roles, behaviours, expressions, and identities of people. It influences how people perceive themselves and each other, how they act and interact, and the distribution of power and resources in society. Gender is usually categorized as woman/girl or man/boy.

While some of the sex differences identified in this article are related to sex—females have smaller coronary arteries; females develop heart disease on average 10 years later than males—some important differences are more gender based. For example, women are less likely to be prescribed medications and are less likely to be referred to cardiac rehabilitation programs. Medication use can be expensive and women are overrepresented among those with lower incomes. The lower use of medications may therefore be driven by women's lower socio-economic status, which is associated with gender, not sex. Lower referral to cardiac rehabilitation may be driven by women's traditional role in child and elder care. If a woman who has just suffered a heart attack is responsible for child care and elder care, and perhaps works full time, it will be very difficult for her to participate in a cardiac rehabilitation program.

In order to improve women's cardiovascular health and close care gaps, both sex and gender need to be considered. This will require not only further research, but also different approaches to care provision, namely, care that recognizes and responds to sex and gender differences in heart disease and integrates care across the continuum, from primary prevention to cardiac rehabilitation, and from primary care in the community to tertiary care in a highly specialized teaching hospital.

References

Anand, S. S., S. Islam, A. Rosengren, M.G. Franzosi, K. Steyn, A. H. Yusufali, & S. Yusuf. (2008). *Risk Factors for Myocardial Infarction in Women and Men: Insights from the INTERHEART Study.* doi: 10.1093/eurheartj/ehn018.

Canadian Institutes of Health Research. (2014). *Definitions of Sex and Gender.* Retrieved from http://www.cihr-irsc.gc.ca/e/47830.html.

Canto, J. G., W. J. Rogers, R. J. Goldberg, E.D. Peterson, N. K. Wenger, V. Vaccarino, & Z. J. Zheng. (2012). Association of Age and Sex with Myocardial Infarction Symptom Presentation and In-Hospital Mortality. *JAMA* 307(8): 813–822. doi: 10.1001/jama.2012.199.

Choi, J., S. S. Daskalopoulou, G. Thanassoulis, I. Karp, R. Pelletier, H. Behlouli, & L. Pilote. (2014). Sex- and Gender-Related Risk Factor Burden in Patients with Premature Acute Coronary Syndrome. *Canadian Journal of Cardiology* 30(1): 109–117. doi: 10.1016/j.cjca.2013.07.674.

Khan, N. A., S. S. Daskalopoulou, I. Karp, M. J. Eisenberg, R. Pelletier, M. A. Tsadok, & L. Pilote. (2013). Sex Differences in Acute Coronary Syndrome Symptom Presentation in Young Patients. *JAMA Internal Medicine* 173(20): 1863–1871. doi: 10.1001/jamainternmed.2013.10149.

Ko, D. T., H. C. Wijeysundera, J. A. Udell, V. Vaccarino, P. C. Austin, H. Guo, & J. V. Tu. (2014). Traditional Cardiovascular Risk Factors and the Presence of Obstructive Coronary Artery Disease in Men and Women. *Canadian Journal of Cardiology* 30(7): 820–826. doi: 10.1016/j.cjca.2014.04.032.

McSweeney, J. C., M. Cody, P. O'Sullivan, K. Elberson, D. K. Moser, & B. J. Garvin. (2003). *Women's Early Warning Symptoms of Acute Myocardial Infarction.* doi: 10.1161/01.CIR.0000097116.29625.7C.

Further Reading

Arthur, H. M., D. M. Wright, & K. M. Smith. (2001). Women and Heart Disease: The Treatment May End but the Suffering Continues. *Canadian Journal of Nursing Research* 33(3): 17–29.

Bairey Merz, C. N., & V. Regitz-Zagrosek. (2014). The Case for Sex- and Gender-Specific Medicine. *JAMA Internal Medicine.* doi: 10.1001/jamainternmed.2014.320.

Brister, S. J., & M. A. Turek. (Eds.). (2001). Canadian Cardiovascular Society Consensus Panel Report: Women and Ischemic Heart Disease. *Canadian Journal of Cardiology* 17(Suppl. D): 1D-69D.

Government of Canada, Health Canada Health Policy Branch, Policy Planning and Priorities Directorate, Bureau of Women's Health and Gender Analysis. (2005, April 22). *Women and Hearth Health.* Retrieved from http://www.hc-sc.gc.ca/hl-vs/pubs/women-femmes/heart-cardiovasculaire-eng.php.

Grace, S. L., R. Fry, A. Cheung, & D. E. Stewart. (2004). Cardiovascular Disease. *BMC Women's Health* 4(Suppl. 1): S15. doi: 10.1186/1472-6874-4-S1-S15.

Heart and Stroke Foundation of Canada. (2007). *Real People, Real Lives, Real Results: Annual Report 2007.* Retrieved from http://www.heartandstroke.ca.

Izadnegahdar, M., J. Singer, M. K. Lee, M. Gao, C. R. Thompson, J. Kopec, & K. H. Humphries. (2014). Do Younger Women Fare Worse? Sex Differences in Acute Myocardial Infarction Hospitalization and Early Mortality Rates over Ten Years. *Journal of Women's Health* 23(1): 10–17. doi: 10.1089/jwh.2013.4507.

Killien, M., et al. (2000). Involving Minority and Underrepresented Women in Clinical Trials: The National Centers of Excellence in Women's Health. *Journal of Women's Health and Gender-Based Medicine* 9(10): 1061–1070.

Mosca, L., et al. (2004). Evidence-Based Guidelines for Cardiovascular Disease Prevention in Women. *Journal of American College of Cardiology* 43(5): 900–921. doi: 10.1016/j.jacc.2004.02.001.

Mosca, L., J. E. Manson, S. E. Sutherland, R. D. Langer, T. Manolio, & E. Barrett-Connor. (1997). Cardiovascular Disease in Women: A Statement for Healthcare Professionals from the American Heart Association (Writing Group). *Circulation* 96(7): 2468–2482.

National Institute of Health. (1991). *Opportunities for Research on Women's Health: Report of National Institutes of Health* (pp. 1–34). Bethesda, MD: Author.

Pilote, L., K. Dasgupta, V. Guru, K. H. Humphries, J. McGrath, C. Norris, & V. Tagalakis. (2007). A Comprehensive View of Sex-Specific Issues Related to Cardiovascular Disease. *Canadian Medical Association Journal* 176(6): S1–S44. doi: 10.1503/cmaj.051455.

Price, J. A. (2004). Management and Prevention of Cardiovascular Disease in Women. *Nursing Clinics of North America* 39(4): 873–884, xi. doi: 10.1016/j.cnur.2004.07.006.

Sawatzky, J. A. (2005). Cardiovascular Health in Canadian Women: The Bigger Picture Revisited. *Canadian Journal Cardiovascular Nursing* 15(3): 53–62.

Shaw, L. R., & Redberg, R. F. (2003). *Coronary Disease in Women: Evidence-Based Diagnosis and Treatment.* Totowa, NJ: Humana Press.

Vaccarino, V., et al. (2005). Sex and Racial Differences in the Management of Acute Myocardial Infarction, 1994 through 2002. *New England Journal of Medicine* 353(7): 671–682. doi: 10.1056/NEJMsa032214.

Wenger, N. K. (2004). You've Come a Long Way, Baby: Cardiovascular Health and Disease in Women: Problems and Prospects. *Circulation* 109(5): 558–560. doi: 10.1161/01.CIR.0000117292.19349.D0.

Zusterzeel, R., et al. (2014). Cardiac Resynchronization Therapy in Women: U.S. Food and Drug Administration Meta-Analysis of Patient-Level Data. *JAMA Internal Medicine.* doi: 10.1001/jamainternmed.2014.2717.

Relevant Websites

Centres for Disease Control—Women and Heart Disease Prevention: www.cdc.gov/women/heart/

Harvard Health Publications—Gender Matters: Heart Disease Risk in Women: www.health.harvard.edu/newsweek/Gender_matters_Heart_disease_risk_in_women.htm

Healthy Women: www.healthywomen.org

Heart and Stroke Foundation—HeartSmart Women: www.heartandstroke.com/site/c.ikIQLcMWJtE/b.4356323/k.89AA/Heart_disease__HeartSmart8482_Women_A_guide_to_living_with_and_preventing_heart_disease_and_stroke.htm

Heart and Stroke Foundation—The Heart Truth Canada: www.thehearttruth.ca

Ontario Women's Health Network—Key to Women's Health: A Health Promotion Framework to Prevent Stroke among Marginalized Women: http://www.owhn.on.ca/stroke/report.pdf

Society for Cardiovascular Angiography and Interventions (SCAI)—Seconds Count: www.scai.org/SecondsCount/Disease/Women.aspx

WomenHeart: www.womenheart.org

Women's Health Matters—Heart Health: www.womenshealthmatters.ca/health-centres/heart-health

Women's Health Matters—Sex Differences and Heart Disease: www.womenshealthmatters.ca/health-centres/heart-health/medical-description

SECTION TWO

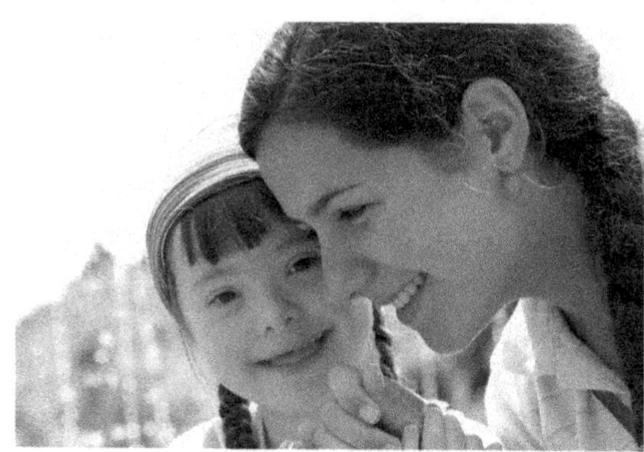

Asking Which Women

While the first section of this text focuses primarily on women as a group in order to emphasize the importance of a gender-based analysis, the second section explores the perspectives of women in different social and physical locations in order to stress the importance of recognizing the diversity, as well as the inequality, among women. Gender intersects with other social and physical locations, often compounding the impact of gender. As a result, we need to keep asking: Which women?

The first chapter in this section describes the pathways into care, specifically in-patient psychiatric services, for women who are mothering and living with serious mental illness. Written by Phyllis Montgomery, Cheryl Forchuk, and Sharolyn Mossey—all nurses with academic positions—this chapter details the challenges that women who have serious mental illness face in being supported to mother. They offer the unique perspectives of women so positioned and call for a shift in care from symptom management to active, deliberate support for women's mothering.

Chapter 6,written by Madeleine Dion Stout, offers a methodological and philosophical challenge to dominant approaches to women's health and women's health research through a discussion of the women whose ancestors were first in the country we now call Canada and who make up one of the largest populations of those identified by Statistics Canada as a visible minority. It is difficult to imagine a more revered expert on the issue of Aboriginal women's health than Madeline Dion Stout, a woman who began her career as a nurse, became a university professor in charge of a program devoted to Aboriginal issues, and moved on to establish a research program on Aboriginal women's health. With the hard evidence of statistics that expose Aboriginal women's poor health, she challenges the soft logic of Aboriginal women as primary health guardians.

In the next chapter, Ito Peng and Caitlin Cassie use their extensive experience studying immigrant women's issues in Canada to explore how the three statuses of age (elderly), immigration/ethnicity (culture, language, religion, etc.), and gender (female) intersect to generate "triple jeopardy" for older immigrant women. Older immigrant women are multi-disadvantaged because of the combined effects of occupying these stigmatized statuses. Their analysis of the research shows that the neglect is not just in the research but also in the practices that create barriers to both health and care.

In Chapter 8, Paula Pinto uses a human rights frame to reveal the barriers to health and care faced by women with disabilities and to challenge notions that see disabilities as simply biologically determined. With such an approach and based on her current international work with disability communities, she offers an analysis that leads to alternatives that take into account the social construction of disabilities.

Chapter 9, by Beverly Leipert and Robyn Plunkett, brings in both a new method and another population of women. In this case, both physical location and age are the basis of identity. Older rural women are the participants in a project that employs an increasingly popular research strategy called photovoice. This method puts cameras in women's hands, teaching them how to use the technology and how to capture their perspectives on health and care. The pictures became the basis of focus group discussions and the focus groups are the basis for the analysis of older rural women's health needs and resources in Ontario.

Chapter 10 considers women whose identity crosses all of the groups considered in this section. Anna Travers is the manager of the lesbian, gay, bisexual, transgendered, and transsexual program in a community health centre. As she explains, it is difficult to write such a chapter because there are challenges in describing the constituencies as well as challenges in presenting the issues these groups face in both getting care and keeping healthy. Nevertheless, she manages to draw a moving portrait of the many health and care issues faced by these constituencies.

The final chapter in this section, written by a team of researchers from across Canada, draws attention to the specific health needs of girls and younger women. Through their research into girls' groups as a site and method for health promotion, Nancy Poole, Christina Talbot, Jennifer Bernier, Cheryl van Daalen-Smith, Tatiana Fraser, and Bilkis Vissandjée share the perspectives of girls in several communities about how girls-only spaces may be important resources for girls' development and well-being.

The chapters in this section are meant to illustrate the importance of recognizing differences and inequities among women and girls, as well as draw our attention to the specifics of health problems experienced by the particular groups of women considered here. In the space available, it is possible to explore only some issues for some women. However, it is possible to demonstrate how intersectional analysis can be done and why it should be done. As you read these chapters, consider the following questions:

1. What, if anything, is similar in the portrayals of diverse groups of women found in this section?
2. What methods do the various authors advocate for understanding the particular group of women they write about?
3. Why do women's health researchers and advocates stress the importance of examining diversity and inequity among women?

CHAPTER 5

Pathways into In-Patient Psychiatric Services for Women Who Are Mothering and Living with Serious Mental Illness

Phyllis Montgomery, Cheryl Forchuk, and Sharolyn Mossey

Introduction

The Mental Health Commission of Canada (2010) reports that annually, over 3.6 million Canadian females live with mental health problems and illnesses. This pan-Canadian survey reports that mental illness occurs across the lifespan for one in five females. One of the highest prevalence rates of any mental illness for women is between the ages of 20 to 29 years, a period associated with coupling and parenting. Although no Canadian statistics exist, international researchers estimate that between 56 and 65 percent of women with a serious mental illness (SMI) are mothers (Campbell et al., 2012; Nicholson, Biebel, Hinden, Henry, & Stier, 2001). The overall fertility rate of women with schizophrenia in Ontario is 14 live births per 1,000 women, representing a modest increase since the mid-1990s (Vigod et al., 2012). Although variable, these statistics suggest a substantive prevalence of mothering in the context of mental illness.

Generated knowledge about mothers with SMI has yet to be comprehensively integrated into service delivery. Mental health structures, in particular, remain predominantly focused on servicing individual women for the purposes of symptom management (Ad Hoc Working Group on Women, Mental Health, Mental Illness, and Addictions, 2006). This orientation limits opportunities to purposefully support women living with SMI as they parent dependent children. Recent research involving mental health care providers has identified the need to ensure parent-sensitive approaches within community-based and in-patient services (Korhonen, Pietilä, & Vehvailäinen-Julkunen, 2010; O'Brien, Brady, Ababd, & Gillies, 2011; White & McGrew, 2013). Collectively this work supports the need for mental health service providers to competently address mothering realities inclusive of their social and economic hardships. Ultimately, standardization of parent-sensitive services could optimize the health outcomes for mothers, their dependent children, and extended family members.

Women with SMI have themselves articulated the need to be acknowledged and valued as mothers while in receipt of services. Evidence is building in relation to the perspectives of women who are mothering and living with SMI, their service needs, and service-seeking practices (Benders-Hadi, Barber, & Alexander, 2013; Blegen, Hummelvoll, & Severinsson, 2012). A recent synthesis of research involving samples of mothers with SMI identified the presence of shared experiences, including stigma, guilt, custodial loss, worry about their children's health, isolation, identity issues, and the overall importance of being a mother (Dolman, Jones, & Howard, 2013; Montgomery, 2005).

In light of the prevalence of mothering within the context of SMI, it is important to understand how mothers enter in-patient psychiatric services for management of acute symptoms. This chapter describes, from the perspective of women who are mothering and living with SMI, the circumstances that preceded their need for in-patient services. The goal of the chapter is to explain the circumstances that influence mothers' pathways into services. The authors hope to extend service providers' understanding of women's clinical presentations to include the possibility of mothering realities. The chapter begins with a brief descriptive review of literature on mothering with SMI. This review establishes a background for the presentation of a subset of data extracted and analyzed from qualitative interviews conducted with mothers who had been discharged from in-patient psychiatric services. These excerpts support earlier findings exploring pathways into in-patient psychiatric services for women who are mothering and living with SMI (Montgomery & Forchuk, 2009). The chapter concludes with a discussion of the implications for practice.

What the Literature Tells Us about Mothering and Serious Mental Illness

Help-seeking involves engaging others to obtain understanding, information, support, or treatment in response to the perception of need (Rickwood, Deane, Wilson, & Ciarrochi, 2005). Help-seeking for mental health needs is typically multi-dimensional and shaped by the interplay of individual, social, and cultural factors (Pescosolido, Gardner, & Lubell, 1998; Thompson, Hunt, & Issakidis, 2004). Individual-level help-seeking predictors are associated with heightened psychological distress, low self-rated mental health, the presence of a psychiatric diagnosis, a chronic medical condition, and a physical disability (Vasiliadis, Lesage, Adair, & Boyer, 2005). Although in a given year Canadian women are three times more likely to seek help for their mental health concerns compared to men (Cox, 2014), this does not equate with women's needs being met. "Moreover, there is not a linear relationship between diagnosis and need for treatment, nor is there a clear definition of what need for service entails" (Holmes-Nelson & Park, 2006, p. 2292).

Some of the diverse barriers to help-seeking for mothers with SMI include their beliefs and perceptions of illness severity, social disadvantage, and structural constraints such as poor service coordination or exclusionary practices (Benders-Hadi et al., 2013; Jeffery et al., 2013; Nicholson et al., 2001). Fear that their child may be removed by services, embarrassment about asking for help, or prior negative help-seeking experiences minimize mothers' involvement in community mental health services that may prevent an in-patient admission (Hearle, Plant, Jenner, Barkla, & McGrath, 1999; Montgomery, Tompkins, Forchuk, & French, 2006). If admitted to an in-patient psychiatric service, women hope to receive compassionate as opposed to "pathologizing" care (Miedema & Stoppard, 1993). A compassionate climate can support the establishment of a partnership with service that safely addresses a mother's unique health needs and contexts.

Although the majority of mothers with SMI want to be responsible for their children, few parenting supports are available to assist them (Hollingsworth, Swick, & Choi, 2011; Krumm, Becker, & Wiegard-Grefe, 2013; Sands, Koppelman, & Solomon, 2004). The stigma of mental illness places mothers with SMI under surveillance. Further, their preference to parent outside of the gaze of formal services, their experience of living with social disadvantage, and the possibility of symptom relapse increases their risk of mothering in isolation. On one hand, preferring to parent without professional intervention is understandable. On the other hand, however, without support, the ability of women with SMI to parent may be jeopardized. Services can mediate the effects of stress in illness and thereby allow mothers to attend to their responsibilities in the community (Blegen et al., 2012; Bybee, Mowbray, Oyserman, & Lewandowski, 2003; Dolman et al., 2013). For example, interviews by Mowbray and associates (2000) with mainly poor African American women living in the United States found that the most frequently reported stressor was a psychiatric crisis within the past year. In addition, daily fatigue, poor health, loss of significant others, problematic interactions with social service providers, and economic challenges compounded their stress. Only a minority of this group of women perceived mental health services as "somewhat helpful."

Investigating a Canadian Experience

The selected data set presented to illustrate a Canadian experience of entry into in-patient psychiatric services was collected from ethically approved qualitative interviews conducted with mothers with SMI. Using purposive and snowball sampling methods, the recruitment strategies involved oral invitations by clinicians and posters placed in health and social service agencies. For the purposes of this chapter, SMI is designated by the combined features of diagnosis, disability, and duration (Ontario Ministry of Health and Long-Term Care, 1999). Aspects of a particular feature may be more apparent than others relative to the interplay of biological, emotional, psychological, and social factors. Excerpts of data were extracted from transcribed interviews with seven consenting mothers who met the following criteria: age 20 to 29 years; formal diagnosis of a major mental illness (such as schizophrenia or a mood disorder); illness duration greater than two years; disability that negatively impacted their daily living; past history of in-patient psychiatric services; resident of northeastern Ontario; and living with or separate from dependent children.

Thematic analysis was used to allow the authors to theorize across the selected interviews. The focus was on the content of each mother's interview and the search for shared patterns within and across the selected interviews. Initial categorization of "what was said" and connections between the categories led to interpretation of data for the identification of themes (Kohler Riessman, 2005; Tatano Beck, 2013). This yielded three themes, which constitute a conceptual description of the circumstances that precipitated mothers' pathways into in-patient psychiatric services.

Who Are the Mothers Who Shared Their Pathways into In-Patient Psychiatric Services?

Individually, the mothers had between one and three children, aged three to 12 years old. Five of the mothers resided with their children. Other family members assumed custodial responsibility for the children of two of the mothers. These mothers maintained ongoing contact with their children. Five of the mothers were living apart from the biological fathers of the children. All of the mothers were unemployed and reported relying on public assistance as their source of income. Each mother was hopeful about entering the paid workforce in the future.

Each of the seven mothers was partnered with a psychiatrist for management of her mental illness symptoms. Several of them had received a variety of diagnoses over time, dating back to as young as 13 years old. Formal diagnoses included schizophrenia, bipolar, and major depression. Three mothers also had a history of illicit substance use. The length of time this group of mothers had lived with illness varied from three to 15 years, with many identifying that their illness symptoms predated formal diagnosis.

What the Mothers Tell Us

The immediate event that precipitated a psychiatric admission varied for each mother. There were, however, commonalities in the mothers' accounts of the experiences that unfolded resulting in their hospitalization. Across the interviews, the mothers described their illness, the impact of their illness on self and others, and the actions undertaken by themselves or others to get help. The three themes that represent pathways to in-patient psychiatric services were intrusive illness symptoms, unrelenting suffering, and seeking relief.

Intrusive Illness Symptoms

Mothers described the symptomatic presentation of SMI as dynamic rather than static. Symptoms typically cycle "in and out" of their lives, are either "up or down," and constantly threaten to "push, pull, or crush" them. Although mothers describe periods of symptom stability, their worry about relapse was a shared concern. The potential presentation of illness symptoms "at any time" was described as a reality that loomed in the backdrop of their lives. This is one mother's description of the pervasiveness of illness throughout her adult life:

> I was depressed "off and on" since I was 13. I didn't know what was wrong. Then when I attempted suicide at 17 and they [the police] put me in the hospital. After that I was "off and on" medication but it didn't really work. I spent years trying different medication but nothing worked. I was sick most of the time. I was very rarely what you would call "stable." Once I was finally diagnosed with bipolar disease and started on the right medication that helped. Being pregnant and postpartum was a breeze, compared to the psychotic mania I had before. I was stable for three years but I always had to be aware of things. I had to keep an eye on my illness. I had to be vigilant. Then I got ill again . . . my child was two.

As the presence of "uncontrolled" symptoms escalates, mothering practices become disrupted. All mothers valued their role as mother and thus feared "the point" that they would no longer be able to independently contain the impact of their illness. This theme is illustrated by the following excerpt:

> For me it starts so slow, I don't always notice that it is even happening. It might start out innocently by missing just one appointment because I have no ride. Then I miss a medication when my prescription runs out. I can become a bit more agitated and a bit more suspicious and I don't trust anyone or even myself. It gets to the point that I don't go out, I don't do anything. It's even hard to play with my son. I have to spend more time in my room and he sees that. That is illness. It's made of anxieties, worries, responsibilities, and the fear that I might cause pain to other people or myself.

Compounding the presence or threat of illness symptoms, the mothers described life contexts characterized by economic and social disadvantage. All engaged in efforts to protect themselves and their children from the cumulative vulnerabilities imposed by illness and socio-economic disadvantage. At times, however, their efforts to protect their children from the intrusiveness of their symptoms were undermined by the severity and duration, as well as by the magnitude of their situational disadvantage. Mothers' struggle to preserve their role as mothers in the presence of illness symptoms precipitated suffering.

Unrelenting Suffering

As pervasive illness symptoms became "monumental," mothers experienced suffering on a daily basis. Depicted as having "nightmares when you are awake," suffering was equated with "emotional torture" and "fleeting terror" in response to the belief that they were in jeopardy. Consumed by unrelenting suffering, mothers become overwhelmed and unable to fulfil basic roles and responsibilities, not only for themselves, but more importantly, from their perspective, for their children. At this critical juncture, mothers could no longer protect their children from their illness. For mothers, this was "hitting bottom." Being trapped in suffering fuelled thoughts, behaviours, and beliefs that were the antithesis of "who we really, really are." For example, one mother shared the following:

> I was crying, and crying, and crying. And my sister said "WHAT is the matter with you?" I didn't know. I didn't know why I was feeling this way, or what was happening, I just knew I wasn't me. I just cried. I remember yelling, out of my mouth came the words "Why don't you all leave and don't come back!" This was really strange. It was so weird, I loved my son, I loved my sister, you know. I didn't really want them to leave. I just balled and balled [*sic*]. I was exhausted. I had NEVER felt like this before and it wasn't going away.

Other mothers had "hit bottom" previously. Each sequential "hit" was described as more despairing, more destructive to their identities as mothers. Suffering was so "deep" it trapped them in time and space, robbing them of their desired lives. An ability to discern reality in the midst of suffering prompted self-questioning regarding their abilities, self-worth, and the essence of their lives.

> You get sick. You get better. You get sick. It's tiring, very tiring. You never win. When I'm really sick I don't think I can take care of my child. I KNOW I can't take care of her on my own. When I was really, really sick I even considered giving her up to protect her. I thought to myself that maybe she shouldn't have me as her mother. It's not logical thinking, I know that now. But other people looked at me and told me "you're crazy." I didn't know who I could talk to about this. You have to be careful who you talk to when you are really, really sick. I could have lost my daughter. I talked to my family, that was scary, but I was lucky, they took care of her. I could have lost her forever because I was not myself at all.

Mothers often suffered in isolation. Increasing symptoms led women to remove themselves from social situations that would expose their illness to others. In other circumstances, mothers described limited social contact because of ongoing conflict with their family of origin. Without a social network, their ability to carry out mothering practices was unsupported and invisible. Increasing deficits in their mothering practices were met with criticism by others, including their older children. They tried as "hard" as they could to care for their children, to uphold external mothering expectations, and as energy permitted, to fulfil their own needs. Juggling these responsibilities, mothers describe being "judged," "misunderstood," "unsupported," "trapped," and "alone." They often felt inadequate, and this increased their suffering.

> I remember a time when I was sick, so sick, and I had no groceries for me and my son. I couldn't go back to the food bank because I was already at my limit. They know me and my son. I hadn't talked to my mother much lately, but I needed help. I didn't want to burden her, but I had to tell her that I needed help. So, I called her. But, she didn't call back. I didn't know who to call next. I had to wait a few more weeks for my cheque to arrive. I wasn't even going to be able to give my son one dollar for pizza at school. I was so, so worried about what people would think.

In the context of unrelenting suffering, limitations on mothering practices were imposed by illness, concerned family members, or service providers. Mothers described being ashamed of or shamed for not being able to care for their children. They often became preoccupied with the creation of a plan to either endure or escape suffering. Plans vacillated between two opposing dialectics, some with extreme consequences: to seek/to avoid in-patient services, to mother/to relinquish mothering, or to live/to die.

> I just wanted to die. Would or wouldn't my son be better off? I got to a point where I just didn't care about anyone or anything. If I died part of me would be relieved because it held the promise of a little bit of peace. I was freighted [*sic*] though to hurt myself, I wished to simply die in my sleep. Somehow child services got involved and I knew something wasn't right.

Prior to in-patient psychiatric admission, taking medication was a viable option for the symptom management while maintaining contact with their children. Unfortunately, medication did not address their suffering; it only "dulled" their illness symptoms. To a point, being near their children helped mothers persevere through suffering. When symptoms did not abate, some mothers deliberately sought, or were taken to, in-patient services. Such services offered the hope of relief from symptoms and suffering. Ultimately, the goal of service for most was a return to their role as mother.

Seeking Relief

The decision to seek in-patient services is difficult for mothers. Some mothers courageously and voluntarily sought in-patient services only to be turned away. They describe being told by a health professional that they were "doing OK" and to keep up with their medications. They felt disheartened, especially in view of their readiness for separation from their children and to "surrender" to illness. Rather than getting the help they wanted, they had to return to their "chaos at home." Their hope for a "light at the end of the tunnel"—relief—was extinguished. As one mother explained:

> I've been sick a lot. I know what to expect from the hospital. I've been there at least 15 times. I just get sick of being sick. I love my children and know when I need help. I HATE the hospital and never want to go back. I'm not going there because I like it. I only go because I need to, so I can be there for my children. So when I show up, don't send me away because I probably haven't eaten, haven't slept, haven't had the right medication, tried everything I can think of, and I can't get it right. I needed their help. But can you believe that they turned me away. They were SO disrespectful.

Whether voluntary or involuntary, mothers' pathways to relief were preceded by a myriad of experiences, including powerlessness, fear, anger, rage, anxiety, profound sadness, fatigue, and psychosis. These emotions and their personal consequences were described as "painful," compounded by the perception that they were "absent," "undeserving," or "bad" mothers due to hospitalization. Separation from their children meant that family and others had to care them. Although comforting to some degree, mothers feared that surrogate caregivers may not validate their successes as mothers or do things the "way I do it." For others, an admission to hospital for psychiatric services was perceived as a real threat to their child custody.

> I wasn't really being a parent before I went into the hospital. I couldn't do things with my son even though I tried every single medication that was ordered for me. Some of the drugs even made me gain weight, some made me so agitated I couldn't sleep, but nothing worked for me. I was still hearing voices, and it was just too hard for me to deal with. I was scared. I couldn't tell the difference between reality and fantasy. I thought someone was going to kill me. I had to go to the hospital, even though it felt like punishment. I know people look down on me because I've been admitted so many times. I hate it there but I wanted desperately to get better. I needed to get better. I didn't want to lose everything. My parents took custody of my children when I couldn't, thank goodness.

All mothers described the centrality of their children in their lives. Separation from the chaos at home, however, while in receipt of in-patient services, offered the opportunity for mothers to come to understand the interplay of mothering and illness, discern their challenges, and address their concerns. Early optimism regarding the potential outcomes of acute care was described by mothers who believed that their children were "taken care of" by someone they "trusted" during their temporary absence. For some mothers, hospitalization was perceived as the last resort for securing safe, timely, and intensive services to support their quest to be "good," "responsible," and "well" mothers, worthy of being with their children.

> My daughter and I were always together. I knew she needed me and I love her so much. But I was having terrible thoughts. I knew I wouldn't kill myself. But I was having really, really bad thoughts. I told my psychiatrist and he said I could [go] in [to the hospital], but I wasn't sure it would help and I didn't want to leave my daughter. I was my own worst enemy. Then it got really, really, really bad. I just wanted it to stop, it was weird. It came to a point that my psychiatrist said "Why don't you come in for a break?" I decided that I couldn't go any further downhill. So I found somebody I trusted to take care of my daughter for me and I went in to the hospital respite to get time away from the world.

Interpreting the Voices

Each mother's voice included in this chapter provides a glimpse into their life and illness events, part of their unique mothering realities. Collectively, their voices detail a common pathway into in-patient psychiatric services. An interweaving of intrusive illness symptoms, unrelenting suffering, and the need to seek relief were consistent among all the women's descriptions. Consumed by illness symptoms, mothers are unable to fulfil desired life roles, including mothering their children. Mothers described this as the lowest point in their lives, analogous to "hitting bottom."

Literature has identified stigma as a barrier to seeking mental health services. Compounding this reality, mental illness is commonly perceived as incompatible with the social ideal of motherhood (Jeffrey et al., 2013; Krumm et al., 2013; Montgomery, 2005). Prior to in-patient admission, mothers explained how they minimized the risk of child removal by limiting their social contact to trusted family members. Avoidance of others, including health care professionals, lessened their perceived risk of having their child taken from them subsequent to a negative assessment of their mothering competencies. Delays in help-seeking and increasing social isolation, however, increased their risk for hitting bottom. For some, delays in seeking services compromised their ability to see how ill they were, and entrenched them at their lowest point in their lives—the bottom. In-patient services, although not preferred, offer the hope of relief from suffering and a return to their rightful place as mother for those in the midst of the bottom.

The term "bottom" has been used in the literature to signify loss of control, not only of illness, but also of one's desired life (DuPont & McGovern, 1992; Montgomery, Mossey, Bailey, & Forchuk, 2011). The bottom for mothers with SMI is indicative of an inability to sustain mothering in illness. Retrospectively, mothers describe the powerlessness they feel over their illness and life circumstances immediately prior to acute hospitalization. The extent of each mother's suffering at the bottom was not exclusively tied to her diagnosis or her symptoms, but to the impact of her illness on her treasured life roles. Situations that severely undermine self-identity and loss of agency have been reported to contribute to suffering (Cox & Holmes, 2000; Oliver, 2001).

Without agency, mothers are unable to fulfil their mothering responsibilities and lose their internal and external identity as a "good" mother. Looking back at their time at the bottom, they described themselves in undesirable terms: "undeserving," "crazy," "weird," and "awful." They realized how far removed they had unintentionally become from their children. Despite their lingering sense of responsibility for their children, they described their depletion of resources and thus choices to support their agency in the midst of suffering.

The availability and accessibility of resources, such as energy, coherent thoughts, support, affects mothers' degree of agency (Blegen et al., 2012). In the presence of mental health symptoms, non-professionals and professionals may not recognize mothers' sense of responsibility to their children and consequently fail to acknowledge and support mothers' agency (Brunette & Dean, 2002; Nicholson & Biebel, 2002). Yet, emerging in the area of psychosocial peer support rehabilitation services are parent-to-parent peer specialist mentoring (Reupert & Maybery, 2011). Mothers, through mutual, strength-based interactions, guide other mothers to promote their parenting, self-care, and social competencies. What remains unknown is the long-term impact of specialized peer support on families' well-being.

The mothers' voices in this chapter recount that acute psychiatric hospitalization occurs during their most vulnerable time, when illness symptoms and mothering collided. Immediately prior to admission, they have difficulty making sense of their suffering and finding the words to express their meaning. According to Younger (1995), crying, yelling, and inarticulate language are characteristic expressions of suffering. In crisis, mothers struggle to articulate the depth of their suffering, which has disrupted their mothering and separates them from their children. Mothers' accounts suggest that they would benefit from interactions with knowledgeable care providers who are competent in gender-informed care to address their suffering. Williams and Paul (2008) identify that gender-informed in-patient service providers are able to create opportunities for mothers to engage in safe conversations about illness and mothering. Such conversations are facilitated through the integration of core principles, including equity, knowledge, commitment, and relational-centredness. Through gender-informed dialogue, providers are able to intervene relative to presenting symptoms, respectfully acknowledge expressed suffering, validate mothers' strengths and challenges, and coordinate multi-agency community supports to sustain their desired role as mother (Williams & Paul, 2008).

Westad and McConnell (2012) contend that Canadian mothers living with SMI who are involved with child-protection services require broad-spectrum, multi-disciplinary services to address gender-specific issues. Prevalent issues experienced by mothers include stigmatization, single parenthood, unresolved emotional and physical trauma from their childhood, ongoing domestic violence, poverty, unstable housing, and guilt for cognitive, emotional, and behavioural issues with their children (Westad & McConnell, 2012). Effective, individualized, and continuity in services may mediate mothers' disadvantage and associated stressors and enable them to re-establish their desired responsibilities for their children (Dolman et al., 2013; Krumm et al., 2013).

With support, mothers are able to regain agency. They develop insight into and are capable of providing guarded testimony about the intrusiveness of their illness symptoms and their suffering that led them to seek in-patient services. The clarity of the mothers' description of illness symptoms and suffering integrated in this chapter is indicative that the mothers had begun to regain agency. They willingly shared their pathway to in-patient services, described as a vital component of their recovery process.

Conclusions

Within the context of SMI, women may struggle to fulfil their responsibilities of mothering, manage their illness symptoms, and avoid suffering. Although delaying in-patient psychiatric services may not be conducive to illness symptom management and may entrench suffering, it can be perceived as a strategy to remain with their children, to retain their identity as mothers, and to fulfil their mothering responsibilities. The pathway into in-patient care, which leads to a temporary separation from her child, although not preferred, becomes necessary in crisis. As described by mothers who had been discharged from in-patient services, their admission was precipitated by the interrelation of intrusive illness symptoms, unrelenting suffering, and the need to seek relief. In-patient services that address the reality of mothering in illness offers the hope of understanding the suffering experienced at the "bottom" and thereby support mothers in challenging contexts.

References

Ad Hoc Working Group on Women, Mental Health, Mental Illness, and Addictions. (2006). *Women, Mental Health, and Mental Illness and Addiction in Canada: An Overview*. Canadian Women's Health Network. Retrieved from www.cwhn.ca.

Benders-Hadi, N., M. Barber, & M. J. Alexander. (2013). Motherhood in Women with Serious Mental Illness. *Psychiatric Quarterly* 84(1): 65–72.

Blegen, N., J. Hummelvoll, & E. Severinsson. (2012). Experiences of Motherhood When Suffering from Mental Illness: A Hermeneutic Study. *International Journal of Mental Health Nursing* 21(5): 419–427.

Brunette, M. F., & W. Dean. (2002). Community Mental Health Care for Women with Severe Mental Illness Who Are Parents. *Community Mental Health Journal* 38(2): 153–165.

Bybee, D., C. T. Mowbray, D. Oyserman, & L. Lewandowski. (2003). Variability in Community Functioning of Mothers with Serious Mental Illness. *The Journal of Behavioral Health Services and Research* 309(3): 269–289.

Campbell, L., M.-C. Halon, A. W. C. Poon, S. Paolini, M. Stone, C. Galletly, H. J. Stain, & M. Cohen. (2012). The Experiences of Australian Parents with Psychosis: The Second Australian National Survey of Psychosis. *Australian and New Zealand Journal of Psychiatry* 46(9): 890–900.

Cox, D. R. (2014). Gender Differences in Professional Consultation for a Mental Health Concern: A Canadian Population Study. *Canadian Journal of Psychology* 55(2): 68–74.

Cox, H. M., & C. A. Holmes. (2000). Loss, Meaning, and the Power of Place. *Human Studies* 23: 63–78.

Dolman, C., I. Jones, & L. M. Howard. (2013). Pre-Conception to Parenting: A Systematic Review and Meta-Synthesis of the Qualitative Literature on Motherhood for Women with Severe Mental Illness. *Archives of Women's Mental Health* 16: 173–196.

DuPont, R. L., & J. P. McGovern. (1992). Suffering in Addiction: Alcoholism and Drug Dependence. In P. L. Starck & J. P. McGovern (Eds.), *The Hidden Dimension of Illness: Human Suffering* (pp. 155–201). New York: National League for Nursing Press.

Hearle, J. K., L. Plant, J. Jenner, J. Barkla, & J. J. McGrath. (1999). A Survey of Contact with the Offspring and Assistance with Child Care among Parents with Psychotic Disorders. *Psychiatric Services* 50(10): 1356.

Hollingsworth, L. D., D. Swick, & Y. J. Choi. (2011). The Role of Positive and Negative Social Interactions in Child Custody Outcomes: Voices of U.S. Women with Serious Mental Illness. *Qualitative Social Work* 12(2): 153–169.

Holmes-Nelson, C., & J. Park. (2006). The Nature and Correlates of Unmet Health Care Needs in Ontario, Canada. *Social Science and Medicine* 62(9): 2291–2300.

Jeffery, D., S. Clement, E. Corker, L. M. Howard, J. Murray, & G. Tornicroft. (2013). Discrimination in Relation to Parenthood Reported by Community Psychiatric Service Users in the UK: A Framework Analysis. *BMC Psychiatry* 13:120.

Kohler Riessman, C. (2005). Narrative Analysis. In C. Riessman Kohler (Ed.), *Narrative, Memory, and Everyday Life* (pp. 1–7). Huddersfield: University of Huddersfield. Retrieved from http://www.medarbetarportalen.gu.se/infoglueCalendar/digitalAssets/1771183328_BifogadFil_Chapter_1_-_Catherine_Kohler_Riessman.pdf.

Korhonen, T., A.-M. Pietilä, & K. Vehvailäinen-Julkunen. (2010). Are the Children of the Clients Visible or Invisible for Nurses in Adult Psychiatry—A Questionnaire Survey. *Scandinavian Journal of Caring Sciences* 24(1): 65–74.

Krumm, S., T. Becker, & S. Wiegand-Grefe. (2013). Mental Health Services for Parents Affected by Mental Illness. *Current Opinion in Psychiatry* 26(4): 362–368.

Mental Health Commission of Canada. (2010). *Making the Case for Investing in Mental Health in Canada*. Ottawa: Author.

Miedema, D., & J. M. Stoppard. (1993). Understanding Women's Experiences of Psychiatric Hospitalization. *Canada's Mental Health* 41(1): 2–6.

Montgomery, P. (2005). Mothers with a Serious Mental Illness: A Critical Review of the Literature. *Archives of Psychiatric Nursing* 19(5): 226–235.

Montgomery, P., & C. Forchuk. (2009). Pathways into In-Patient Psychiatric Services for Women Who Are Mothering and Living with Serious Mental Illness. In P. Armstrong & J. Deadman (Eds.), *Women's Health: Intersections of Policy, Research, and Practice* (pp. 61–76). Toronto: Women's Press.

Montgomery, P., S. Mossey, P. Bailey, & C. Forchuk. (2011). Mothers with Serious Mental Illness: Their Experience of "Hitting Bottom." *International Scholarly Research Network*. Article ID 708318, 8 pp.

Montgomery, P., C. Tompkins, C. Forchuk, & S. French. (2006). Keeping Close: Mothering with Serious Mental Illness. *Journal of Advanced Nursing* 54(1): 20–28.

Mowbray, C., S. Schwartz, D. Bybee, J. Spang, A. Rueda-Riedle, & D. Oyserman. (2000). Mothers with a Mental Illness: Stressors and Resources for Parenting and Living. *Family in Society: The Journal of Contemporary Human Services* 8(2): 118–129.

Nicholson, J., & K. Biebel. (2002). Commentary on "Community Mental Health Care for Women with Severe Mental Illness Who Are Parents"—The Tragedy of Missed Opportunities: What Providers Can Do. *Community Mental Health Journal* 38(2): 167–172.

Nicholson, J., K. Biebel, B. Hinden, A. Henry, & L. Stier. (2001). *Critical Issues for Parents with Mental Illness and Their Families*. Retrieved on from http://mentalhealth.samhsa.gov/publications/allpubs/KEN-01-0109/default.asp.

O'Brien, L., P. Brady, M. Ababd, & D. Gillies. (2011). Children of Parents with Mental Illness Visiting Psychiatric Facilities: Perceptions of Staff. *International Journal of Mental Health Nursing* 20(5): 358–363.

Oliver, K. (2001). *Witnessing: Beyond Recognition*. Minneapolis: University of Minnesota Press.

Ontario Ministry of Health and Long-Term Care. (1999). *Making It Happen: Operational Framework for the Delivery of Mental Health Services and Supports*. Toronto: Queen's Printer.

Pescosolido, B. A., C. B. Gardner, & L. M. Lubell. (1998). How People Get into Mental Health Services: Stories of Choice, Coercion, and "Muddling Through" from "First-Timers." *Social Science and Medicine* 46(2): 275–286.

Reupert, A., & D. Maybery. (2011). Programmes for Parents with a Mental Illness. *Journal of Psychiatric and Mental Health Nursing* 18(3): 257–264.

Rickwood, D., F. P. Deane, C. J. Wilson, & J. Ciarrochi. (2005). Young People's Help-Seeking for Mental Health Problems. *Australian e-Journal for the Advancement of Mental Health* (AeJAMH) 4(3) (Suppl.): 1–34.

Sands, R. G., N. Koppelman, & P. Solomon. (2004). Maternal Custody Status and Living Arrangements of Children of Women with Severe Mental Illness. *Health and Social Work* 29(4): 317–325.

Tatano Beck, C. (2013). *Routledge International Handbook of Qualitative Nursing Research*. New York: Routledge Taylor and Francis Group.

Thompson, A., C. Hunt, & C. Issakidis. (2004). Why Wait? Reasons for Delay and Prompts to Seek Help for Mental Health Problems in an Australian Clinical Sample. *Social Psychiatry and Psychiatric Epidemiology* 39: 810–817.

Vasiliadis, H.-M., A. Lesage, C. Adair, & R. Boyer. (2005). Service Use for Mental Health Reasons: Cross-Provincial Differences in Rates, Determinants, and Equity of Access. *Canadian Journal of Psychiatry* 50(10): 614–619.

Vigod, S. M., M. V. Seeman, J. G. Ray, G. M. Anderson, C. L. Dennis, S. Grigoriadis, A. Gruneir, P. A. Kurdyak, & P. A. Rochon. (2012). Temporal Trends in General and Age-Specific Fertility Rates among Women with Schizophrenia (1996–2009): A Population-Based Study in Ontario, Canada. *Schizophrenia Research* 139(1–3): 169–175.

Westad, C., & D. McConnell. (2012). Child Welfare Involvement of Mothers with Mental Health Issues. *Community Mental Health Journal* 48: 29–37.

White, L. M., & J. H. McGrew. (2013). Parents Serviced by Assertive Community Treatment: Prevalence, Treatment Services, and Provider Attitudes. *Journal of Behavioral Health Services and Research* 40(3): 263–278.

Williams, J., & J. Paul. (2008). *Informed Gender Practice: Mental Health Acute Care That Works for Women.* National Institute of Mental Health Care in England. Retrieved from https://www.google.ca/search?q=pdf+care+service+a+move+from+whats+wrong&ie=utf-8&oe=utf-8&aq=t&rls=org.mozilla:en-US:official&client=firefox-a&channel=np&source=hp&gfe_rd=cr&ei=i7K6U_fOI-HL8geQ3YCoDg#.

Younger, J. B. (1995). The Alienation of the Sufferer. *Advances in Nursing Science* 17(4): 53–72.

Further Reading

Benders-Hadi, N., & M. E. Barber (Eds.). (2014). *Motherhood, Mental Illness, and Recovery: Stories of Hope.* New York: Springer.

Ostler, T. (2008). *Assessment of Parenting Competencies in Mothers with Mental Illness.* Baltimore: Paul H. Brooks Publishing Co.

Reupert, A., & P. D. Maybery. (2007). Families Affected by Parental Mental Illness: A Multiperspective Account of Issues and Interventions. *American Journal of Orthopsychiatry* 77(3): 362–369.

Relevant Websites

Canadian Mental Health Association: http://ontario.cmha.ca/network/remodelling-the-village-supporting-parents-with-mental-illness/ and http://www.cmha.bc.ca/get-informed/personal-stories/visions-journal/parenting

Canadian Women's Health Network: http://www.cwhn.ca/

Centre for Addiction and Mental Health: http://www.camh.ca/en/hospital/about_camh/mission_and_strategic_plan/Pages/mission_and_strategic_plan.aspx

Centres of Excellence for Women's Health: http://www.cewh-cesf.ca/

Mental Health Commission of Canada: www.mentalhealthcommission.ca

Ontario Ministry of Health and Long-Term Care: www.health.gov.on.ca

CHAPTER 6

Healthy Living and Aboriginal Women: The Tension between Hard Evidence and Soft Logic

Madeleine Dion Stout

Introduction

Two narratives define Aboriginal women and healthy living: hard evidence documents our poor health status while soft logic passes us off as primary health guardians. Understanding this tension requires an insight into the health and social disparities we experience and a description of the linkages between these realities and healthy living policies. Key demographics, biological indicators, lifestyle behavioural issues, and social conditions that aggravate Aboriginal women's health have to be weighed against the totality of our environments and our desire and potential to contribute as health guardians. Ultimately, "healthy living" for Aboriginal women depends, to a great extent, on meaningful, appropriate, and responsive policies.

Hard Evidence: Aboriginal Women's Health Status

In 2001, there were about 499,605 Aboriginal women in Canada out of a total Aboriginal population of 976,305. Roughly 62.9 percent of these women self-identified as North American Indian, 29.2 percent as Métis, 4.5 percent as Inuit, and 2.6 percent as belonging to more than one group. In absolute terms, Ontario and British Columbia had the largest populations of Aboriginal women (97,180 and 86,805 respectively).

Aboriginal women made up the greatest share of the general female population in three territories and two provinces: Nunavut (86.8 percent), Northwest Territories (51.7 percent), Yukon (23.6 percent), Manitoba (13.7 percent), and Saskatchewan (13.7 percent). Meanwhile, the number of Aboriginal peoples over 65 years is growing three times faster than any other age group (Native Women's Association of Canada, 1997). Notably, in 2001 Aboriginal

	Total Aboriginal	North American Indian	Métis	Inuit	Total non-Aboriginal
			%		
Females aged					
Under 15	31.7	33.4	28.1	38.0	18.1
15 to 24	17.1	16.8	18.0	17.9	12.8
25 to 44	31.2	30.6	32.3	29.8	30.5
45 to 65	15.7	14.9	17.2	11.4	24.7
65 and over	4.3	4.3	4.5	2.8	13.8
Total	**100.0**	**100.0**	**100.0**	**100.0**	**100.0**
Total Population	**499,605**	**314,420**	**146,130**	**22,510**	**14,575,150**

Table 6.1: Age Distribution of Female Aboriginal Population, by Group, 2001

Source: Statistics Canada, 2006, *Women in Canada: A Gender-Based Statistical Report* (Ottawa: Author), retrieved from www.statcan.ca/english/freepub/89-503-XIE/0010589-503-XIE.pdf.

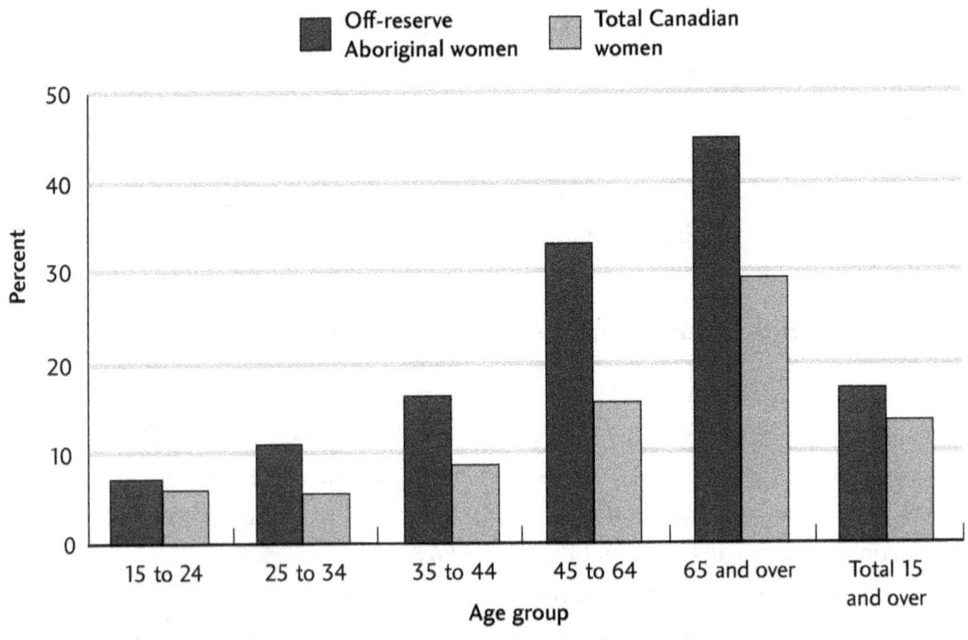

FIGURE 6.1: Percentage of off-reserve Aboriginal and all Canadian women reporting fair or poor health, by age, 2001

Source: Statistics Canada, 2006, *Women in Canada: A Gender-Based Statistical Report* (Ottawa: Statistics Canada), retrieved from www.statcan.ca/english/freepub/89-503-XIE/0010589-503-XIE.pdf.

	Females		Males		Females as a percent of the total Aboriginal population group in region	Aboriginal females as a percent of the total female population in region
	Number	%	Number	%		
Newfoundland and Labrador	9,375	1.9	9,400	2.0	49.9	3.6
Prince Edward Island	715	0.1	635	0.1	53.0	1.0
Nova Scotia	8,690	1.7	8,320	1.7	51.1	1.9
New Brunswick	8,335	1.7	8,655	1.8	49.1	2.3
Quebec	40,410	8.1	38,995	8.2	50.9	1.1
Ontario	97,180	19.5	91,135	19.1	51.6	1.7
Manitoba	77,015	15.4	73,030	15.3	51.3	13.7
Saskatchewan	66,895	13.4	63,295	13.3	51.4	13.7
Alberta	80,275	16.1	75,950	15.9	51.4	5.5
British Columbia	86,805	17.4	83,220	17.5	51.1	4.4
Yukon Territory	3,355	0.7	3,190	0.7	51.3	23.6
Northwest Territories	9,370	1.9	9,355	2.0	50.0	51.7
Nunavut	11,195	2.2	11,520	2.4	49.3	86.8
Canada	**499,605**	**100.0**	**476,700**	**100.0**	51.2	3.3

TABLE 6.2: Female and Male Aboriginal Populations, by Province and Territory, 2001

Source: Statistics Canada, 2006, *Women in Canada: A Gender-Based Statistical Report* (Ottawa: Author), retrieved from www.statcan.ca/english/freepub/89-503-XIE/0010589-503-XIE.pdf.

women aged 65 and over made up 4.3 percent of all Aboriginal seniors even though proportionally to youth, fewer Aboriginal women were seniors (Statistics Canada, 2006).

Recent data from the Canadian Population Health Initiative (CPHI, 2004) demonstrate that Aboriginal peoples are the unhealthiest group in Canada. Aboriginal women, however, are experiencing a disproportionate burden of ill health compared to Aboriginal men and other Canadian women (Statistics Canada, 2006).

For example, diabetes among First Nations and Inuit men is reported to be three times the rate for all Canadian men; for First Nations and Inuit women, however, the diabetes rate is five times the rate for all Canadian women (First Nations and Inuit Regional Health Steering Committee, 1999). Compared to about 4 percent in the general population, 40 percent of First Nations women have gestational diabetes (Health Canada, 2000a). One study revealed that rates of gestational diabetes increased with maternal age such that there was a 46.9 percent prevalence rate in women who were over 35 years of age (Harris et al., 1997).

On the eve of International Women's Day, the Canadian Aboriginal AIDS Network issued a press release with bleak statistics on Aboriginal women and HIV and AIDS:

> In Canada, Aboriginal people are significantly over-represented for both HIV/AIDS, seeing an estimated 91 percent increase (1,430 to 2,740) during a three year period, between 1996–1999 alone, for HIV infections. AIDS cases among Aboriginal women are almost three times higher than non-Aboriginal women (23.1 percent versus 8.2 percent). Various social, economic, and behavioral issues are believed to be influencing this health concern. In addition, Aboriginal women can experience a triple layer of marginalization, based on gender, race, and HIV status. With injection drug use accounting for two-thirds of the new HIV infections among Aboriginal populations, Aboriginal women face further challenges. AIDS figures reveal that injection drug use as a risk factor is six times more common among Aboriginal women than their counterparts (35.9 percent versus 6.3 percent). (Canadian Aboriginal AIDS Network, 2004)

As for reproductive patterns, 55 percent of Aboriginal mothers are under 25 years of age and 9 percent are under 18 years of age. Among non-Aboriginal mothers, roughly 28 percent are less than 25 years old, and only 1 percent are under 18 years of age (Health Canada, 2000b). Given the relative youthfulness of Aboriginal women, they have a higher fertility rate than non-Aboriginal women and larger families (Statistics Canada, 2006).

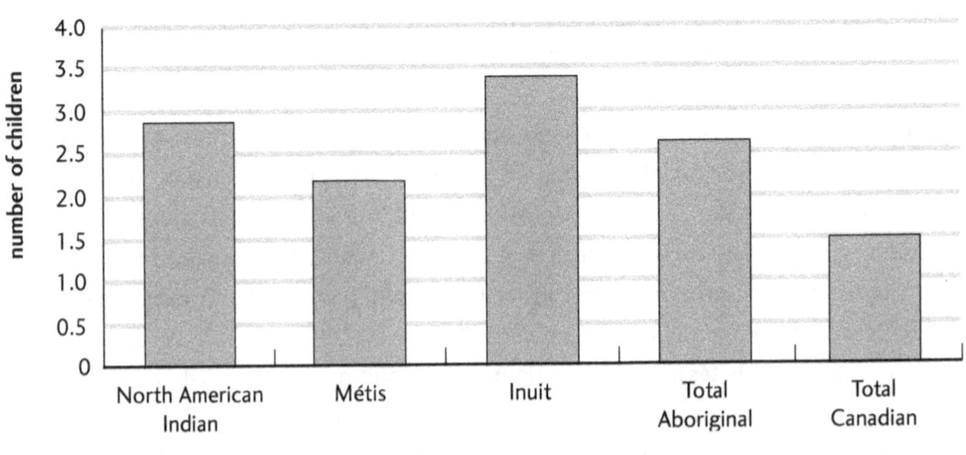

FIGURE 6.2: Fertility rates of Aboriginal and all Canadian women, by group, 1996–2001

Source: Statistics Canada, 2006, *Women in Canada: A Gender-Based Statistical Report* (Ottawa: Author), retrieved from www.statcan.ca/english/freepub/89-503-XIE/0010589-503-XIE.pdf.

The Canadian Population Health Initiative (2004) reports that "chlamydia rates are higher in Nunavut than for First Nations on-reserve, and the prevalence among these two populations is six times higher than the prevalence in the all-Canadian population" (p. 84). As well, more Aboriginal women are dying from cervical cancer than non-Aboriginal women, with the mortality rate of First Nations women in British Columbia being six times that of non-First Nations women (Botwinick, 1999). Likewise, Inuit women in Nunavik have three times the rate of cervical cancer than the general population (Hodgins, 1997).

Clearly, Aboriginal women have serious sexual and reproductive health problems. In addition, our health challenges are particularly relevant to the discussions in the Integrated Pan-Canadian Healthy Living Strategy.

For example, Aboriginal women face a high risk of obesity. In 1999, a study in northern Ontario deemed 60 percent of adult First Nations women obese. Research on adult Cree and Ojibwa Indians living in northern Canada found a high proportion to be overweight in all age and sex groups, with almost 90 percent of women ages 45–54 having a body mass index (BMI) of at least 26. According to Health Canada (2000a), BMI levels between 25 and 27 may lead to health problems in some people. First Nations and Labrador Inuit women are more likely to report chronic diseases such as arthritis, hypertension, and heart problems. First Nations women are more likely to die from ischemic heart disease and stroke at a rate that is much higher than that of non-Aboriginal Canadian women (Dion Stout, Kipling, & Stout, 2001). According to the 2001 Aboriginal Survey, a higher percentage

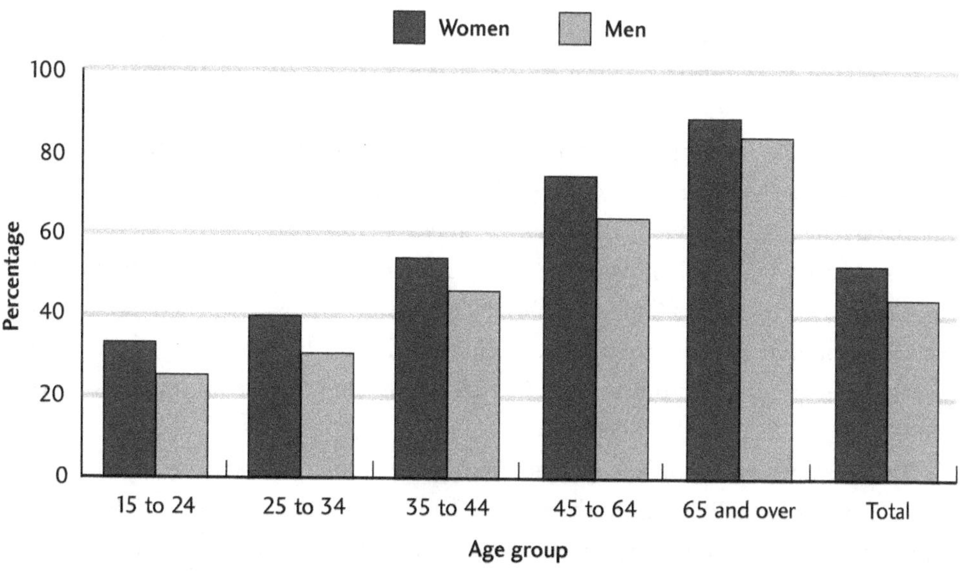

FIGURE 6.3: Percentage of Aboriginal women and men living off-reserve diagnosed with at least one chronic health condition, by age, 2001

Source: Statistics Canada, 2006, *Women in Canada: A Gender-Based Statistical Report* (Ottawa: Author), retrieved from www.statcan.ca/english/freepub/89-503-XIE/0010589-503-XIE.pdf.

of Aboriginal women than men are diagnosed with at least one chronic health condition (Statistics Canada, 2006).

Inuit women are particularly hard hit by environmental hazards according to the CPHI:

> In 2003 Inuit mothers had levels of oxychlordane and trans-nonachlor pesticides that were 6–12 times higher than those in Caucasians, Dene (First Nations), Métis, or other ethnicities. Inuit mothers have markedly higher levels of mercury in their blood than other ethnic groups. Inuit mothers have higher levels of polychlorinated biphenyls than Caucasian, Dene (First Nations), and Métis mothers. (Canadian Population Health Initiative, 2004)

Injuries, poisonings, and suicides exact a heavy toll in Aboriginal communities. The Report of the Advisory Group on Suicide Prevention (2001) revealed that youth suicide rates in First Nations differ by gender, with young men committing suicide more often than young women, but that Native young women are eight times more likely to commit suicide than their non-Aboriginal cohort.

A review of our social circumstances brings into sharper relief the multiple health burdens of Aboriginal women. Naomi Adelson, in a report from the International Think Tank on Reducing Health Disparities and Promoting Equity for Vulnerable Populations held in September 2003, observed that Aboriginal women are at a particular disadvantage:

> The colonial legacy of subordination of Aboriginal people has resulted in a multiple jeopardy for Aboriginal women who face individual and institutional discrimination, and disadvantages on the basis of race, gender, and class. (see Adelson, 2004)

In 2001, while Aboriginal women fared poorly in educational attainment compared to non-Aboriginal women, we were slightly more likely to have a university degree than Aboriginal men, 4.5 percent of whom have completed university.

Also, Aboriginal women were less likely to be employed, let alone full-time, than Aboriginal men (Statistics Canada, 2006). Notably, we were twice as likely as Aboriginal men to be employed in low-paying occupations, and almost twice as likely as Aboriginal men to be employed as professionals: 22 percent versus 12 percent (Statistics Canada, 2000).

Statistics Canada (2006) reported that Aboriginal women are less likely than non-Aboriginal women to be living in husband–wife families, are twice as likely to be living in common-law relationships, and are more likely to be lone parents. In 2001, 19.4 percent of Aboriginal women were lone parents.

Violence is a particular problem for Aboriginal women. From all accounts, most Aboriginal women have experienced domestic violence (Aboriginal Nurses Association of

	Aboriginal peoples		Non-Aboriginal peoples	
	Women	Men	Women	Men
			%	
Highest Level of Schooling				
Less than high school graduation certificate	40.1	44.1	29.2	28.2
High school graduation certificate only	9.1	9.0	15.3	12.4
Some post-secondary education	13.4	11.6	8.8	8.7
Trades certificate or diploma	11.3	18.9	8.4	16.0
College certificate or diploma	17.3	10.6	18.4	13.6
University certificate or diploma below bachelor's degree	2.2	1.2	3.2	2.3
University degree	6.6	4.5	16.6	18.9
Total	**100.0**	**100.0**	**100.0**	**100.0**
Total population 25 years and over	**255,520**	**227,765**	**10,065,140**	**9,364,735**

TABLE 6.3: Highest Level of Schooling of Aboriginal and Non-Aboriginal Women and Men Aged 25 and Over, 2001

Source: Statistics Canada, 2006, *Women in Canada: A Gender-Based Statistical Report* (Ottawa: Author), retrieved from www.statcan.ca/english/freepub/89-503-XIE/0010589-503-XIE.pdf.

	Total Aboriginal		North American Indian		Métis		Inuit		Total non-Aboriginal	
	Women	Men	Women	Men	Women	Men	Women	Men	Women	Men
People aged										
15 to 24	35.0	37.6	28.0	30.4	48.7	52.2	33.5	32.6	56.6	56.9
25 to 44	58.0	64.7	53.7	59.2	66.7	75.7	59.6	61.0	75.8	86.2
44 to 64	49.8	56.9	46.3	52.6	56.0	63.4	49.8	58.7	61.0	75.1
65 and over	5.6	10.6	5.4	9.1	6.0	12.9	10.3	15.5	4.8	13.0
Total	**47.1**	**52.5**	**42.5**	**47.0**	**55.9**	**63.0**	**48.0**	**49.2**	**56.3**	**67.6**

TABLE 6.4: Percentage of Aboriginal and Non-Aboriginal Peoples Employed, by Age and Group, 2001

Source: Statistics Canada, 2006, *Women in Canada: A Gender-Based Statistical Report* (Ottawa: Author), retrieved from www.statcan.ca/english/freepub/89-503-XIE/0010589-503-XIE.pdf.

	Total Aboriginal	North American Indian	Métis	Inuit	Total non-Aboriginal
			%		
Living with family					
With husband or wife	31.7	29.7	35.2	32.1	48.7
With common-law partner	17.1	18.0	14.5	23.0	9.2
Lone parent	19.4	21.3	16.0	16.9	8.4
Child living with parents	15.4	15.3	15.8	18.5	13.9
Living with extended family members	3.4	3.8	2.7	3.1	2.6
Total living with family	87.0	88.2	84.2	93.6	82.9
Not living with family					
Living alone	8.7	8.1	10.2	3.9	13.8
Living with non-relatives	4.3	3.7	5.6	2.5	3.3
Total not living with family	13.0	11.8	15.8	6.4	17.1
Total	**100.0**	**100.0**	**100.0**	**100.0**	**100.0**
Total population (000s)	**340.1**	**208.8**	**104.8**	**13.9**	**11,890.8**

TABLE 6.5: Family Status of Aboriginal Women Aged 15 and Over, by Group, 2001

Source: Statistics Canada, 2006, *Women in Canada: A Gender-Based Statistical Report* (Ottawa: Author), retrieved from www.statcan.ca/english/freepub/89-503-XIE/0010589-503-XIE.pdf.

Canada and Royal Canadian Mounted Police, 2001; Lane, Bopp, & Bopp, 2003). An initiative concerning Missing Women, the Sisters in Spirit Campaign, was launched on March 22, 2004,

> to draw attention to the tragedy of 500 missing Aboriginal women in Canada and to the travesty that there is so little awareness of this. Here in BC, 32 women have gone missing from the Highway of Tears between Prince Rupert and Prince George. Over the past 20 years, approximately 500 Aboriginal women have gone missing in communities across Canada. Yet government, the media, and Canadian society continue to remain silent. In Vancouver, more than 50 women went missing in that city's Downtown Eastside. Sixty percent were Aboriginal, and most were young. These were poor women involved in the sex trade. They struggled with drugs and alcohol. Some suffered from the effects of Fetal Alcohol Syndrome and many were victims of childhood sexual abuse. Every one of them grew up in a foster home. In other words, their lives bore all of the markings of the violence of colonization. (Status of Women Action Group, 2004)

Aboriginal women are reacting angrily about the politics of justice in Canada or, more fittingly, the lack of justice in politics. Similarly, a recent publication from the National Aboriginal Health Organization (NAHO) criticizes current policies that focus on changing individual lifestyle behaviours rather than dealing with historically determined power relations that have adversely affected the health of Aboriginal peoples. Myriad studies show that obesity, smoking, and physical inactivity have a lesser impact on health status than income and education (National Aboriginal Health Organization, 2003).

Conclusions: Soft Logic—Aboriginal Women as Health Guardians

Aboriginal women are critical players in the health development of our communities whether we are taking care of families, maintaining cultures, conducting research, or assuming leadership roles—all this in spite of our poor health prospects. Aboriginal women view health holistically and view social and cultural conditions as integral to the health of our communities. For example, childbirth in the North and midwifery in Inuit communities go hand in hand and are the heart of women working to keep culture alive and well.

As was suggested earlier, there is a link between the poor health of Aboriginal women and the health stewardship roles we play in the health of Aboriginal communities, yet only soft logic tries to locate this link and the immediate and intermediate health outcomes that arise from it. It is important to press hard evidence into service here for the following reasons. First, it recognizes a different context for healthy living policies where Aboriginal women are concerned, given the poor health and often deadly health determinants that impact us. Second, it reorients healthy living policies toward an emphasis on the positive realities of Aboriginal women's struggle for health development. Increasingly, we are identifying our human agency, pragmatism, and resilience as key strengths in this process. We also want to repair our efforts with Aboriginal men for the sake of our families and communities. Finally, it brings about a policy focus on Aboriginal women as nurturers of families, keepers of cultures, researchers, and leaders, and it recognizes the fluid and complex factors that affect our health and determine our capacity to take up and keep up the mantle of improving community health along with maintaining traditional roles.

The Women's Health Bureau of Health Canada stated: "While Aboriginal women play an essential role in community health, often under difficult social and economic conditions, their own health status is poorer than that of women in the general Canadian population" (Health Canada, Women's Health Bureau, 2003, p. 23). Therefore, as a strategy, "Healthy Living" has to be meaningful, appropriate, and responsive to Aboriginal women. It has to pay attention to the root causes of obesity, physical inactivity, and poor nutrition among Aboriginal women, along with the policies and programs that are all too often fractured and exclusive of the full range of health determinants. While healing and wellness programs have their place in the short term, it is economic and social reforms that will bring lasting change. Above all, healthy living has to be inclusive of mental, emotional, physical, and spiritual aspects and must be based on culture and tradition and be flexible to meet community needs and priorities. It needs both a gender analysis and an Aboriginal analysis. In addition, a healthy living strategy must consider the net effects of colonization and discrimination if it is to be meaningful to Aboriginal women. Finally, healthy living must be considered in light of the context of Aboriginal women's lives and their cultural, socio-economic, and political aspirations.

References

Aboriginal Nurses Association of Canada and Royal Canadian Mounted Police. (2001). *Family Violence in Aboriginal Communities: A Review.* Ottawa: Aboriginal Nurses Association of Canada.

Adelson, N. (2004). Reducing Health Disparities and Promoting Equity for Vulnerable Populations. Aboriginal Canada: Synthesis Paper. Edmonton: Institute of Gender and Health.

Botwinick, O. (1999). Gynecological Health Care. In J. M. Galloway, B. W. Goldberg, and J. S. Alpert (Eds.), *Primary Care of Native American Patients* (pp. 247–257). Woburn: Butterworth Heinemann.

Canadian Aboriginal AIDS Network. (2004). Aboriginal Women Continue to Face Major Challenges as International Women's Day Approaches. Press Release. Retrieved from www.caan.ca.

Canadian Population Health Initiative (CPHI). (2004). *Improving the Health of Canadians.* Ottawa: Canadian Institute for Health Information. Retrieved from www.cihi.ca.

Dion Stout, M., G. Kipling, & R. Stout. (2001). *Aboriginal Women's Health Research Synthesis Project: Final Report.* Winnipeg: Centres of Excellence for Women's Health.

First Nations and Inuit Regional Health Survey National Steering Committee. (1999). *First Nations and Inuit Regional Health Survey, National Report.* St. Regis, QC: Akwasasne Mohawk Territory.

Harris, S., L. Caulfield, & M. Sugamori. (1997). The Epidemiology of Diabetes of Pregnant Native Canadians. *Diabetes Care* 20(9): 1422–1425.

Health Canada. (2000a). *Diabetes among Aboriginal People (First Nations, Inuit, and Métis) in Canada: The Evidence.* Ottawa: Health Canada, First Nations and Inuit Health Branch.

Health Canada. (2000b). *Facts and Issues: The Health of Aboriginal Women.* Retrieved from www.hc-sc.gc.ca/english/women/facts_issues/facts_aborig.htm.

Health Canada. Women's Health Bureau. (2003). Aboriginal Women and Healthy Communities. *Health Policy Research Bulletin* 5: 23–26.

Hodgins, S. (1997). *Health and What Affects It in Nunavik: How Is the Situation Changing?* Kuujuaq, QC: Nunavik Regional Board of Health and Social Services.

Lane, P., Jr., J. Bopp, & M. Bopp. (2003). *Aboriginal Domestic Violence in Canada.* Ottawa: Aboriginal Healing Foundation.

National Aboriginal Health Organization. (2003). *Analysis of Aboriginal Health Careers: Education, and Training Opportunities.* Ottawa: Author.

Native Women's Association of Canada. (1997). *"Hear Their Stories": 40 Aboriginal Women Speak*. Ottawa: Author.

Report of the Advisory Group on Suicide Prevention. (2001). *Acting on What We Know: Preventing Youth Suicide in First Nations*. Ottawa: Health Canada, First Nations and Inuit Health Branch. Retrieved from http://www.hc-sc.gc.ca/fnih-spni/alt_formats/fnihb-dgspni/pdf/pubs/suicide/prev_youth-jeunes_e.pdf.

Statistics Canada. (2000). *Women in Canada 2000: A Gender-Based Statistical Report*. Ottawa: Author.

Statistics Canada. (2006). *Women in Canada 2005: A Gender-Based Statistical Report*. Ottawa: Author.

Status of Women Action Group. (2004). *Aboriginal Women's Health List*. Retrieved from awhrig-l@list.web.net.

Further Reading

Bolaria, B. Singh, & R. Bolaria (Eds.). (1994). *Racial Minorities in Medicine and Health*. Halifax: Fernwood.

DesMeules, M., D. Stewart, A. Kazanjian, H. McLean, J. Payne, & B. Vissandjée. (2003). *Women's Health Surveillance Report*. Ottawa: CIHI.

Dion Stout, M., G. D. Kipling, & R. Stout. (2001). *Aboriginal Women's Health Research Synthesis Project: Final Report*. Winnipeg: Centres of Excellence for Women's Health. Retrieved from www.cwhn.ca.

Network Magazine 4/5(4/1) (Fall/Winter 2001/2002).

Pauktuutit Inuit Women's Association of Canada. *Inuit Women's Health: A Call for Commitment*. Retrieved from www.cwhn.ca.

Relevant Websites

The Assembly of First Nations: www.afn.ca

CIHR Guidelines for Health Research Involving Aboriginal People: www.cihr-irsc.gc.ca/e/29134.html

Ethics of Health Research Involving First Nations, Inuit, and Métis People: http://www.cihr-irsc.gc.ca/e/29339.html

Prairie Women's Health Centre of Excellence: www.pwhce.ca/

CHAPTER 7

Older Immigrant Women's Health:
From the Triple Jeopardy to Cultural Competency[1]

Ito Peng[2] and Caitlin Cassie

Introduction

Canada's population is becoming older and more diverse. The proportion of Canadians over the age of 65 was 14.8 percent in 2011, up from 10.1 percent in 1981 (Statistics Canada, 2014a). It is projected that this proportion will increase to between 23 percent and 25 percent by 2036 (Statistics Canada, 2010). According to the 2011 National Household Survey, 30.15 percent of elderly Canadians (1.37 million people or 54.18 percent of total elderly population) are immigrants.[3]

	45–64 Years	65–74 Years	75 Years and over
		%	
United States	4.0	4.0	5.8
Central and South America	5.0	2.3	1.5
Caribbean and Bermuda	6.0	3.4	2.4
Europe	**50.0**	**65.6**	**72.0**
Africa	4.0	2.6	1.7
Asia	**30.0**	**21.4**	**16.1**
Oceania and other	1.0	0.7	0.6
Immigrant population	**100.0**	**100.0**	**100.0**

TABLE 7.1: Place of Birth for Immigrant Seniors in Canada, 2001

Source: I. Peng, 2006, *Older Immigrant Health and Its Policy Implications*, report presented at Institute for Life Course and Aging, Toronto.

Over one-tenth (12.7 percent or approximately 437,000) of the immigrant elderly immigrated to Canada between 2001 and 2011. The elderly Canadian population is also becoming more ethnically and culturally diverse. In 2001, about a third of all elderly immigrant Canadians had been born in countries other than in Europe. By 2011, this percentage had increased to 57.6 percent. Furthermore, among immigrant seniors who immigrated to Canada between 2006 and 2011, 86.3 percent of them came from countries outside of Europe, with 63.5 percent born in Asia (Statistics Canada, 2014b). In large cities such as Toronto, Montreal, and Vancouver, immigrants make up a significantly larger proportion of the population compared to the proportion suggested by the Canadian Census figure for the country. For example, according to the 2011 National Household Survey, nearly half of Toronto residents (49 percent) are immigrants, and over half of Toronto residents (51 percent) are born outside of Canada, with the majority from non-European countries. Moreover, a third (33 percent) of immigrants living in Toronto arrived between 2001 and 2011 (City of Toronto, 2013).

	45–64 Years	65–74 Years	75 Years and over
		%	
United States	3.0	3.1	3.7
Central and South America	5.0	2.8	1.9
Caribbean and Bermuda	7.0	4.1	2.8
Europe	53.0	68.5	75.2
Africa	4.0	2.0	1.3
Asia	28.0	19.2	14.9
Oceania and other	0.4	0.3	0.3
Immigrant population	**100.0**	**100.0**	**100.0**

TABLE 7.2: Place of Birth for Immigrant Seniors in Ontario, 2001

Source: I. Peng, 2006, *Older Immigrant Health and Its Policy Implications*, report presented at Institute for Life Course and Aging, Toronto.

Given the size and the ethnic and cultural diversity of the immigrant population, we can anticipate greater diversity of health care issues and concerns among the older Canadian population. As well, we can expect issues and concerns that relate to cultural differences and linguistic barriers to health care to become more prominent (Peng & Lettner, 2004).

Despite the demographic trend, however, little is known about immigrant health, and even less is known about the health of older immigrant women. In this chapter we survey existing literature on older immigrant women's health in Canada.[4] We focus on two areas of concern that are particularly important to understanding the health of older immigrant women: the ideas of the triple jeopardy and cultural competency. In what follows, we first discuss the idea of triple jeopardy and how it leads to health disparities experienced by older immigrant women. In the second part, we shift our attention to understanding how experiences of cultural dislocation and immigration may impact older immigrant women and their health. We build on the idea of triple jeopardy to examine how factors such as age, gender, ethnicity, and immigration interact to create stressors, buffers, and barriers to health care for individuals. Following this examination, we discuss buffers that are currently being employed and some ways in which professionals, organizations, and institutions can develop greater cultural competency in dealing with older immigrant women patients.

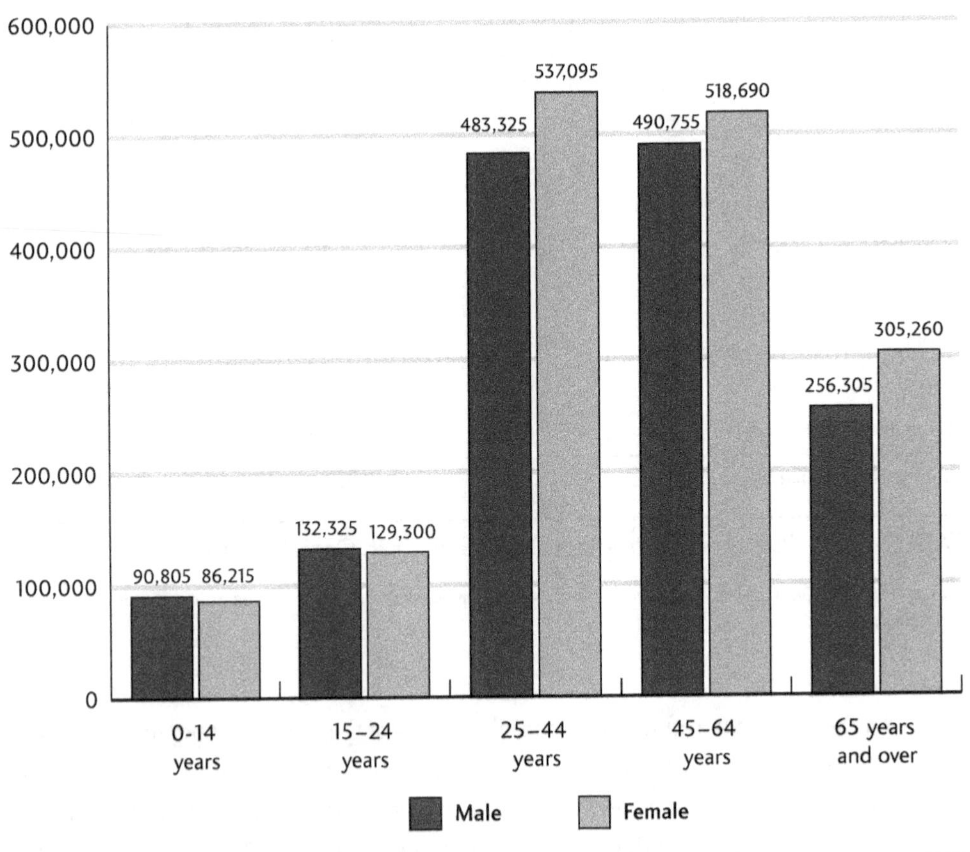

FIGURE 7.1: Immigrants by age and sex, Ontario, 2001 Census

Source: I. Peng, 2006, *Older Immigrant Health and Its Policy Implications*, report presented at Institute for Life Course and Aging, Toronto.

The Triple-Jeopardy Perspective to Older Immigrant Women's Health in Canada

It is now widely accepted in population health study that variables such as age, sex, income, education, disability, and ethnicity are important determinants of health. Researchers often use these variables to classify individuals, and to compare them to the general population to determine how these factors impact on health outcomes (Durst, 2005). This multiple determinants approach to population health has its theoretical root in sociological research on structural inequality. In the 1970s and the 1980s, feminist scholars and women of colour began to challenge the theoretical limitations of traditional social stratification theory that focused primarily on class-based inequalities, and began to theorize about the compounding effects of gender and ethnicity. They argued that women of colour faced double disadvantages because of their sex and their race/ethnicity.

The theory of double jeopardy that emerged out of this debate underscored the cumulative effects of multiple disadvantages (Beal, 1970; Chow, 1987; Garcia, 1989). Building onto the concept of double jeopardy, the triple-jeopardy hypothesis argues that status-based disadvantages are indeed cumulative. As Havens and Chappell point out, "the combined negative effects of occupying three stigmatized statuses are greater than occupying any one status or even two such statuses" (1983, p. 119). Researchers have applied the concept of triple jeopardy to study a variety of disadvantaged groups and people in different social locations, for example, older women of colour, women of colour with HIV/AIDS, women of colour with disabilities, and older people with HIV/AIDS or other illnesses. In our study, we focus on statuses of age (elderly), immigration/ethnicity (culture, language, religion, etc.), and gender (female). Older immigrant women are multi-disadvantaged because of the combined effects of occupying these stigmatized statuses.

Traditionally, studies examining population health related to age, ethnicity, and gender have been conducted primarily in the United States, and particularly in relation to African American, Hispanic, and Aboriginal populations, or by making distinctions between white and non-white people (Havens & Chappell, 1983). Canadian studies, such as this one, differ from American studies in that they tend to focus on more ethnically diverse groups, and are more likely to include people of Asian and South Asian origins.[5]

Impacts of Immigration on Older Immigrant Women's Health: Stressors and Barriers

Literature shows that older immigrant women in Canada face numerous health disadvantages because of their race/ethnic backgrounds, sex, and age. As the triple-jeopardy perspective suggests, race, sex, and age have compounding negative effects on older immigrant women's health. These effects are expressed in terms of higher levels of depressive symptoms and other forms of mental health issues, difficulties reconciling their paid work and caregiving responsibilities, higher rates of breast and cervical cancers, underutilization of preventive services such as cancer screening and breast self-examination, and difficulties accessing health care services and managing illnesses. These issues often arise from, and are compounded by, institutional racism and a lack of cultural understanding among health practitioners; sexism that neglects or marginalizes women's health priorities; and multiple stresses that are often associated with immigration and settlement, such as the lack of language competency, loss of social network, isolation, cultural dislocation, economic hardship, changes in family dynamics, and loss of personal autonomy. These overlapping challenges point to the need to develop effective strategies to address the health care concerns of older immigrant women at the institutional, service, community, and individual levels.

In this section, we first describe how the triple jeopardy of older immigrant women in Canada is evidenced through five multifaceted stressors: (1) migration stresses: immigration/resettlement; (2) age-related stresses; (3) gender-related stresses; (4) stress related to changing a socio-cultural environment; (5) and mental health stresses. Following this discussion, we examine a number of structural, organizational, and clinical barriers to health care that older immigrant women face.

We then use the framework of cultural competency to identify buffers elderly immigrant women use to cope with and/or reduce stressors and overcome the barriers to health care that they face. We elaborate on some strategies that could potentially help minimize stressors and barriers even further, supporting the empowerment of older immigrant women. A comprehensive framework of cultural competency is necessary in order to truly address the complex and nuanced realities faced by older immigrant women.

Pearlin et al. (2005) identify stressors as the "dogged hardships, demands, conflicts, and frustrations that may be instrumental in structuring people's experiences across time and to events that disrupt the continuities of their lives" (p. 205). They argue that exposure to different stressors contribute to the relationship between status inequalities and disparate health outcomes. Stressors can range from environmental or physical factors, such as weather conditions and urban setting and a fast-paced lifestyle that inhibit older immigrant women's mobility and social networks, to much more pervasive structural problems such as racism. The stressors identified in this review do not solely affect the older immigrant women population, nor are they experienced uniformly within this group. However, the fact that older immigrant women experience multiple stressors that are specific to their age, race/ethnicity, socio-economic status, and sex makes their situation unique. Furthermore, similarities of conditions and corroborating experiences of older immigrant women are identified in the literature, and therefore do suggest important trends with regard to direct health impacts on older immigrant women.

Migration Stresses: Immigration/Resettlement

In their studies, Meadows and her colleagues (2001) found that immigration affects the health of these women in multiple ways. The process of migrating itself was initially stressful, but a number of the women also reported more enduring health consequences. Some experienced improvements in their post-migration health, including reductions in migraines, flu, colds, and allergies. This was associated with better working conditions, improved air quality, and higher standards of living in their host country. But others found that their health had suffered after their moves. Both mental and physical factors were believed to play a role in the aches, pains, sleeplessness, and depression experienced by these women (Meadows et al., 2001). Other studies have also found that economic hardship, loss of status, downward mobility, homesickness, isolation, loneliness, and loss of social support associated with immigration sometimes led to depression and physical and emotional fatigue (Ahmad et al., 2004; Elliott & Gillie, 1998).

Immigration and resettlement experiences have specific impacts on the health outcomes of older immigrant women. Choudhry (2001) identifies four themes related to immigration and problems associated with resettlement for older immigrant women: "isolation and loneliness, family conflict, economic dependence, and settling in and coping" (p. 376). Feelings of isolation and loneliness result from decreased social support, children who have busy lives and no time for their mothers, and language barriers. Family conflict often arises from an erosion of traditional values, for example, what parents perceive to be their children's lack of respect for their parents, the independence of daughters-in-law, and the Westernization of grandchildren. Lack of personal income, widowhood, and ineligibility for an old age pension also create economic dependence. On the other hand, participating in spiritual activities and building social networks seemed to help older immigrant women adapt to life in Canada (Choudhry, 2001).

Many older immigrant women who come to Canada through the family reunification program may find themselves particularly dependent on their sponsoring children. When family conflicts arise, these women become vulnerable, as they may have little access to resources or options for independent living. In Canada, sponsoring older family members is a 10-year commitment, while the sponsorship commitment for a spouse or a child older than 22 years is three years (Koning & Banting, 2013, p. 592). During this long period, sponsored immigrants are not eligible for social assistance. Indeed, when the Ontario government learned that 7,500 sponsored immigrants were receiving social assistance in 2004, they informed the sponsors that this money was now considered a debt to the Government of Ontario. Despite legal proceedings going all the way to the Supreme Court, the sponsors were forced to pay (Koning & Banting, 2013, p. 592). In summary, achieving financial independence can be incredibly difficult for older immigrant women who are sponsored by their adult children, and the situation can become particularly precarious if familial relationships break down.

Nevertheless, women are more likely to put their family's well-being before their own. When interviewed about their health and well-being, most older immigrant women would identify issues related to physical health, adjusting to immigrant life, and restarting their lives in a new country, minimizing psychological and emotional stresses (Meadows, Thurston, & Melton, 2001). Although women define their health in holistic terms, involving physical, mental, and spiritual elements, when describing their individual health, they tend to focus more on physical and functional aspects. The latter relates to their roles as mothers, spouses, caregivers, and/or employees as sources of their families' well-being. Women are often hesitant to talk about non-physical or psychological aspects of their health, but they do discuss mental health if asked about it in a general sense while describing everyday life. The family also plays an important role in determining the well-being of older immigrant women by acting as a mediator for health concerns. Often, the overall health of the family influences the health of the women, particularly when older immigrant women are in the process of adjusting to life in a new country.

Age-Related Stresses

While immigration experience, loneliness, and the corresponding loss of connectedness present multiple stresses on an individual, there is no question that age is also an important factor. Stress is typically high among those in the advanced stages of life. People who immigrate later in life must deal with aging in an unfamiliar context with neither the accumulated life experiences nor the family or social networks that they likely have fostered over a lifetime in their countries of origin. Their experiences and knowledge may no longer be relevant in their new socio-cultural context. For the women who migrated from India to live with their adult children, isolation and loneliness were major sources of stress. These women had lost the companionship of the extended family and friends who helped them to deal with the everyday problems and issues they encountered in India. Their loneliness and isolation were compounded by feelings of being on the sideline of their children's hectic lives and being unable to communicate with those around them due to language difficulties (Choudhry, 2001). While younger immigrant women can often lessen their sense of isolation and derive financial and social benefits from participating in paid labour (Hyman et al., 2004), elderly immigrant women, who do not tend to work outside the home, are more dependent on their families and adult children.

Gender-Related Stresses

Men and women often have culturally prescribed roles and responsibilities that change in a new socio-cultural context. Immigrant women can experience stress related to maintaining "homeland" gender roles in a host country where conditions, structures, and supports may not be conducive to maintaining these roles. Elliott and Gillie (1998) note the propensity among South Asian Fijian immigrant women to define themselves according to their "traditional" familial roles. For many, however, economic necessity requires that they take on work outside the home in addition to maintaining their traditional caregiving and familial roles. As a result, these women performed their multiple roles as wives, mothers, caregivers, and waged workers while living in an unfamiliar environment with varying levels of social support. Many service providers are therefore concerned about these women being overburdened and compromising their health (Elliott & Gillie, 1998). Choudhry (1998) and Ahmad et al. (2004) concur that maintaining traditional gender roles in the new country is a significant source of stress for middle-aged and elderly immigrant women.

Moreover, older women are more likely than younger women to be expected to play the gender roles they filled before immigrating to Canada. In interviews with heterosexual married couples who had migrated from Ethiopia, Hyman et al. (2004) found that the older women were more likely than the younger women to accept "traditional" gender roles. For example, the older women did not expect their husbands to share household tasks, even when the women also participated in paid labour. The researchers found that older women were "reluctant to ask for help, citing their partner's age and/or consideration for his social status back in Ethiopia" (p. 84). As a result, gender and advanced age evidently work together to compound gender role-related stresses more acutely than if either one of these characteristics was experienced on its own.

Shifting gender roles and changing balances of power between men and women in the new country can create further stress in immigrant families. Interviews with elderly women from India who had been sponsored by their children revealed that conflict with their daughters-in-law was "the most frequent source of strain and stress for the participants" (Choudhry, 2001, p. 386). While women of the older generation expected to be respected and revered in their sons' homes based on their past experience as "dutiful daughters-in-law" to their husbands' parents, instead, these women had to be "passive and undemanding in their daughters-in-law's house" (Choudhry, 2001, p. 386).

Stresses Related to Changing Socio-Cultural Environment

Immigrants often face the challenge of adapting long-held lifestyle beliefs and activities, including their health regimes, into new physical and socio-cultural environments. Different contexts may be more or less hospitable to this task. The Canadian weather, for example, was frequently mentioned as an area of adjustment for new immigrant women (Ahmad et al., 2004; Choudhry, 1998; Elliott & Gillie, 1998). Women reported that the colder temperatures often limited their physical movement, which had consequences for their physiological as well as their mental health.

Choudhry (1998) shows that the middle-aged and older women who migrated from India were quite knowledgeable about how to maintain good health. For example, to stay healthy the women in the study claimed that they needed to regulate their weight, eat fresh fruit and vegetables, as well as take regular walks and remain active. However, many were unable to continue these health practices after moving to Canada because of social and physical factors that constrained them from pursuing these activities. For instance, the colder Toronto weather prevented them from going for regular walks, as was their custom in India. The lack of independent means of transportation and constraints to mobility also restricted their opportunities to go out and buy fresh fruit and vegetables on a regular basis, which limited them physically as well as socially since such activities had also contributed to social interaction in India.

Nutrition-related health ailments, such as diabetes and high blood pressure, were also a problem for older South Asian Fijian immigrant women in British Columbia (Elliott & Gillie, 1998). This was linked to socio-cultural conditions experienced in their new environment, including a relatively cold climate that restricted time spent outdoors; less physical movement due to living in an unfamiliar urban setting; and cultural traditions that place women in the home, focusing their role on the preparation of food for both the family and the community (Elliott & Gillie, 1998).

Spitzer et al.'s (2003) study of family caregiving among South Asian and Chinese immigrant communities in Canada shows that many immigrant women saw caregiving to be a central part of their lives. These women perceived themselves as primary caregivers because they regard women as the natural and more appropriate ones to provide care for their families. Furthermore, their gender-role assumptions for women were not limited to their duty to act as caregivers. Many of these women believed that the *process* of caregiving also helped them to solidify and reinforce their cultural and ethnic identity. These personal beliefs were, however, often at odds with the reality of their lives in Canada. The women in the study found that their paid work often created competing demands on them and took time away from their personal roles as unpaid caregivers. To preserve their cultural values and traditions, women seldom renegotiate their caregiving responsibilities, nor do they consider such renegotiation possible. The study thus highlights how the act of caregiving may, on the one hand, strengthen immigrant women's sense of cultural identity, but on the other, create enormous conflicts for them in attempting to reconcile their caregiving and paid work responsibilities.

The study also points to the fact that caregiving may be more costly for these women in Canada than in their countries of origin because of the lack of kin support, women's low wages not permitting the hiring of outside help, and the difficulties associated with balancing caregiving and paid work in the Canadian social context. These issues are further compounded by the lack of public support for immigrant caregivers (Stewart et al., 2006). Indeed, U.S. studies show that immigrant caregivers are less likely to receive support services such as home care and meal delivery, partly because of the caregivers' inability to negotiate the complex bureaucracy associated with receiving public services, and partly because of the lack of English language proficiency (Hong, 2004; Choi, 2001). As well, many social service providers also have cultural expectations that certain ethnic groups should provide more family care (Brotman, 2003). These studies suggest that not only are gender and ethnicity important factors determining the caregiving roles performed by immigrant women, but that socio-culturally based gender-role expectations also contribute to the triple-jeopardy situation older immigrant women face.

Mental Health Stresses

The importance of social and family connectedness in maintaining mental health is evident from studies such as Gee (2000), which found that widowed Chinese women living alone were significantly less satisfied with their health, accommodations, food, spiritual life, and self than those who lived with their children or those who were not widowed. The lone widows not only had lower scores on the well-being scale, but they were also much less likely to have a confidante—having a number of close friends was positively correlated with the women's life satisfaction. Gee (2000) also found that both health and English-speaking ability were positively correlated with a sense of well-being and life satisfaction, while age had a negative effect on these Chinese widows' sense of well-being. These findings indicate that age, gender, and ethnicity have a combined effect on individual mental health.

Lai's (2000, 2004a) studies of the mental health of elderly Chinese in Calgary found that women were more prone to mild to severe levels of depression (28.8 percent as compared to only 10 percent of men). The studies found that the women were more likely to report the following depressive symptoms: afraid that something bad is going to happen; feel unhappy most of the time; frequently worry about the future; and frequently get upset over little things. In addition, older Chinese women fared poorly compared to their male counterparts with regard to physical functioning. It was also found that those who identify more closely with traditional Chinese cultural values were more likely to experience depressive symptoms. The oldest group of Chinese women (75 years of age or older) fared poorly in the areas of social functioning and mental health compared to their counterparts in the overall Canadian population. This finding supports U.S. data that show suicide rates among elderly Chinese women were 10 times higher than among elderly Caucasian women (Lai, 2000). They also underscore the interaction of age, gender, and ethnicity effects on older Chinese women's health, and point to the importance of understanding multiple factors affecting older immigrant women's health.

In their research on the provision of mental health care services to immigrant women O'Mahony and Donnelly (2007) note that "immigrant women face many difficulties when accessing mental health services due to cultural and social stigma, and due to their unfamiliarity with Western biomedicine." They also discovered that "spiritual beliefs and practices influence immigrant women's mental health care practices," and that "the health care provider-client relationship exerts great influence on the ways in which immigrant women seek mental health care" (O'Mahony & Donnelly, 2007, pp. 459–460). The authors recommend a holistic approach to mental health care provision for immigrant women, whereby health care providers develop women-centred models for patient care that interrogate the complex relationships between culture, environment, and the interpretation of illness, recognize the systemic issues at play, and focus upon more nuanced interactions in order to improve health outcomes (O'Mahony & Donnelly, 2007, pp. 468–469).

A recent review of common mental problems among immigrants and refugees corroborates the triple-jeopardy perspective on older immigrant women's health (Kirmayer et al., 2011). It highlights risk factors for psychological distress among newly arrived older immigrants, including "female sex, less education, unemployment, poor self-rated health, chronic diseases (heart disease, diabetes, asthma), widowhood or divorce, and a lack of social support or living alone" (Kirmayer et al., 2011, p. 962). Thus, by virtue of being female, older immigrant women are at higher risk for psychological distress. Furthermore, the risk factors are compounded by socio-economic status. Since older immigrant women are often in a position of financial dependency or vulnerability when they arrive in Canada, the risk of them experiencing psychological distress presumably increases proportionately.

Further Mental Health Stresses Due to Racism, Economic Hardship, and Loss of Social Network

Compounding the effects of economic hardship, social isolation, uprootedness, and the loss of social networks, discrimination also significantly contributes to mental health issues among immigrants. A study of refugees in British Columbia that included people from China, Vietnam, and Laos found that depressive symptoms were higher among those who felt that they had experienced discrimination in Canada—more than a quarter of the sample identified as having been discriminated against (Noh et al., 1999).

Ethnic minority immigrants also have reported experiencing discrimination when using health care services. In Beiser, Simich, and Pandalangat's study (2003), 11 percent of the Tamils surveyed reported previous experiences of discrimination in the health care system. Brotman's (2003) interview study with older ethnic women and health care workers revealed that elderly ethnic women were often subject to discriminatory acts. The perceptions of what constitutes discrimination, however, differ between immigrant women and health care providers. Interviews with South Asian women immigrants and with their health care providers reveal that these two groups had very different perceptions of their interactions with each other. Johnson et al. (2004), for example, claim that female patients talked openly about their experiences with race, racism, and discrimination, while the health care workers described their encounters with South Asian women in terms of equal treatment and cultural "appropriateness." As the authors point out, the institutional practices that emphasize providing "uniform and efficient services" can often disadvantage South Asian women who do not easily fit into perceived "norms." As a result, they become "othered" in the health care system, thus reinforcing their sense of marginality (Johnson et al., 2004).

Barriers to Health Care for Older Immigrant Women

Betancourt et al. (2003) identify three levels of socio-cultural barriers that contribute to racial/ethnic health and health care disparities: structural, organizational, and clinical. Structural barriers occur when patients face barriers to health care due to system design that makes it difficult for racial/ethnic groups to access services or care. Structural barriers typically result from the health care system's failure to acknowledge and accommodate the needs and beliefs of a diverse population, resulting in patients feeling alienated, isolated, or neglected by the health care system. Factors include perceived cultural differences, perceptions of illness and treatments, language, discrimination and racism, and lack of access to information.

Perceived Cultural Differences

Many immigrant women feel that their cultural and ethnic backgrounds are not or would not be understood in the health care system. They are further deterred by the lack of health care professionals who share the same or similar ethnic and cultural background as them (Beiser et al., 2003). Lai (2004b) contends that among elderly Chinese women, perceived cultural-related barriers to health are associated with a higher risk of depression.

Perceptions of Illness and Treatments

Patients' perceptions and beliefs surrounding illness and health can also serve as barriers to health and health care. For example, the idea that breast cancer is a source of shame, moral dysfunction, or stigmatization can lead women to avoid having mammograms. Zhang and Verhoef (2002) found that the Chinese immigrants they interviewed did not view arthritis as a serious disease; hence, they did not seek treatment until the condition worsened. It is also not uncommon for immigrants to use a combination of self-care remedies, including consulting both Western and Chinese medicine doctors. In their study of illness management practices among Chinese immigrants, Zhang and Verhoef (2002) found that none of the respondents believed that Western medicine could completely cure or significantly improve their conditions. Instead, many believed that Western medicine might harm their internal organs, which could, in turn, lead to more serious problems than arthritis. Moreover, patients had positive attitudes about Chinese medicine and believed that it is more effective than Western medicine because of its holistic approach. Even if patients had not had good results with Chinese medicine in the past, they still retained faith in it.

Language

Language difference is an important barrier to health care. For example, Meadows et al. (2001) found that the language proficiency of immigrant women helped to determine the quality of their interaction with the health care system. Choudhry's study (1998) shows that the immigrant women from India who did not know English could not access printed or audiovisual health information, and instead had to rely on family members for interpretation, while female immigrants from India who were proficient in English used the available printed and audiovisual materials to become more informed. Zhang and Verhoef (2002) also found that Chinese immigrants with arthritis who had difficulty reading English tended to ignore informational materials if they were written in English.

English-speaking family members are often called on to facilitate elderly immigrant women's ability to understand and communicate concerns while interacting with health care providers. This situation, however, might inhibit women from talking about personal or private health matters (Meadows et al., 2001), as the family members could potentially be a source of stress, and thus part of the health problem. It might also be arduous for a family member who is called on to interpret, and there is no guarantee that he or she will translate and communicate the information accurately (Elliott & Gillie, 1998).

In the management of diabetes, it was found that the lack of effective communication between patients and health care providers can present a significant barrier to care, leading to differential health outcomes (Anderson et al., 1995). Interview surveys with Euro-Canadian, Chinese, and South Asian women revealed that some of these women did not fully understand the information that their health care practitioners had conveyed to them, and many of them did not have a clear understanding of their illness or their treatment (Anderson et al., 1995). This had an important effect on how well the women complied with the prescribed treatment. The study found that providing interpreters led to a noticeable improvement in the women's diet and medication self-management.

Discrimination and Racism

Discrimination and racism were also identified as barriers and possible deterrents to accessing health care (Brotman, 2003; Beiser et al., 2003). It is important that institutions recognize the structural constraints that might inhibit older immigrant women's access to and ability to benefit from available health care services. Anderson (1998) points out that

> illness meanings, and decisions about how to manage an illness are enmeshed in many layers of cultural and spiritual meanings, priorities within the family, the relationship of the family to the community, and the economic context of a woman's life—the job she is able to get, and the resources that are available to her. (p. 201)

Even when patients and providers shared the same language, patients can be restricted by conditions in their lives that limit their ability to use the conveyed information (Anderson, 1998).

To understand barriers to health care more fully, it is therefore important to move beyond barriers at the individual level, such as language proficiency and cultural incompatibility, to examining institutional and structural barriers, such as racism, discrimination, socio-economic disparities, and the lack of institutional understanding of cultural nuances. Racism is often viewed as an individual rather than institutional problem for patients and workers alike. This in turn inhibits discussions about people's experiences with racism and the development of anti-racist agendas within health care institutions. In fact, most patients and workers do not even use the term "racism" to describe their experiences. This leaves institutions to decipher and interpret experiences of discrimination based on race and ethnicity. To address more pervasive forms of institutional racism, it is therefore important that institutions understand that both ethnic minority patients and workers can experience racism, and begin to develop ways to address these issues. The *Ontario Women's Health Status Report* (Stewart et al., 2002) also points to a variety of cultural and institutional barriers to health care for immigrant women. It notes that immigrant women have less access to health care services because of their social isolation, culturally specific beliefs, and poverty. This is further reinforced by institutional barriers such as the language barrier, the lack of culturally sensitive services, and the under-representation of health care professionals from different ethnocultural backgrounds.

Lack of Access to Information

Kinch and Jakubec (2004) refer to the "politics of poverty" and "politics of access to information and services" where a woman's financial situation and/or her ability to access information and services impacts the care she receives. For instance, this research found that "[s]ome of the more educated women with resources and initiative sought information from television, the Internet, and wellness centres in shopping malls (which they highly recommended), but the Ismaili and First Nations women had no such points of reference" (p. 103). With regard to Aboriginal women, poverty and neglect were the primary causes of their lack of access to health care, while lack of access to information and services (largely due to language barrier) specifically affect Ismaili women.

Interpretation services might help alleviate information access problems for immigrant women, but Brotman (2003) warns that this is not always the best solution. Specifically, she identifies the following problems when immigrant women try to access health care: language barriers between patients and providers; the overreliance on patients' families and ethnic staff for interpretation due to lack of institutional resources; inconsistencies in deciding which services require interpretation; and service providers not understanding the role that culture plays in interpretation. Brotman also argues that viewing individual communication and language barriers as the primary problem associated with health care access can be inherently discriminatory because it frames the problem as being individual rather than systemic. As well, it excludes certain groups who do not experience language barriers (e.g., people of African origin who speak English or French) but who also have trouble accessing health care (Brotman, 2003).

The power of collective advocacy (women getting together to strive toward a common goal) can be a viable solution to the challenges encountered when accessing health care. In general, the women manage their health care privately with the support of family, friends, and voluntary organizations (usually of a faith-based, cultural, or Internet-access nature). Ironically, the same means that they use to access health care also keeps their specific issues out of public and political arenas and debates. In sum, being marginalized in multiple ways—being older, women, and members of visible minorities—constituted significant challenges to accessing care. Moreover, marginalization also makes it difficult to draw sustained attention to structural and organizational barriers (Kinch & Jakubec, 2004).

Organizational barriers refer to health care systems and structural processes that do not necessarily reflect the racial/ethnic composition, needs, and experiences of the serviced population. A good illustration of an organizational barrier is when health care institutions silence and make invisible the difficulties older immigrant women face in accessing health care by reducing the issue to an individualized language barrier (Brotman, 2001, 2003). Excessive focus on language as a barrier can inappropriately allocate the responsibility for differential treatment at an individual level rather than at an institutional one, thus leading to further oppression. Indeed, Brotman (2003) argues that health care institutions often silence and make invisible the experiences of older immigrant women, thus contributing to their experience of oppression and racism. For example, institutional assessment forms often do not identify the cultural background of patients, and many health care institutions also lack ethnic minority representation in their health care workers, thus making it more difficult for institutions to identify institutional racism and implement institutional change.

Finally, clinical barriers refer to situations when socio-cultural differences between health care providers and patients or their families are not fully accepted, appreciated, explored, or understood. Clinical barriers occur during the interaction between the health care provider and the patient. They include barriers on the part of the provider and resistance on the part of the patients. Meana et al. (2001b) found that physicians often do not screen for breast cancer (e.g., order mammography and/or perform clinical breast examination) for older Tamil women because patients refuse or feel too embarrassed or because they have language, communication difficulties, and cultural issues. In Hyman et al.'s (2001) survey asking physicians about mammography referrals for older Caribbean women, it was found that male physicians in particular would not refer patients for screening because of their perception that patients were uncomfortable with the intervention and would therefore refuse to go. Health care providers' cultural understanding is believed to directly affect their treatment plans. Kobayashi (2003) cites research that found that male Vietnamese physicians do not advise their older female patients to go for testing because they do not believe their advice will be followed.

Meana et al. (2001b) also identify the following beliefs as barriers to breast cancer screening: the belief that one should go to see a doctor only when one feels sick and that medical procedures are performed only on ill people or people suspected of being ill; the belief that God will protect one's health so one does not need to engage in breast cancer screening practices; and the view that breast cancer is outside of one's control. Other common barriers include ideas such as: breast cancer is associated with shame in the community and leads to questions about one's moral character and social stigmatization; breast cancer is seen as a form of divine retribution for past or current wrongs; and if it becomes known that one is having a mammogram, people will think that one already has breast cancer. Still other barriers include women's embarrassment about exposing their breasts or having them manipulated by a health care professional. Meana et al. (2001a) found that women who had never had a mammogram tended to be less educated, to have immigrated more recently, and to be less acculturated compared to those who had undergone at least one mammogram.

The triple jeopardy is also evident with regard to rates of cervical cancer. Factors related to low rates of Pap testing include place of birth, never having been married, living a shorter time in North America, not being fluent in English, having lower education and household income, and living in subsidized housing. As well, women who had undergone a hysterectomy were less likely to have been screened recently. These findings concur with the 2002 *Ontario Women's Health Status Report*, which notes that immigrant women are more likely to underutilize preventive and mental health services than native-born Canadian women (Hyman, 2002).

Volume 2, Ontario Women's Health Equity Report—Improving Health and Health Equity in Ontario, published by Project for an Ontario Women's Health Evidence-Based Report (POWER), provides supporting evidence for the triple-jeopardy perspective, particularly with regard to barriers to cervical cancer screening. For example, by focusing specifically on social determinants of health and populations at risk, the report points out that immigrants and recent Ontario Health Insurance Plan (OHIP) registrants have lower cervical cancer screening rates than Canadian citizens or long-term residents (Bierman et al., 2012). Among the women who identified themselves as immigrants, women of South Asian, Middle Eastern, and North African descent have the lowest rates of cervical cancer screening, whereas women of Latin American and Caribbean descent have the highest rates (Bierman et al., 2012). The report also identifies that women aged 50–66 are less likely to have had at least one Pap test in a three-year period than women aged 18–49 (Bierman et al., 2012). Socio-economic status also affects the regularity of cervical cancer screenings, with women living in the lowest income neighbourhoods getting screened less often than women living in the highest income neighbourhoods (Bierman et al., 2012). Thus, the findings suggest older immigrant women living in low-income neighbourhoods are the least likely to be regularly screened for cervical cancer, which corroborates the triple-jeopardy perspective.

Patients' perceptions about their interaction with care providers also affect their treatment and care. Gender matching was seen as an issue for a number of immigrant groups. For example, Morioka-Douglas et al. (2004) found that same-sex health care providers were important for Afghan women. Meana et al. (2001b) noted that Tamil women's embarrassment while having a mammogram could prevent them from going for the test, though their embarrassment could be overcome by having a female technician. Previous experiences with health care providers could also be a factor in accessing care. For example, many

Chinese immigrants with arthritis had negative feelings about "Western treatment" because of their previous interactions with rheumatologists and physicians (Zhang & Verhoef, 2002).

The above describes different levels of socio-cultural barriers to health care for older immigrant women. Many organizations dealing with older people have adopted a "multicultural" strategy, which includes expanding their workers' cultural repertoires to increase their knowledge about different ethnic groups (Brotman, 2003). Although it is important to understand how cultural differences affect a group's access and interaction with health care services, culture is only one aspect of the barriers older immigrant women experience when accessing health care. Patients encounter stresses and barriers that are not related to their culture or specific to their ethnic group. As a result, calls for increased cultural competency and cultural sensitivity have been accompanied by an insistence that health care providers also take into account the structural and socio-economic factors that impact patients' lives. According to Guberman and Maheu (2003/2004), "[t]rue cultural competency rests on an analysis that, while taking into account cultural differences, situates the analysis within the socioeconomic context of the groups in question and within the larger picture of dominant social relations" (p. 43).

Toward Cultural Competency

Elderly immigrant women often suffer worse health outcomes than their male counterparts and Canadian-born women. How can health care providers reduce these health disparities? What is clear from the literature is the multiplicity of stressors and barriers experienced by elderly immigrant women in Canada that can affect their health and inhibit their access to effective care. On the positive side, older immigrant women often marshal their personal and cultural resources to create buffers to cope with stressors. The question, then, is: How can the health care system minimize the stressors that contribute to ill health and address the barriers that prevent this population from accessing care, while simultaneously increasing support to this population? In this section, we first examine a number of buffers that are currently being employed as coping mechanisms, and then point to a few strategies to aid in accomplishing this goal.

Buffers

Thus far we have focused on factors that have detrimental effects on the health and well-being of older immigrant women. It would be wrong, however, to simply view these women as passive victims. While the idea of triple jeopardy does suggest multiple disadvantages, it would be misleading to think that being old or having an ethnic background is fundamentally problematic and can only adversely affect women's health. Rather, older immigrant women often use coping mechanisms and mobilize social support to minimize the stresses they face or to overcome the barriers associated with their position within the triple jeopardy. The transitions experienced by elderly immigrant women and the associated stresses are not necessarily negative in the long term. As Pearlin and Mullan (1992) point out, even transitions that start off as losses can lead to gains.

Cultural Beliefs as a Source of Support

Noh et al. (1999) assert that the use of the culturally congruent coping techniques can be an effective buffer against the depression associated with perceived discrimination. For example, they found that Southeast Asian refugees who practised "forbearance," described as "cognitive and behavioural responses that may be characterized as passive acceptance and avoidance," were less likely to have depressive symptoms (p. 201). But this was only among immigrants who had strong attachments to traditional ethnic values and practices.

Studies show that while immigrant women are often disadvantaged in terms of access to social and health care services, and that the process of immigration and settlement are significant stressors, certain culturally specific health beliefs and practices can have a positive impact on immigrant women's health. George's (1988) exploratory study of Indo-Canadian Sikh women's perceptions of menopause, for example, found that these women tended to view menopause as a positive event in their lives. This is because menopause means that they will no longer have pads and mess to deal with and can be "clean and free." Menopause is also considered the "final cleansing event in their lives" and the only concern expressed is related to its timing. If it starts too early it may be perceived as unhealthy since it may cause problems such as headaches due to "blood going to the head." On the other hand, if it starts too late it may cause one to become weak by exhausting all of one's energy. The study shows that in Sikh tradition, menopause is considered a liberating and transitional event into elderhood; maintaining this belief before and after immigration can help women maintain positive views of menopause and life-stage transition.

Faith and Religion as a Source of Support

Religious and spiritual beliefs can also contribute to immigrant women's ability to maintain and manage their health (Choudhry, 1998; Kinch & Jakubec, 2004; Meadows et al., 2001). In a study involving a diverse group of older women, respondents reported that their faith and religious affiliation were significant to their health management, providing support and comfort during times of sickness and adversity (Kinch & Jakubec, 2004). For middle-aged and elderly immigrant women from India, Choudhry (1998) notes "a deep sense of faith helps these women come through difficult and stressful times" (p. 5). As well, many of the immigrant women interviewed by Meadows et al.'s (2001) study cited their faith and religion as a central resource for their health management. For example, "[c]hurches were perceived as a place for prayer, in addition to [being] a place of support, relaxation and place to confide. Women spoke of this time for spirituality as nurturing or as part of their health practices" (p. 1454).

Social Supports

Social supports are also important for older immigrant women's overall well-being. As Elliott and Gillie (1998) contend, "family support systems play an important role in facilitating a positive migration experience. When support is withdrawn or if family ties are not strong, problems occur" (p. 334). A study of older Chinese and Korean immigrants in the United States (Wong, Yoo, & Stewart, 2005) shows that these immigrant elders had multiple support needs, including financial and other material aid, information/advice, emotional support, language support, and companionship. These men and women received aid from a number of different sources, depending on the kind of support they needed. Many of these seniors turn to their adult children for help in providing rides or carrying groceries, for example. Adult children were also called upon for language support and, to a lesser extent, for companionship. Friends were the most common source of information and advice, and also provided the most companionship.

For Chinese immigrants in Calgary suffering from osteoarthritis or rheumatoid arthritis, arthritic friends were an important source of information about treatment (especially about family doctors and Chinese healers). This information was obtained by elderly immigrants during social activities that they attended to make friends (Zhang & Verhoef, 2002). Having "trusted individuals" who can give them health information is particularly important for immigrant women. The majority of older ethnic women in Brotman's (2001) study accessed health information through their informal networks. They used connections with trusted individuals to find out the best place to go and access services or the best service provider to see. The "trusted individuals" can help these women find caring practitioners who can help them understand Western medical processes, who can speak their language, and who are familiar with and respectful of their cultural heritage (Brotman, 2001).

Overcoming Stresses and Barriers Faced by Older Immigrant Women

Building on the buffers outlined above, we identify a few strategies to help overcome stresses and address barriers that older immigrant women face.

Increase Social Support

The research highlights the importance that social support plays in successful immigrant adaptation. Programs should be developed to provide social support and strengthen community networks for older immigrant women. Ahmad et al. (2004) suggest that a host program can be established that links newcomers with more settled residents. This type of program could be specifically adopted for older immigrant women, in order to connect them with others who can provide social support as well as companionship.

Provide Safe Places and Opportunities for Older Immigrant Women to Discuss Their Issues and Concerns

In-Patient–Provider Interactions

Older immigrant women are often marginalized and silenced in the public arena, and their concerns are not well heard; as a result, practitioners working with these groups need to learn more about these women's health care experiences and issues. Practitioners can do this by creating opportunities for women to talk about their experiences and voice their concerns in a clinical setting. Creating such a space will require critically scrutinizing the interaction between health care practitioners and patients, and further developing actionable ways in which this interaction can improve.

In a Group Setting

Programs can also be developed for older immigrant women to work in groups with health care professionals, in order to support one another and to ensure that their needs are acknowledged and their health care requirements are met. Kinch and Jakubec (2004) developed a research method that incorporated focus group discussions involving small groups of peers. They write: "The notion of women supporting each other at new levels was evident in the interviews. . . . It became clear that this supportive approach was beneficial for the participants during the group meetings . . ." (p. 96). This statement was confirmed by reports that one group requested a follow-up meeting and then suggested that they would like to meet again. The participants suggested that this way of meeting was a "new and powerful experience for them" (p. 104).

Service providers need to work directly with elderly immigrant women to understand their sources of stress as well as the barriers that prevent them from receiving care. Furthermore, they should find ways to empower these women to receive the support they need in order to protect their health.

Develop Policies to Combat Institutional/Organizational Barriers

While the onus to deal with health care disparity problems are often left to health practitioners and health care workers at a clinical level, a more comprehensive policy to address health care barriers to older immigrant women at the organizational level is absolutely necessary. While many studies reviewed in this chapter have pointed to the problems of organizational barriers to access (Beiser et al., 2003; Lai, 2004a; Meadows et al., 2001; Zhang & Verhoef, 2002), Brotman's study (2003) explicitly addresses this issue. Policies to combat organizational barriers need to begin with recognition of the organization's role in creating barriers to health care, and the commitment to minimize and remove these barriers. Organizational policies would then need to address: (1) ways to identify barriers; (2) mechanisms to minimize and reduce barriers, including training workers, adding more resources and staff, and monitoring the process of change; and (3) ways to maintain and mainstream culturally competent practice in health care services.

Building Knowledge and Understanding of Older Immigrant Women and Their Health Issues

While research on women's health is beginning to accumulate, the issue of older immigrant women's health continues to remain marginal to health research. In addition, studies of older immigrant women's health are also uneven. While the amount of Canadian research related to East, Southeast, and South Asian women has grown over the last decade, there has been very little research attention paid to the health of older immigrant women of Caribbean, African, and Latin American origins. A significant amount of knowledge and data already exists within communities, but much of this information is not published in official or academic journals. Researchers and practitioners would benefit a great deal by working with communities and front-line professionals to disseminate this knowledge to broader research and policy communities.

Understanding and Addressing Older Immigrant Women's Health Issues from a Comprehensive Societal Perspective

Finally, to interrogate older immigrant women's health from solely a health practice/clinical perspective would be missing an important aspect of the triple jeopardy: that health of older immigrant women is firmly embedded in the larger social, economic, and cultural contexts. Therefore, to address health care barriers, policy focus cannot be directed to health care services and health care institutions alone. Such policies would be rendered ineffectual if resettlement and environmental stresses (i.e., living arrangements, language and communication problems, and social welfare concerns) in older immigrant women's lives were not properly addressed. As Hyman (2002) points out, health of immigrant women is "largely determined by environmental and living conditions and often changes in response to pressures associated with poverty, marginalization, and class inequality" (p. 338). Any policy strategy aimed at improving the health of older immigrant women would therefore have to begin with a global societal perspective to health that would embed older immigrant women's health within the context of the community and society in which they live.

Conclusion

In this chapter, we described the health status and health needs of older immigrant women in Canada from the perspective of the triple jeopardy. As the review of literature reveals, older immigrant women face multiple disadvantages as a result of their age, sex, and ethnicity/immigrant status. We emphasize that the process of immigration and settlement creates a significant amount of stress on older immigrant women. Although older immigrant women are often able to marshal their personal and cultural resources to buffer themselves from these stresses, given their often limited resources and constrained circumstances, their ability to buffer is often compromised. To ensure that adequate social and health services are provided to these women, we recommend the integration of a cultural competency model in social and health services at all levels, from front-line service delivery to organizational and policy development.

Notes

1. An earlier version of this literature review was compiled for a community-based research project, Health Status and Health Needs of Older Immigrant Women: Individual, Community, and Societal and Policy Links, in partnership with Ontario Women's Health Network, South Riverdale Community Health Centre, Women's Health in Women's Hands, and Stonegate Community Health Centre in Toronto. We would like to thank Public Health Agency Canada for the research grant for this project.
2. Author names are listed in alphabetical order. For further information on this report, please contact: Ito Peng, Professor of Sociology and Public Policy, Department of Sociology, University of Toronto, 725 Spadina Avenue, Toronto, Ontario (itopeng@chass.utoronto.ca).
3. Statistics Canada defines immigrants as individuals who were born outside of Canada, and "recent immigrants" as individuals who have immigrated to Canada within the last 10 years.
4. In our study we define "older immigrant women" as women who were born outside of Canada, and who are over the age of 50.
5. From our contacts and discussions with online professionals and health service organizations, we know that health and social service professionals are beginning to document and accumulate information and data about the health status of older immigrant women of Caribbean, African, and Latin American origins. However, because much of these data are not published, we were unable to pick up this information through a literature search. We are therefore extremely conscious of the fact that we will not be able to extend our literature analysis of published Canadian research related to older immigrant women much beyond those from ethnic backgrounds other than Asia and South Asia.

References

Ahmad, F., A. Shik, R. Vanza, A. M. Cheung, U. George, & D. E. Stewart. (2004). Voices of South Asian Women: Immigration and Mental Health. *Women & Health* 40(4): 113–130.

Anderson, J. M. (1998). Speaking of Illness: Issues of First Generation Canadian Women—Implications for Patient Education and Counselling. *Patient Education and Counselling* 33(3): 197–207.

Anderson, J. M., S. Wiggins, R. Rajwani, A. Holbrook, C. Blue, & M. Ng. (1995). Living with a Chronic Illness: Chinese-Canadian and Euro-Canadian Women with Diabetes—Exploring Factors That Influence Management. *Social Science and Medicine* 41(2): 181–195.

Beal, F. M. (1970). *Double Jeopardy: To Be Black and Female*. Detroit: Radical Education Project.

Beiser, M., L. Simich, & N. Pandalangat. (2003). Community in Distress: Mental Health Needs and Help-Seeking in the Tamil Community in Toronto. *International Migration* 41(5): 233–245.

Betancourt, J. R., A. R. Green, J. E. Carrillo, & O. Ananeh-Firempong. (2003). Defining Cultural Competence: A Practical Framework for Addressing Racial/Ethnic Disparities in Health and Health Care. *Public Health Reports* 18(4): 293–302.

Bierman, A. S., A. Johns, B. Hyndman, C. Mitchell, N. Degani, A. R. Shack, & M. I. Creatore. (2012). Chapter 12: Social Determinants of Health and Populations at Risk. In *Project for an Ontario Women's Health Evidence-Based Report: Vol. 2*. Toronto: St. Michael's Hospital and the Institute for Clinical Evaluative Sciences.

Brotman, S. (2001). Accessing Care through a Trusted Individual: Help Seeking Patterns of Ethnic Minority Elderly Women. *Vital Aging* 7(1): 1–4.

Brotman, S. (2003). The Limits of Multiculturalism in Elder Care Services. *Journal of Aging Studies* 17(2): 209–229.

Choi, N. G. (2001). Frail Older Persons in Nutrition Supplement Programs: A Comparative Study of African American and Hispanic Participants. *Journal of Gerontological Social Work* 36(1–2): 187–207.

Choudhry, U. K. (1998). Health Promotion among Immigrant Women from India Living in Canada. *Image: Journal of Nursing Scholarship* 30(3): 269–274.

Choudhry, U. K. (2001). Uprooting and Resettlement Experiences of South Asian Immigrant Women. *Western Journal of Nursing Research* 23(4): 376–393.

Chow, E. N. (1987). The Development of Feminist Consciousness among Asian American Women. *Gender & Society* 1(3): 284–299.

City of Toronto. (2013). *2011 National Household Survey: Immigration, Citizenship, Place of Birth, Ethnicity, Visible Minorities, Religion and Aboriginal Peoples.* Retrieved from http://www1.toronto.ca/city_of_toronto/social_development_finance__administration/files/pdf/nhs_backgrounder.pdf.

Durst, D. (2005, June 17). Aging amongst Immigrants in Canada: Policy and Planning Implications. In the *12th Biennial Canadian Social Welfare Policy Conference: Forging Social Futures*. Retrieved from www.ccsd.ca/cswp/2005/durst.pdf.

Elliott, S. J., & J. Gillie. (1998). Moving Experiences: A Qualitative Analysis of Health and Migration. *Health and Place* 4(4): 327–339.

Garcia, A. M. (1989). The Development of Chicana Feminist Discourse, 1970–1980. *Gender & Society* 3(2): 217–238.

Gee, E. M. (2000). Living Arrangements and Quality of Life among Chinese Canadian Elders. *Social Indicators Research* 51(3): 309–329.

George, T. (1988). Menopause: Some Interpretations of the Results of a Study among a Non-Western Group. *Maturitas* 10(2): 109–116.

Guberman, N., & P. Maheu. (2003/2004). Beyond Cultural Sensitivity: Universal Issues in Caregiving. *Generations* 27(4): 39–43.

Havens, B., & N. Chappell. (1983). Triple Jeopardy: Age, Sex, and Ethnicity. *Canadian Ethnic Studies* 15(3): 119–132.

Hong, L. (2004). Barriers to and Unmet Needs for Support Services: Experiences of Asian American Caregivers. *Journal of Cross-Cultural Gerontology* 19(3): 241–260.

Hyman, I. (2002). Immigrant/Visible Minority Women. In D. E. Stewart, A. M. Cheung, L. E. Ferris, I. Hyman, M. M. Cohen, & J. I. Williams (Eds.), *Ontario Women's Health Status Report* (pp. 338–358). Toronto: Ontario Women's Health Council.

Hyman, I., S. Guruge, R. Mason, J. Gould, & N. Stuckless. (2004). Post-Migration Changes in Gender Relations among Ethiopian Couples Living in Canada. *Canadian Journal of Nursing Research* 36(4): 74–89.

Hyman, I., M. Singh, F. Ahmad, L. Austin, M. Meana, U. George, L. M. Wells, & D. Stewart. (2001). The Role of Physicians in Mammography Referral for Older Caribbean Women in Canada. *Medscape Women's Health* 6(5): 6.

Johnson, J. L., J. L. Bottorf, A. J. Browne, & S. Grewal. (2004). Othering and Being Othered in the Context of Health Care Services. *Health Communication* 16(2): 253–271.

Kinch, J. L., & S. Jakubec. (2004). Out of the Multiple Margins: Older Women Managing Their Health Care. *Canadian Journal of Nursing Research* 36(4): 90–108.

Kirmayer, L. J., et al. (2011). Common Mental Health Problems in Immigrants and Refugees: General Approach in Primary Care. Canadian Guidelines for Immigrant Health. *Canadian Medical Association Journal* 183(12): E959–E967.

Kobayashi, K. M. (2003). Do Intersections of Diversity Matter? An Exploration of the Relationship between Identity Markers and Health for Mid- to Later Life Canadians. *Canadian Ethnic Studies* 35(3): 85.

Koning, E. A., & K. G. Banting. (2013). Inequality below the Surface: Reviewing Immigrants' Access to and Utilization of Five Canadian Welfare Programs. *Canadian Public Policy* 39(4): 581–601.

Lai, D. W. L. (2000). Prevalence of Depression among the Elderly Chinese in Canada. *Canadian Journal of Public Health* 91(1): 64–66.

Lai, D. W. L. (2004a). Impact of Culture on Depressive Symptoms of Elderly Chinese Immigrants. *Canadian Journal of Psychiatry* 49(12): 820–827.

Lai, D. W. L. (2004b). Health Status of Older Chinese in Canada: Findings from the SF-36 Health Survey. *Canadian Journal of Public Health* 95(3): 193–197.

Meadows, L. M., W. E. Thurston, & C. Melton. (2001). Immigrant Women's Health. *Social Science and Medicine* 52(9): 1451–1458.

Meana, M., T. Bunston, U. George, L. Wells, & W. Rosser. (2001a). Influences on Breast Cancer Screening Behaviors in Tamil Immigrant Women 50 Years and Over. *Ethnicity and Health* 6(3/4): 179–188.

Meana, M., T. Bunston, U. George, L. Wells, & W. Rosser. (2001b). Older Immigrant Tamil Women and Their Doctors: Attitudes toward Breast Screening. *Journal of Immigrant Health* 3(1): 5–13.

Morioka-Douglas, N., T. Sacks, & G. Yeo. (2004). Issues in Caring for Afghan American Elders: Insights for Literature and a Focus Group. *Journal of Cross-Cultural Gerontology* 19(1): 27–40.

Noh, S., M. Beiser, V. Kaspar, F. Hou, & J. Rummens. (1999). Perceived Racial Discrimination, Depression, and Coping: A Study of Southeast Asian Refugees in Canada. *Journal of Health and Social Behavior* 40(3): 193–207.

O'Mahony, J. M., & T. T. Donnelly. (2007). The Influence of Culture on Immigrant Women's Health Care Experiences from the Perspectives of Health Care Providers. *Issues in Mental Health Nursing* 28(5): 453–471.

Pearlin, L. I., & J. T. Mullan. (1992). Loss and Stress in Aging. In M. L. Wykle, E. Kahana, & J. Korval (Eds.), *Stress and Health among the Elderly* (pp. 117–132). New York: Springer.

Pearlin, L., S. Schieman, E. M. Fazio, & S. C. Meersman. (2005). Stress, Health, and the Life Course: Some Conceptual Perspectives. *Journal of Health and Social Behavior* 46(2): 205–219.

Peng, I., & M. Lettner. (2004). *Socio-Economic Inclusion: Demographic Aging among Immigrant Populations and Its Implications for Health Policy in Ontario*. Report Prepared for Health Canada, Ontario/Nunavut Region.

Spitzer, D., A. Neufeld, M. Harrison, K. Hughes, & M. Stewart. (2003). Caregiving in Transnational Context: My Wings Have Been Cut; Where Can I Fly? *Gender and Society* 17(2): 267–286.

Statistics Canada. (2010). *Population Projections for Canada, Provinces, and Territories, 2009 to 2036*. Ottawa: Author.

Statistics Canada. (2014a). *Census of Canada, 2011*. Ottawa: Author. Retrieved from http://www12.statcan.gc.ca/census-recensement/index-eng.cfm.

Statistics Canada. (2014b). *National Household Survey—Data Products 2011*. Ottawa: Author. Retrieved from http://www12.statcan.gc.ca/nhs-enm/2011/dp-pd/index-eng.cfm.

Stewart, D. E., A. M. Cheung, L. E. Ferris, I. Hyman, M. M. Cohen, & J. I. Williams (Eds.). (2002). *Ontario Women's Health Status Report*. Toronto: Ontario Women's Health Council.

Stewart, M. J., A. Neufeld, M. J. Harrison, D. Spitzer, K. Hughes, & E. Makwarimba. (2006). Immigrant Women Family Caregivers in Canada: Implications for Policies and Programmes in Health and Social Sectors. *Health and Social Care in the Community* 14(4): 329–340.

Wong, S. T., G. J. Yoo, & A. L. Stewart. (2005). Examining the Types of Social Support and the Actual Sources of Support in Older Chinese and Korean Immigrants. *International Journal of Aging and Human Development* 61(2): 105–121.

Zhang, J., & M. J. Verhoef. (2002). Illness Management Strategies among Chinese Immigrants Living with Arthritis. *Social Science and Medicine* 55: 1795–1802.

Further Reading

Hyman, I. (2004). Setting the Stage: Reviewing Current Knowledge on the Health of Canadian Immigrants. What Is the Evidence and Where Are the Gaps? *Canadian Journal of Public Health* 95(3):14–18.

Lai, D. (2004). Health Status of Older Chinese in Canada. Findings from the SF-36 Health Survey. *Canadian Journal of Public Health* 95(3): 193–197.

Mulvihill, M. A., L. Mailloux, & W. Atkin. (2001). *Advancing Policy and Research Responses to Immigrant and Refugee Women's Health in Canada*. Winnipeg: Centres of Excellence in Women's Health. Retrieved from www.cewh-cesf.ca/PDF/cross_cex/im-ref-health.pdf.

Statistics Canada. (2006). *Women in Canada 2005: A Gender-Based Statistical Report* (5th ed.). Cat. no. 89-503-XIE. Ottawa: Author.

Relevant Websites

Canadian Women's Health Network: www.cwhn.ca
Centre of Excellence for Women's Health: www.cewh-cesf.ca
Ontario Council of Agencies Serving Immigrants (OCASI): www.ocasi.org/index.php
Ontario Women's Health Network: www.owhn.on.ca
Women's Health Matters: www.womenshealthmatters.ca

CHAPTER 8

Women, Disability, and the Right to Health

Paula C. Pinto

Introduction

Few studies have examined intersections of gender and disability, especially in their implications for women. In fact, both the disability and feminist movements have been criticized for ignoring the issues facing disabled women (Begum, 1992; Gerschick, 2000; Lloyd, 2001; Morris, 1995; Nixon, 2009; Traustadottir, 1990). Disability analyses are typically gender-blind, portraying disabled people as a homogeneous group. Therefore, the distinct ways in which gender affects the lives of women and men with disabilities are rarely investigated or discussed; in practice, however, disability studies have mostly echoed male-centric perspectives while the specific realities and concerns of disabled women have remained obscured. Disability has also been largely disregarded in feminist thought, even after relationships between gender and other forms of oppression such as race and class were acknowledged and investigated. In short, the particular needs and perspectives of women with disabilities are hardly reflected in either the disability or the feminist literatures.

This chapter sets out to overcome this double marginalization by examining how gender and disability intersect to shape disabled women's health experiences. Naturally, with Nasa Begum (1992), I recognize that women with disabilities are themselves a diverse group and in this sense, multiple identities related to race, age, sexuality, and class are likely to compound or alleviate the forms of oppression they are subjected to. While addressing the complexity of all these interactions is beyond the scope of this chapter, it remains important not to overlook their significance.

In gendering disability and health, I want to avoid the pitfall of talking about disabled women experiencing a "double disadvantage." As pointed out by Jenny Morris (1995), this is neither truthful nor useful and leads to social constructs of these women as "passive victims of oppression" (p. 63). Feminist research on disabled women, on the contrary, must be empowering. By placing "women's subjective reality at its core" (p. 63), research must expose the prejudice that permeates social relations involving disabled women. At the same time it must recognize "the source of strength, celebration, or liberation" (p. 63) that disabled women find in their struggle to transform demeaning images of their lives. In an attempt to apply these principles here, the arguments throughout this chapter will be illustrated with stories of disabled women, including quotations from a pilot project in which I have been involved conducted with women with disabilities in Ontario, Canada.[1] The decision to frame arguments in the language of human rights, with particular reference to the right to health, is also a deliberate intent to emphasize the humanness that fundamentally underlies disabled women's health experiences and needs—in other words, it highlights that what women with disabilities demand is nothing less than what all human beings are entitled to just by nature of their membership in the human family. Moreover, it is what the Canadian government (and many others all over the world) have subscribed and legally committed to under international human rights law, notably the recent Convention on the Rights of Persons with Disabilities.

Box 8.1

The Right to the Highest Attainable Standard of Health

The international human rights system comprises a number of legally binding instruments enacted under the patronage of the United Nations and other international organizations. The right to the highest attainable standard of health, commonly known as the *right to health*, is codified in several of them, including:

- the Covenant on Economic, Social, and Cultural Rights (CESCR)
- the Convention on the Rights of the Child (CRC)
- the Convention on the Elimination of Discrimination Against Women (CEDAW)
- the Convention on the Rights of Persons with Disabilities (CRPD)

Canada is signatory to all of these treaties, thus subscribing to a broad conception of the right to health that encompasses access to timely and appropriate health care and also involves the underlying preconditions for a healthy life, such as access to safe drinking water and adequate sanitation, proper nutrition and housing, to mention just a few. Under current human rights law the international community recognizes that everyone has a right to health, which involves the right to access without discrimination the resources and conditions that enable each individual to enjoy "the highest attainable standard of health conducive to living a life with dignity." In the specific context of disability, the CRPD further highlights the importance of taking into account gender specificities in access to health care.

Source: United Nations, 2000, Convention on Economic, Social, and Cultural Rights.

According to official statistics (Statistics Canada, 2011), 1.7 million Canadian women aged 15 and over have a disability[2] compared to just under 1.5 million men. The experience of disability is thus more common among women than among men. The gap is particularly wide among seniors, as females tend to live longer than males and are therefore more likely to develop age-related chronic conditions that prevent them from participating in social activities. Disabled women are thus likely to face distinct and unique challenges. It therefore becomes crucial to understand how the simultaneous experience of disability and gender (Lloyd, 2001) affects women's lives.

This chapter will explore this theme by addressing four main topics: (1) access to health care and wellness; (2) sexual and reproductive rights; (3) gender-based violence; and (4) poverty. Not surprisingly, these are important topics for any discussion about women's health in general. In fact, as Carol Gill (1997) pointed out, "the needs and concerns of women with disability are less exotic than many non-disabled people might think" (p. 1). Certainly, some health issues for disabled women are amplified or given a particular emphasis because of the unique features that surround the experience of disability in our culture; nevertheless, in essence, they remain basic women's health issues.

Defining Disability and Gender

Before we can address the intersections of disability and gender we need to define what we mean by those concepts. Two broad models have shaped understandings of disability

	Female		Male	
	With Disability[1]	Without Disability	With Disability	Without Disability
Achieved less than high school (percent)	27.1*	17.1	25.0*	17.4
Employed last week (percent)	60.2*	80.6	66.6*	88.9
Main source of personal income (percent)[2]				
Paid work or self-employed	34.7*	68.4	44.9*	78.2
Pensions, investments	28.3*	12.0	30.3*	12.0
Old age security, guaranteed income support, social assistance	21.1*	6.8	13.4*	3.4
Average personal income (dollars)	24,000	32,100	41,200	51,000

Notes:
1. Disability equated in the survey with activity limitation.
2. Includes only those who reported income.
* Statistically significant differences from same sex without disability at $p < .05$.

TABLE 8.1: Quick Facts: Adults with Disabilities (Age 15 and over) in Canada

Source: Statistics Canada, *Participation and Activity Limitation Survey 2006*, Tables (Part V), retrieved from http://www5.statcan.gc.ca/olc-cel/olc.action?objId=89-628-X&objType=2&lang=en&limit=1.

in Western societies. Traditional conceptions define disability as "a personal tragedy," the consequence of individual impairments and functional incapacities. Giving rise to actions aimed at repairing or eliminating individual impairments through therapeutic interventions, this approach became known as the "medical model" of disability. Over the last two decades, however, a vast number of disability scholars, many of whom are people with disability (Barnes, 1990; Finkelstein, 1980; Oliver, 1983, 1996; Rioux & Valentine, 2006), have been calling attention to the ways in which social, economic, and political structures, processes, and institutions disadvantage, oppress, and *disable* some members of the human family. By placing the problem outside the person and in society, this approach became known as the "social model" of disability. It is also the paradigm that informs this chapter. In this sense, the terms "disabled women" and "women with a disability" will be used interchangeably throughout this chapter, both to reflect an understanding of disability as socially created and to emphasize the human nature, rather than the impairment, of those disabled by society. In population surveys, the concept of activity limitation is increasingly being used to measure the prevalence of disability. The category is constructed using a set of five questions and the respondents are classified as having an activity limitation if they answer "often" to at least one of them.

Much like disability, gender is socially construed through social and economic processes, practices, and relations. These relations are fundamentally unequal, marked by unequal access for women and men to material and non-material resources (Sen, George, & Östlin, 2002). Gender norms, values, and expectations become entrenched in particular roles, attributes, and responsibilities that are distinctly assigned to women and men in the family and in society. Given the fundamental inequalities that signal the roles and relations between women and men, gender is, above all, a powerful form of stratification that both influences and is influenced by all other physical and social markers such as class, race, sexual orientation, and disability.

In short, both disability and gender are *socio-political realities*, and as such they need to be understood in the context of social relations of power and control. In Western societies, disability status and female gender are usually associated with greater vulnerability and powerlessness, and therefore women with disabilities are potentially at greater risk than disabled men of facing discrimination and having their human rights violated (World Health Organization, 2011).

Access to Health Care and Well-Being

Gender inequities are widespread within health care systems globally. They may involve differential access to health care resources by women and men as well as discrepancies in the way the system responds to their health needs. These disparities tend to reflect broader and more profound socio-economic inequalities that distinguish the lives of women and men in most societies. Drawing on data from the Canadian Community Health Survey—CCHS 2009—a Statistics Canada report, "Women in Canada" shows that working-age women with disabilities visit health professionals more often than other women, yet they report poorer general health and lower mental health.

Disabled women's discrimination in the health care system is pervasive. Despite women's numerical supremacy, rehabilitation medicine has traditionally focused on the needs of men—the soldiers, the male workers, or the athletes who had acquired disabilities (Gill, 1997;

	Female		Male	
	With Disability[1]	Without Disability	With Disability	Without Disability
Self-rated mental health (percent)				
Poor to fair	17.1*	3.9	17.1*	3.5
Good	30.1*	20.3	29.1*	19.6
Very good	29.7*	38.1	29.3*	36.8
Excellent	23.1*	37.7	24.5*	40.0
Self-rated general health (percent)[2]				
Poor to fair	43.8*	7.2	43.2*	7.0
Good	34.7*	27.4	30.8	28.3
Very good	17.3*	40.9	18.4*	39.5
Excellent	4.2*	24.5	7.6*	25.1
Perceived life stress (percent)				
Low	28.3*	33.1	30.5*	36.9
Medium	37.5*	43.4	37.4*	42.8
High	34.2*	23.5	32.1*	20.3
Had visited health professional in past 12 months (percent)	98.7*	96.0	97.8*	91.2
Visits to a medical doctor (percent)				
Low range (0 to 1)	9.6*	33.4	17.1*	50.0
Mid-range (2 to 4)	30.6*	41.1	33.3	34.4
High range (5 or more)	59.8*	25.4	49.6*	15.5

Notes:
1. Disability equated in the survey with activity limitation.
2. Not only absence of disease or injury but also physical, mental, and social well-being.
* Statistically significant differences from same sex without disability at $p < .05$.

TABLE 8.2: Perceptions of Health Status and Health Behaviours

Source: Adapted from Statistics Canada, *Women in Canada: A Gender-Based Statistical Report*, 2011 (data from the Canadian Community Health Survey, 2009).

Morrow, 2000; Tuck & Wallace, 2000). Therefore, conditions that affect mostly women, such as, for instance, chronic fatigue syndrome, continue to be less investigated and are less understood than those that typically affect men (i.e., spinal cord injury). Because disabled women's lives have been rendered invisible, the examination of how different disabilities impact general female health conditions and needs has also been neglected (Frazee, Gilmour, & Mikytiuk, 2006; Gill, 1997; Morrow, 2000). Not surprisingly, then, in several studies (Frazee et al., 2006; Masuda, 1999; Morrow, 2000; Odette et al., 2003) women with disabilities have identified a lack of information on issues so diverse, such as routine health care, nutrition, and safe sex as a barrier to health and wellness.

While many disabled women go without needed care, women's experiences in clinical encounters have also been problematic. In health settings, as Gill (1997) explains, disabled women are not just rendered invisible, they are often de-gendered and dehumanized too, viewed only from the prism of their disability or impairment. In one study (Thomas, 2001), Sarah, a woman with cerebral palsy shares the following:

> My experiences of having a disability and being in need of hospital treatment for an illness or condition other than my Cerebral Palsy has been that I seemingly pose a "problem" [. . .] It seems that their dilemma is whether to relate to me solely in terms of my Cerebral Palsy, so that I am "the Cerebral Palsy Patient," even when I have, for example, toothache! [. . .] It seems then, that if the physical disability is seen by the hospital staff as the patient's point of definition and also the major problem in their view, then the patient, as in my case, is going to experience difficulties. (pp. 252–253)

So for Sarah, as for many disabled women, medical practices are often oppressive rather than supportive. Women find themselves stigmatized and deprived of any privacy and dignity, as when, for instance, they are required to appear undressed in front of a group of health providers who examine them as if they were "a scientific experiment" (Frazee et al., 2006).

The professional gaze that may assume forms of "public stripping" (Gill, 1997) is certainly not an exclusive experience of women with disabilities, but "gender exacerbates the power difference between doctor and patient, making resistance or refusal to participate more difficult" (Frazee et al., 2006, p. 244). Moreover, due to prevailing normative standards and representations of the female body, even beyond medical settings disabled women are caught between the intense "visibility" of their different bodies and the "invisibility" of their selves, desires, and needs as women and human beings. As Hilde Zitzelsberger (2005) has found in her qualitative study of women with physical disabilities and differences, this paradoxical experience constantly challenges disabled women's ability to build healthy lives and identities. For instance, Hope, a woman Zitzelsberger (2005) interviewed, noted:

> So the focus was on being physically visible. Not emotionally being visible because a person could stare at me and see my crutches, but they would not go any further than that. They would not go and think that I could be visible in many different ways. I could be visible as a woman that could have a relationship, as a woman that could be a friend to someone, as a woman that could be seen in a workplace, as a woman that could be a mother one day. (p. 394)

In addition to experiencing heightened in/visibility (Zitzelsberger, 2005), disabled women's access to health and wellness is further compromised by physical barriers and obstacles inscribed in the way health care is organized and delivered, which often does not take into account their varying needs and characteristics (Gill, 1997). Stairs and narrow doors, inaccessible medical equipment (making routine exams difficult or impossible), lack of staff to assist with transfers and communication, and tight scheduling (limiting time available to understand needs, explain procedures, and build reciprocal trust) are some of the most common obstacles disabled women have to put up with in their encounters with the health care system (Gill, 1997; Odette et al., 2003; Rajan, 2012). But it is the increasingly unpredictable access to medical services that women most fear. As Shirley Masuda (1999) found in her study, in contexts of fiscal restraint, disabled women are likely to experience the deterioration in health care and are concerned that financial policies will continue to affect the provision of care for them. One woman summarized: "Threatened cutbacks are very distressing. We live in fear of pain. Do they replace joints or do we have to pay?" (p. 9). In sum, disabled women are facing stigmatization and discrimination in the health care system, and their medical needs are not being adequately met. This represents a clear violation of their right to the highest attainable standard of health and a serious threat to their dignity and well-being.

Sexual and Reproductive Rights

Sexual and reproductive rights are of critical importance to all women, yet among those with disabilities, the term acquires a new and broader meaning. Non-disabled feminists fight sexist ideologies that reduce the lives of women to the role of mothers and nurturers; their arguments tend to focus on women's right to be free from unwanted pregnancy. But for disabled women, who have been sterilized without consent and denied the opportunity to mothering, the right to become pregnant and have a child—including a disabled child—and the right to refuse forced sterilization are equally or even more important (Kallianes & Rubenfeld, 1997; Pinto, 2008).

Social representations of the sexuality of disabled women are filled with contradictions. Construed as dependent, "eternal children," women with disabilities are often presumed to be asexual beings, with no desires, no sexual needs nor capacities. As such, they are not seen as in need of information about birth control, sexuality, and child-bearing (Traustadottir,

1990). But at the same time, efforts have always been made to block disabled women from participation in the sexual sphere. Historically, the reproductive abilities of disabled women, particularly those with learning disabilities, have been tightly controlled through institutionalization, forced sterilization, and social control. Many have lost custody of their children in divorce and others have had their children removed from their care by welfare agencies (Gill, 1997; Kallianes & Rubenfeld, 1997; O'Toole, 2002; Traustadottir, 1990). Therefore, for disabled women the choice of child-bearing is a political act that defies the social oppression they have been subjected to (Morris, 1995). They claim the right to be recognized as sexual, whether in lesbian or heterosexual relationships, and the power to control their fertility and to bear children if they so decide. They also demand access to necessary resources in support of their parenting role (DAWN Ontario, n.d.b). Yet they struggle to find sensitive and informed health providers to help them fully achieve these rights (Gill, 1997; Kallianes & Rubenfeld, 1997).

Little research has been conducted on the sexual health of disabled women (Rajan, 2012; Basson, 1998; Gill, 1997). Health providers receive insufficient training about disability and many fail to assess and adequately respond to women' concerns and needs. Providers' attitudes are often shaped by popular beliefs that portray women with disabilities as not sexually active, and in consequence disabled women may not receive appropriate medical care (Rajan, 2012; Barile, 2003; Riddel et al., 2003). This may have devastating consequences for their health.

Lack of knowledge about disability and its interacting effects with women's sexual and reproductive health may also reinforce health providers' disablist attitudes as Irene, a woman interviewed by Lipson and Rogers (2000), has experienced. She recounted:

> Well, they told me I couldn't get pregnant first off, because of hemorrhaging. He didn't think that the hips, my pelvic area, and my lower back would support the weight of a child. And they didn't feel confident that with all the pelvic and hip fractures that I would be able to accommodate birth. And then after I got pregnant, they tried to tell me that I shouldn't keep him because he'd be brain damaged from all the Prozac and the drugs they were giving me. And I said I didn't care; he was a gift. (p.18)

Despite the anxieties of health providers, Irene's baby was born healthy and without any known disabilities. Yet her story powerfully speaks of the many barriers facing disabled mothers—in particular, society's fears that they can only produce defective babies, and the increasing acceptance (inclusive within the women's movement) of selective abortion (the abortion of fetuses identified as disabled), which is seen by disabled people as an indication of how their lives are devalued in our society.

Women with disabilities who become pregnant and give birth seem also more likely to be subjected to high-tech procedures and have their pregnancies assumed to be "high-risk"

(Lipson & Rogers, 2000). This again indicates the prevalence of the medical model in health providers' perceptions of and responses to disability.

As with other areas of health, barriers to appropriate sexual and reproductive care for women with disabilities further include the physical inaccessibility of many medical facilities and equipment (Rajan, 2012; Barile, 2003), which prevent them from being assessed and receiving care. Different disabilities require different things: for those with physical impairments, it is important that physicians' offices, examination tables, and other screening technologies are accessible; for those who are blind, deaf, or deal with learning disabilities, the lack of alternative formats to convey information may become an excluding barrier. But for all, finding responsive, sensitive providers is critical (Rajan, 2012; Kallianes & Rubenfeld, 1997; Riddel et al., 2003). Reports of disabled women being abused during clinical assessments have been collected (Thomas, 2001). Access to gynecological care may be particularly constrained for women who have experienced sexual trauma. For these women, the consequences of not finding practitioners sensitive to their needs may even lead to avoidance of treatment (Rajan, 2012; Riddel et al., 2003).

Women with disabilities are not a homogeneous group, but they are all sexual beings with the potential to build relationships that include sexual aspects (Basson, 1998). As any other women, all are entitled to basic sexual and reproductive rights, including the right to enjoy their sexuality, the right to bear children, and the right to access appropriate care and resources to give birth to and raise their children.

Gender-Based Violence

Violence against women is a persistent and pervasive phenomenon in contemporary societies (World Health Organization, 2005). Women with disabilities face the same risks as all other women, but they are also exposed to specific vulnerabilities related to their disability (Rajan, 2011; Nosek, Howland, & Rintala, 2001; Tilley, 1998). The issue of violence and abuse is therefore central for discussions of disabled women's health and well-being.

It has been reported (e.g., Barrett et al., 2009) that women with disabilities experience interpersonal violence almost twice as often as women without disabilities. Violence against disabled women encompasses a wide range of injurious acts, including deliberate physical, psychological, or sexual maltreatment or abuse, as well as more passive forms of neglect such as denial of food or medical care (DAWN Ontario, n.d.a). Verbal abuse, intimidation, social isolation and confinement, economic deprivation or exploitation, and abuse by the system, including refusal or unwillingness to provide needed care have also been described as typical forms of abuse of disabled women (Rajan, 2011; Mays, 2006). As in the non-disabled community, most of the abusive acts are perpetrated by men who tend to be close and well known to their victims (Mays, 2006; World Health Organization, 2005) and yet, because investigators rarely assume that disabled women have intimate partners, intimate partner violence often goes undetected (Barnett, Miller-Perrin, & Perrin, 2005)

A number of factors have been identified as contributing to disabled women's increased vulnerability to violence and abuse. First, it has been suggested that an increased dependency on a variety of people to provide assistance with daily activities greatly increases opportunities for abuse (Rajan, 2011; DAWN Ontario, n.d.a; Nosek, Howland, & Rintala, 2001; Nosek, Foley, Hughes, & Howland, 2001; Tilley, 1998). Receiving care often involves intimate and emotional contact, and many women have experienced violence at the hands of their caregivers, including spouses and boyfriends, personal assistants, physicians, and therapists. Abuse from caregivers has been reported to involve inappropriate touch, physically rough treatment, refusal to respect women's choices, or even theft of their money and property (Nosek, Foley et al., 2001). In one study a woman shared: "The orthotist told me he had to put his finger in my vagina to be sure the (artificial) leg fit right" (Nosek, Foley et al., 2001). Dependency on perpetrators for daily survival activities accentuates the vulnerability of women with disabilities, who may feel compelled to tolerate acts of abuse, as this other woman in the same study confided: "The father of a girlfriend kissed and fondled me. This was in exchange for helping me up and down steps and the like . . ." (p. 184). Low self-esteem and systematic denial of their human rights are said to produce feelings of powerlessness and over-compliance among many disabled women (Rajan, 2011; Nosek, Howland et al., 2001; Nosek, Foley et al., 2001), diminishing their ability to escape abusive relationships. Lack of money, not knowing where to go for support, and lack of help from service providers can also result in women staying in abusive relationships for longer periods (Rajan, 2011).

A feminist approach, however, must go beyond acknowledging disabled women's vulnerabilities, or it will do little to challenge their stigmatization and marginalization (Mays, 2006). Rather, it must be able to place analyses of violence in the broader context of the oppressive relations of disablism and sexism that encircle the lives of many of these women. It must stress that abuse of disabled women is strongly linked to gendered inequalities in power, and the historical, social, and material conditions that perpetuate and reinforce the subordinate position of people with disabilities in our society. For disabled women, these translate into limited economic opportunities and lack of independence, persisting demeaning images, stereotypes, and gender norms that justify and legitimate the control of their lives by others, especially men. From this perspective, the abuse of women with disabilities is clearly a socio-political issue (Mays, 2006) with potentially devastating consequences for women's health and well-being.

Consequences may be even harsher because a woman with disability may find it particularly difficult to leave a situation of abuse and find adequate support—neither disability-related programs nor existing services for victims of abuse are adequately prepared to respond to disabled women's needs in this area. While disability workers have traditionally disregarded issues of violence and abuse among their clients, many women's shelters do not accommodate

Box 8.2

Women with Disabilities Speak Out

The following are excerpts taken from interviews conducted by the author with women with disabilities, in Ontario, Canada:

On gender and disability:

"We are a male-dominant society, there are . . . there are a lot of issues that are women's issues that are magnified if you're a woman with disabilities." (Susan)

On women and poverty:

"I think that women are more likely to live in poverty than men, simply because men are expected to be bread-winners and . . . if a man and a woman apply for the same job . . . well will give it to him 'cause after all he's got a family to support. I've lost jobs where that thing was said to me . . . 'Well, . . . you know, . . . your application looks really good, but this fellow has to support a family. . . .' Whereas . . . you know, women are expected to stay at home and look after the kids. 'You'll be alright, dear, you have a husband to look after you.'" (Laura)

On current practices of social services:

"They keep you afraid of fraud charges, you're afraid of losing your benefits, you're afraid if your mother comes and gives you $50 for your birthday because it's gonna get taken off your cheque, you're afraid that any minute the phone's gonna ring and you're gonna be audited. . . . If you have an anxiety disorder that makes you ill." (Laura)

On the role of policy:

"For those of us with disabilities there are a lot of barriers that are there, just by the nature of our disabilities. And I think that the policy should be there to ensure that these barriers are removed . . . whether [it] be for participation at society, everything from I can go to a coffee shop and have a coffee to I can compete and hopefully successfully obtain a high-paying job!" (Emma)

women who are in wheelchairs or who need assistance with daily care and medication (Nosek, Howland et al., 2001; Nosek, Foley et al., 2001). Disabled women may also fear they will not be heard or believed when they speak out. Research conducted in Canada (Rajan, 2011) and in Sidney, Australia (Keilty & Connelly, 2001), has shown that disabled women, particularly those with learning disabilities, face numerous barriers when reporting to the police, including prevailing stereotypes that portray them as sexually promiscuous and unable to provide credible accounts, and police officers' lack of time to engage and effectively communicate with victims. Similar barriers are likely to be faced in other contexts by women experiencing different disabilities, further contributing to their social isolation and reinforcing abusers' assumptions that disabled women are "easy prey" (Nosek, Howland et al., 2001). Not surprisingly then, research has also found that disabled women experience abuse and violence for significantly longer periods of time than women without disabilities (Nosek, Howland et al., 2001). For some, suicide might be the only possible escape (DAWN Ontario, n.d.a).

Poverty

All of the barriers to health and well-being highlighted so far are further compounded by disabled women's lack of adequate income. Research in the general population has shown that, on average, people with better income enjoy better health. Among the population with a disability, a strong relationship between income and health has also been found. Disabled women in Canada are more likely than men to experience economic deprivation (Statistics Canada, 2008a, 2008b) and thus are at higher risk for ill health, too.

The problematic income situation of women with disabilities is linked to all the other issues they face, particularly the discrimination they experience in education and the labour market (Statistics Canada, 2008a). Official statistics in Canada show that the unemployment rate of people with disabilities is higher than that of adults without disabilities, disabled women being the least likely group to be employed (Statistics Canada, 2008a).

Women who are able to access work earned in 2006 an average income of $22,213, lower than that of non-disabled women ($28,942) and disabled men ($30,748) (Statistics Canada, 2008b). Many may end up with after-tax household incomes below Statistics Canada's low-income cut-off, defined as comprising people living in "straitened conditions."

The rate of low income is often related to the source of one's income. In the current disability income system, disabled women are particularly disadvantaged (Jongbloed, 1998). Programs linked to labour force attachment, such as employment insurance or workers' compensation, usually offer better benefits than social assistance, but women with disabilities are more likely to have government transfers as their primary source of income. It has been recognized that the great majority (70 percent) of those on social assistance live in low-income households (Office for Disability Issues, 2004); thus, disabled women face an increased risk of poverty. Even if they do receive benefits based on employment earnings, women experience discrimination because they tend to have been paid less than men and are more likely to have taken time off or worked part-time because of their traditional domestic roles. Yet, restrictions imposed on welfare programs over the last decade discourage many of them from exploring the possibility of a job to supplement their income for fear of losing their meagre, but secure, disability benefits (Jongbloed, 1998; Masuda, 1998).

In fact, over the last 20 years women have experienced increased difficulties in accessing the benefits and services they need, which makes their lives ever more difficult (Masuda,

1998). Cuts in home care and homemaking services, for instance, are leaving many disabled women with basic daily needs unmet. Reduced availability and repair of required technical devices, and less help for child care impact disabled women's ability to live independent lives and perform family roles. Cuts to staff in hospital and institutions jeopardize the quality of care to them, especially those who need extra help. All of these have negative consequences for women's health and well-being (Masuda, 1998).

Without an adequate income, disabled women become socially isolated (Schur, 2004). Many cannot access a secure place to live or buy healthy food. Adults with disabilities are twice as likely as those without disabilities to have experienced food insecurity, a risk particularly high among lone mothers. In fact, more than one in every three lone mothers with disabilities runs out of money for food at least once a year (Office of Disability Issues, 2004). Their health, and that of their children, is certainly impacted and their human rights and dignity are further eroded.

Conclusion

Women with disabilities are an under-studied and underserved group. Like other women, their lives are constricted by social and economic disadvantages that undermine their dignity as human beings and their capacity for self-determination. Because of prevailing sexist and disablist ideologies, they experience high poverty rates, severe ratios of violence and abuse, and systematic denial of their sexual, reproductive, and health rights. All these affect their physical and mental health and well-being.

More research is needed to fully understand the interconnections of gender and disability and their health impacts on disabled women. Integrated approaches that combine insights from feminist and critical disability theories can be very useful to uncover structures and social relations of power and control that constrain disabled women's lives. Bringing together women with disabilities, researchers, and social activists, such efforts are elemental not only to an understanding of the inequalities facing disabled women, but also to political processes aiming at ending their discrimination and advancing their human rights.

Notes

1. This study, which received ethics approval by the York University Human Participants Review Committee, involved seven in-depth interviews with women with disabilities living in rural and urban communities of Ontario, Canada. Participants included women with a diversity of impairments recruited through disability organizations. The interviews took place between July and November 2004. The study was conducted in partial fulfillment of the requirements for the Ontario Training Centre's Diploma in Health Services and Policy Research, which the author completed.
2. Disability is equated with activity limitation caused by a long-term health condition or problem.

References

Barile, M. (2003). *Access to Breast Cancer Screening Programs for Women with Disabilities.* Montreal: Action des femmes handicappées de Montréal.

Barnes, C. (1990). *Cabbage Syndrome: The Social Construction of Dependence.* Lewes: Falmer Press.

Barnett, O., C. L. Miller-Perrin, & R. D. Perrin. (2005). *Family Violence across the Life Span: An Introduction* (2nd ed.). Thousand Oaks, CA: Sage.

Barrett, K., B. O'Day, A. Roche, & B. L. Carlson. (2009). Intimate Partner Violence, Health Status and Health Care Access among Women with Disabilities. *Women's Health Issues* 19: 94–100.

Basson, R. (1998). Sexual Health of Women with Disabilities. *Canadian Medical Association Journal* 159(4): 359–362.

Begum, N. (1992). Disabled Women and the Feminist Agenda. *Feminist Agenda* 40: 70–84.

DAWN Ontario. (n.d.) (a). *Family Violence against Women with Disabilities.* Retrieved from dawn.thot.net/violence_wwd.html.

DAWN Ontario. (n.d.) (b). *Women with Disabilities and Reproductive Rights: Plain Language Fact Sheet.* Retrieved from dawn.thot.net/wwd_reproductive_rights.html.

Finkelstein, V. (1980). *Attitudes and Disabled People.* New York: World Rehabilitation Fund.

Frazee, C., J. Gilmour, & R. Mikytiuk. (2006). Now You See Her, Now You Don't: How Law Shapes Disabled Women's Experience of Exposure, Surveillance, and Assessment in the Clinical Encounter. In D. Pothier & R. Devlin (Eds.), *Critical Disability Theory: Essays in Philosophy, Politics, Policy, and Law* (pp. 223–247). Vancouver: UBC Press.

Gerschick, T. (2000). Toward a Theory of Disability and Gender. *Signs: Journal of Women in Culture and Society* 25(4): 1263–1268.

Gill, C. (1997). *Last Sisters: Health Issues of Women with Disabilities.* Retrieved from dawn.thot.net/cgill-pub.htm#top.

Jongbloed, L. (1998). Disability Income: The Experiences of Women with Multiple Sclerosis. *Canadian Journal of Occupational Therapy* 65(4): 193–201.

Kallianes, V., & P. Rubenfeld. (1997). Disabled Women and Reproductive Rights. *Disability & Society* 12(2): 203–221.

Keilty, J., & G. Connelly. (2001). Making a Statement: An Exploratory Study of Barriers Facing Women with an Intellectual Disability when Making a Statement about Sexual Assault to the Police. *Disability & Society* 16(2): 273–291.

Lipson, J. G., & J. G. Rogers. (2000). Pregnancy, Birth, and Disability: Women's Health Care Experiences. *Health Care for Women International* 21(1): 11–26.

Lloyd, M. (2001). The Politics of Disability and Feminism: Discord or Synthesis? *Sociology* 35(3): 715–728.

Masuda, S. (1998). *The Impact of Block Funding on Women with Disabilities.* Ottawa: DisAbled Women's Network (DAWN) Canada.

Masuda, S. (1999). *Women with Disabilities: We Know What We Need to Be Healthy!* Vancouver: British Columbia Centre of Excellence for Women's Health and DAWN Canada.

Mays, J. M. (2006). Feminist Disability Theory: Domestic Violence against Women with a Disability. *Disability & Society* 21(2): 147–158.

Morris, J. (1995). Creating a Space for Absent Voices: Disabled Women's Experience of Receiving Assistance with Daily Living Activities. *Feminist Review* 51(Autumn): 68–93.

Morrow, M. (2000). *The Challenges of Change: The Midlife Health Needs of Women with Disabilities*. Vancouver: British Columbia Centre of Excellence for Women's Health.

Nixon, J. (2009). Domestic Violence and Women with Disabilities: Locating the Issue on the Periphery of Social Movements. *Disability & Society* 24(1): 77–89.

Nosek, M. A., C. C. Foley, R. B. Hughes, & C. A. Howland. (2001). Vulnerabilities for Abuse among Women with Disabilities. *Sexuality and Disability* 19(3): 177–189.

Nosek, M. A., C. Howland, & I. Rintala. (2001). National Study of Women with Physical Disabilities: Final Report. *Sexuality and Disability* 19(1): 5–39.

Odette, F., K. K. Yoshida, P. Israel, A. Li, D. Ullman, A. Colontonio, H. Maclean, & D. Locker. (2003). Barriers to Wellness Activities for Canadian Women with Physical Disabilities. *Health Care for Women International* 24(2): 125–134.

Office for Disability Issues. (2004). *Advancing the Inclusion of Persons with Disabilities: A Government of Canada Report*. Ottawa: Social Development Canada.

Oliver, M. (1983). *Social Work with Disabled People*. Basingstoke: Macmillan.

Oliver, M. (1996). *Understanding Disability: From Theory to Practice*. London: Macmillan.

O'Toole, C. J. (2002). Sex, Disability, and Motherhood: Access to Sexuality for Disabled Mothers. *Disability Studies Quarterly* 22(4): 81–101.

Pinto, P. (2008). Re-Constituting Care: A Rights-Based Approach to Disability, Motherhood, and the Dilemmas of Care. *Journal of the Association for Research on Mothering*, 10(Spring/Summer): 119–130.

Rajan, D. (2011). *Women with Disabilities and Abuse: Access to Services*. Ottawa: DAWN.

Rajan, D. (2012). *Women with Disabilities and Breast Cancer Screening: An Environmental Scan. Identified Problems, Strategies, and Recommended Next Steps*. Ottawa: DAWN and Canadian Breast Cancer Network.

Riddel, L., K. Greenberg, J. Meister, & J. Kornelsen. (2003). *We're Women Too: Identifying Barriers to Gynaecological and Breast Health Care for Women with Disabilities*. Vancouver: British Columbia Centre of Excellence for Women's Health.

Rioux, M. H., & F. Valentine. (2006). Does Theory Matter? Exploring the Nexus between Disability, Human Rights, and Public Policy. In D. Pothier & R. Devlin (Eds.), *Critical Disability Theory: Essays in Philosophy, Politics, Policy, and Law* (pp. 47–69). Vancouver: UBC Press.

Schur, L. (2004). Is There Still a "Double Handicap"? Economic, Social, and Political Disparities Experienced by Women with Disabilities. In B.G. Smith & B. Hutchison (Eds.), *Gendering Disability* (pp. 253–271). New Brunswick, NJ: Rutgers University Press.

Sen, G., A. George, & P. Östlin. (2002). Engendering Health Equity: A Review of Research and Policy. In G. Sen, A. George, & P. Östlin (Eds.), *Engendering International Health: The Challenge of Equity* (pp. 1–33). Cambridge, MA: MIT Press.

Statistics Canada. (2008a). *Participation and Activity Limitation Survey 2006: Labour Force Experiences of People with Disabilities in Canada*. Retrieved from http://www5.statcan.gc.ca/olc-cel/olc.action?objId=89-628-X&objType=2&lang=en&limit=1.

Statistics Canada. (2008b). *Participation and Activity Limitation Survey 2006: Tables (Part V)*. Retrieved from http://www5.statcan.gc.ca/olc-cel/olc.action?objId=89-628-X&objType=2&lang=en&limit=1.

Statistics Canada. (2011). *Women in Canada: A Gender-Based Statistical Report*. Retrieved from http://www.statcan.gc.ca/pub/89-503-x/89-503-x2010001-eng.htm.

Thomas, C. (2001). Medicine, Gender, and Disability: Disabled Women's Health Care Encounters. *Health Care for Women International* 22(3): 245–262.

Tilley, C. M. (1998). Health Care for Women with Physical Disabilities: Literature Review. *Sexuality and Disability* 16(2): 87–102.

Traustadottir, R. (1990). *Obstacles to Equality: The Double Discrimination of Women with Disabilities*. Retrieved from dawn.thot.net/disability.htm.

Tuck, I., & D. Wallace. (2000). Chronic Fatigue Syndrome: A Women's Dilemma. *Health Care for Women International* 21(5): 457–466.

World Health Organization. (2005). *Multi-Country Study on Women's Health and Domestic Violence against Women: Summary Report of Initial Results on Prevalence, Health Outcomes, and Women's Responses*. Geneva: Author.

World Health Organization. (2011). *World Report on Disability*. Geneva: Author.

Zitzelsberger, H. (2005). (In)visibility: Accounts of Embodiment of Women with Physical Disabilities and Differences. *Disability & Society* 20(4): 389–403.

Further Reading

Disability & Society (peer-reviewed international journal).

Thomas, C. (1999). *Female Forms: Experiencing and Understanding Disability*. Buckingham, UK/Philadelphia: Open University Press.

Walsh, P. (2002). *Health of Women with Intellectual Disabilities*. Oxford: Blackwell Publishing Ltd.

Relevant Websites

DAWN Canada—DisAbled Women Network Canada: www.dawncanada.net

Disabled Women's Network Ontario: dawn.thot.net

DRPI—Disability Rights Promotion International: www.yorku.ca/drpi

Women with Disabilities Australia (WWDA): www.wwda.org.au

CHAPTER 9

Rural Older Women's Health-Promotion Needs and Resources:
Two Variations on a Photovoice Theme

Beverly D. Leipert and Robyn Plunkett

What happened to our ideal retirement place?
—RURAL RESEARCH PARTICIPANT

Introduction

In 2011, Canada's population over the age of 65 represented 14.3 percent of the population, or approximately 5 million individuals, a number that is expected to double in the next 25 years (Statistics Canada, 2011). Older women are one of the fastest-growing segments of the female population (Ministry of Industry, 2006), yet older rural women have inadequate access to health resources, which is placing their health at risk (Keating, Keefe, & Dobbs, 2001; Leipert, Leach, & Thurston, 2012). Gendered ideologies, expectations, and practices that shape women's work and life (Dolan & Thien, 2008), including a culturally constructed obligation to serve in the community, may pose additional health vulnerabilities for older rural women because their own health may be neglected as they care for others. Enhanced knowledge of health-promotion needs and resources for older rural residents is an urgent national need (Ministerial Advisory Council on Rural Health, 2002); however, little is known about the nature of health resources that rural women need. For example, in many small rural communities, sports such as curling are a main, if not the only, source of social connection and recreational activity during the long winter months (Morrow & Wamsley, 2013), especially for those with limited transportation (Leipert, et al., 2011). Engaging in recreation and team sport activities is one way that older rural women may be able to provide and obtain important resources of practical, emotional, affirmational, and social support (Trussell & Shaw, 2007).

This chapter reports on two research studies that address gaps in knowledge regarding older rural women's health promotion, which can be defined as the ability to gain control over their own health, thereby improving it (World Health Organization, 2014). In study one, the Southwest Ontario Study (SWO study), two objectives guided the research: (1) to explore health-promotion needs and resources of older rural women from the perspective of the women themselves, and (2) to pilot test the appropriateness and effectiveness of an innovative qualitative data-collection method, photovoice (Wang & Burris, 1997). In study two, the National Canadian Curling Study (NCC study), the objectives were to: (1) examine the influence of curling on the social lives and health of rural women; and (2) determine how sport and recreation are experienced and understood within the broader contexts of gender and rural community. For both of these studies, rural was defined as living "outside of commuting zones of urban centres with 10,000 or more population" (du Plessis, Beshiri, Bollman, & Clemenson, 2001, p. 1), and older was defined as 65 years of age or older, a commonly used definition of older/senior in health research (Canadian Institute for Health Information, 2011).

Why Rural Senior Women?

Senior women often outlive their husbands, and in rural areas where few family members reside, these women are particularly vulnerable to social isolation (Clark & Leipert, 2007). Furthermore, frailty, which can be broadly defined as a decrease in health reserves, including cognitive and physical abilities leading to significant health consequences (Rockwood et al., 2005), has been documented as a gendered and geographic concept, predominantly affecting rural senior women, who tend to outlive senior men (Song, MacKnight, Latta, Mitnitski, & Rockwood, 2007). In a large Canadian study, frailty indices were higher for older rural women than for older rural men, and rural dwellers experienced increased frailty indices compared to their urban counterparts (Song et al., 2007). Senior women also tend to be poorer financially than senior men (Ministry of Industry, 2006) and on average have less education than their urban counterparts (Gilmore, 2010). The combination of lower levels of education and income gives rural women less ability to purchase services and negotiate complex bureaucracies to get those services (Keating et al., 2001). These burdens, combined with women's caring for others (Keating et al., 2001), limited availability of rural health resources (Romanow, 2002), and ever-increasing costs of essential products and services (National Advisory Council on Aging, 2002), suggest that older rural women have health needs, but may not be able to articulate them. In addition, the hardiness, self-reliance, and resilience that are expected in rural settings may discourage older residents from asking for or accepting help (Leipert, 2013; Standing Senate Committee on Agriculture and Forestry [Senate Committee], 2006).

The limited research that explores older rural women's health promotion indicates that the ability to remain in one's home (Hinck, 2004), maintain health and social relationships (Cerhan & Wallace, 1993), and sustain self-reliance and connections with community structures such as recreation resources (Leipert, et al., 2011) and the church (Plunkett & Leipert, 2013) figure significantly in older women's health and health-promotion activities. Further research is needed to determine how social support can be improved for this population

(Cerhan & Wallace, 1993), and to inquire into interventions that empower rural older women to be more knowledgeable about and able to adopt health-promoting behaviours (Pullen, Walker, & Fiandt, 2001). These requirements form the basis of the two studies reported here.

Conversely, the strength, resilience, and knowledge of older rural women can help them to have the confidence and resources to promote their health. Older women contribute significantly to the socio-cultural life of their rural communities. They tend to survive their male partners, often prefer to age in place, and comprise a large cohort of people in depopulated rural areas (Keating et al., 2001). Older rural women provide substantial services and supports to rural communities, including active farming activities, social support, food, and health care (Hinck, 2004; Leipert, 2013; Leipert, Leach, & Thurston, 2012). In other words, they are a major resource in the promotion of health and in the sustainability of underserved communities. Moreover, they provide inspiration to each other and to other rural dwellers through their interests, abilities, role modelling, and commitment to the rural community, in addition to serving as a rich source of historical knowledge.

Research into rural recreation has shown that "sporting clubs are usually the last organizations to fold in small declining communities, often lasting longer than local shops, pubs and churches" (Tonts, 2005, p.142). Thus, despite demographic change and economic strain in rural communities, sport and recreation remain important, especially for the predominantly senior population that resides there. Benefits include providing opportunities for physical activity and social interaction, skill development, and providing a mentoring system for young and old alike to remain engaged (and residing) in rural communities (Mair, 2007, 2009). However, challenges such as the withdrawal of government support for sport and recreation have significantly increased responsibility for the maintenance of rural facilities by rural community members, many of whom are senior women (Leipert, Scruby, & Meagher-Stewart, under review; Warner-Smith & Brown, 2002).

The role of recreation, leisure, and sport in the lives of women living in rural areas is dramatically understudied. A few researchers have explored rural women's involvement in sport and leisure and the extent to which it has been shaped and limited by domestic roles such as caregiving and ideologies of wifehood, motherhood, and femininity (Aitcheson, 2003; Leipert, Scruby, & Meagher-Stewart, under review; Morrow & Wamsley, 2013). Women's traditional labours of cooking and cleaning are often transferred to sports facilities through expectations that they bring home-baked foods for concession areas and social activities. In addition, women's lesser access to funds and playing time, compared to men, may also impact the nature of their involvement in sport. In the case of curling, for example, women may still be less able to pay fees for ice time in curling rinks or be more limited in their ability to engage in the sport due to caregiving and other family responsibilities (Leipert et al., 2011). Thus, the traditional gendered understandings and expectations of women and their roles typical of rural settings can result in more limited sport options and experiences, with concomitant effects on women's physical, mental, and social health. However, the exploration of older rural women's health as a consequence of their experiences in sport in general and curling in particular is an area of study that has received virtually no research attention to date.

Rural women often remark that they are left out of research and that there is a need for more research about rural women's health (Leipert, 2013; Sutherns, McPhedran, & Haworth-Brockman, 2004). In addition, since women live longer and experience aging differently than men (Thomeer, 2013), it is crucial to understand and support aging women's health needs. Rural Canada is aging and it is likely that there are proportionally more elderly women in rural regions than in urban regions, a situation that will probably become more pronounced over time (Standing Senate Committee on Agriculture and Forestry, 2006). Consequently, it is important to conduct research that addresses rural perspectives and that captures the multi-dimensionality and complexity of older rural women's lives.

Why Photovoice?

The photovoice method was originally developed for research with rural women in China (Wang, Burris, & Ping, 1996). Photovoice photographs can act as a creative catalyst for discussion, especially with populations with low literacy abilities, by visually documenting difficult-to-describe situations (such as rural isolation and rural recreation), and the photographs can also promote empathy and understanding that foster social change (Wang, 1999; Wang & Burris, 1997). This unique method encourages greater depth and authenticity and, hence, validity in the interpretation of qualitative findings (Prosser, 2011).

Photovoice is a unique participative action research strategy "by which people create and discuss photographs as a means of catalyzing personal and community change" (Wang, Yi, Tao, & Carovano, 1998, p. 75). Community residents are provided with disposable cameras to take photographs related to the research question. Thus, residents significantly control the data that are generated and are able to provide powerful visual representations of community issues that can be used to influence policy-makers as well as local residents themselves (Wang et al., 1998). Community residents may also become more aware of issues facing their community as they view and discuss photographs taken by themselves and fellow residents. Photovoice is aligned with the principles of health promotion and Paulo Freire's theoretical model of education for critical consciousness whereby information can awake awareness and facilitate understanding (Butler & Xet-Mull, 2001). We began with the assumption that this innovative method could be important for rural women in general, and older rural women in particular, who, due to literacy limitations and cultural and political undervaluation of their health needs and strengths, may find it difficult to realize and articulate their health needs and resources (Leipert, 2013; Sutherns, McPhedran, & Haworth-Brockman, 2004).

By placing a camera in the hands of older rural women and using their photographs as the basis for dialogue, the photovoice method provided these women with the means to highlight features of the rural context that they viewed as important to their health. Photovoice can also help study participants to reveal data that would not likely be disclosed or that are difficult to adequately describe. Furthermore, because residents have the camera for weeks at a time, there is an opportunity for deepened reflection. In addition, the collection of data is influenced by emotional states over several points in time, which promotes increased representation of the data as a temporal reality. Because data are collected in a natural environment directly by study participants, its proximity to lived experiences invariably contributes to its authenticity. Photovoice allows for the identification and elaboration of perspectives, which may empower older rural women to reflect on and voice health points of view, increase collective knowledge about their health, and inform policy-makers about rural health issues (Leipert, 2013; Wang et al., 1996).

The studies reported in this chapter were guided by a feminist theoretical perspective. The authors understand rural older women's health in terms of power and control as these relate to personal and collective health, and in terms of individual, socio-cultural, economic, and contextual factors that influence healthy aging (Olesen, 2011; Ward-Griffin & Ploeg, 1997). A feminist perspective fits well with the critical and empowering philosophical basis of photovoice (Wang, 1999; Wang & Burris, 1997). Feminist research values women's experiences from their perspectives and seeks to ensure that diverse women's experiences are represented (Olesen, 2011). The purpose of feminist research is to foster change at individual and societal levels.

Using Photovoice

Study One: The Southwest Ontario Study

Following approval from the University of Western Ontario Research Ethics Board, this study was conducted in two rural communities in Huron and Perth counties in southwest Ontario. Both counties include agricultural, recreational, and retirement communities that have limited resources and high percentages of isolated rural populations (Turner & Gutmanis, 2005). Huron is the most rural county in southwest Ontario and does not include any urban centres.

After providing written consent, 11 women participants ranging in age from 66 to 96 years attended a camera-orientation session in their rural communities. Five women attended in one rural community, and six attended in another rural community. At these sessions, which were approximately one hour in length, the purpose and nature of the research was explained and the women were given disposable cameras with instructions regarding their use (Wang & Burris, 1997). A discussion on ethical picture-taking ensued. These sessions served to build rapport between researchers and participants as well as among participants. Participants were invited to provide a brief introduction of themselves, in addition to any initial thoughts they had on health needs and resources in their rural community. They were then asked to take pictures in their neighbourhood, town, or farm that depicted health-promotion needs and resources of older rural women and to obtain written consent from individuals whose pictures they wished to take. In addition, each participant was provided with a notebook to keep a log of what she photographed and of what she decided not to photograph. One week after receiving these materials, participants were contacted to determine and encourage progress. At this time, one woman withdrew from the study for health reasons. Cameras and logbooks were retrieved two weeks later, and printed photographs (one copy for participants and one copy for the researchers) as well as digital versions were then obtained. Collectively the women took approximately 100 photos.

In the audio-recorded focus groups that followed, each participant was asked to select, from her own prints, one that best represented a health-promotion need and one that best represented a health-promotion resource. These images formed the basis of the focus group discussion (Wang & Burris, 1997). These focus groups, lasting approximately two hours in length, were semi-structured, which allowed participants to share what was most meaningful to them and to their health. Examples of discussion topics included: descriptions of what participants saw in their photographs, why images mattered to their health or to the health of others in their community, as well as the titling of photographs. The appropriateness and fit of the photovoice method and the significance of the images were also discussed.

Study Two: The National Curling Study

Forty-five women and three youth, ranging in age from 12 to 75 years with an average age range of 50 to 60 years, in seven rural communities in Ontario, Manitoba, Nova Scotia, and the Northwest Territories participated in the study. Participants were present female members of rural curling clubs. Following ethical approval from respective participating universities, participants were provided with disposable cameras and asked to take pictures that illustrated the effect of curling on their physical, mental, social, or other forms of health, and record perspectives in logbooks. Collectively participants provided 955 photos. These photos and logbook recordings formed the basis of subsequent group interviews, similar to the SWO study. (See Leipert et al. [2011] for additional details about this study.) In this chapter, only data from this study related to older women's health will be referenced. For both studies, participants were mailed a booklet of the study findings and provided again with the researchers' contact information in the event that they wished to offer additional thoughts on the research.

What Does Photovoice Reveal?

Analysis in photovoice research is conducted collaboratively by participants and researchers together (Wang & Burris, 1997), and can be supplemented with analysis by researchers alone. In these studies, analysis proceeded when participants identified key data by selecting their photos, and they contextualized data by explaining the meaning of photos. In addition, researchers and participants collaborated to identify issues, concepts, themes, and theories (Wang & Burris, 1997). For example, a participant's selection of a photo of a person rather than an object would indicate the primacy in importance of people and social elements rather than inanimate objects. The participant then would explain the meaning of her photo and identify issues or themes related to concepts, such as kinship or professional relationships, that this photo represented. The audio tape of this process provided material for further analysis by the researchers alone.[1]

Photographic analysis (Oliffe, Bottorff, Kelly, & Halpin, 2008) included revealing individuals' intentions and meaning in the photographs. This analytic step largely took place in the second focus group in which participants not only described their photographs, but also explained why they took certain photographs. Data, including pictorial and narrative data, were then analyzed collectively, incorporating participant and researcher perspectives, and themes were developed and then reconnected with the theoretical bases of the study, including rural (Leipert, 2013) and feminist perspectives (Olesen, 2011). Pictorial and logbook data and interview transcripts in both studies revealed valuable information about the health-promotion needs and resources of older rural women, and about the appropriateness and fit of photovoice for exploring these needs and resources. Findings were rich and detailed and, as a result, only a summary and selected photos can be presented here.

Health-Promotion Needs of Older Rural Women

Women took pictures and spoke about several health-promotion needs in their rural communities. Needs for ramps into public buildings such as post offices and churches, transportation issues, challenges related to weather, safety issues, needs for increased access to health care and other resources, and the effects on health of depopulation and other changing rural demographics were all exposed as problems.

Not having ramps made it difficult for women to attend church services and events in halls that were important venues for social support, or to easily retrieve mail or to do other public business. One participant explained, "A church is the centre of a rural community. [Impeding access to and] closing a church means no social catching up after the Sunday services, no gatherings and working together at church suppers, no community support at funerals. No central place to meet and pray." Women who did not have vehicles, who could not afford to drive, or who had compromised vision needed to depend on others. A participant noted, "It must be very difficult for some women sitting at home day after day, having to depend on someone to come." Challenging weather, especially in winter, made travel difficult or impossible, especially for older women— "Winter driving leaves me frightened"—thereby causing some women to postpone needed health care for weeks or months until the weather improved. Such postponement caused anxiety as well as potentially exacerbating illness conditions. In addition, when the weather is bad, one woman stated, "On those days we pray we are healthy and have no appointments. If you are to see a specialist, you'll have to wait months to get another appointment." Many small communities, several participants noted, "do not have a train, bus, or taxi service." Study participants also raised safety issues related to machinery such as snow blowers and tractors, which some women on farms needed to use; driving in inclement weather and in isolated areas; and rodents and raccoons, which boldly invaded rural spaces.

In part due to limited access to transportation, participants described isolation as a significant health concern for themselves and for other women in their rural communities. One participant recalled her initial experience of isolation: "I came from the city to the rural area... the first year up here was [unbearable]... if I had money, if I had a car, if I had transportation, I'd be gone...." An additional health need that was addressed with much feeling was the lack of access to resources, especially to a primary care provider (such as a nurse practitioner or physician), and to grocery, banking, and other community services (Figure 9.1).

Comments included:

> "We now have no doctor in town.... Without doctors, the need for a drugstore lessened until it closed ... this means we now must travel [for these services]."
>
> "Seniors needing help in their homes find it frustrating. Services by the Community Care Access Centre have been cut back to such short hours of services that much-needed assistance is lacking. [This is due to] government budget cuts."
>
> "No driving [means] no food or supplies. My [temporary] inability to drive was a wake-up call. ... Moving to [a larger community with more resources] will be the only solution in the future."

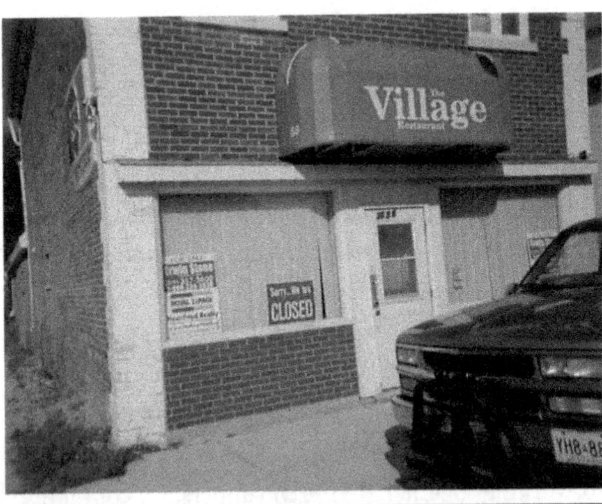

FIGURE 9.1: Closed rural resources

Participants often attributed the closure of services to the depopulation of rural areas and to government misunderstanding or undervaluing of rural community needs. In addition, women noted that changing rural demographics exacerbated their needs for social support and services. Comments included:

> "A [new] family is building a new house down the road from us [but] there's no connection with [our community]." "They rent, they're here, they're gone." "People don't need each other like they used to . . . there's money to do things on your own [now]." "[We used to have] a much more close-knit community because you depended on each other, you helped each other . . . that's gone now."

Factors that the women worried about in terms of compromising their ability to drive and be independent included loss of vision, inclement weather, poor road conditions, vehicle costs, and the loss of partners, family, and neighbours whom they could depend on if their own driving was not possible. Some of these factors are reflected in the following participant comments:

> "Here is a picture of my car. . . . It probably will be my last vehicle because of cost both of purchase and upkeep. My vehicle allows me independence. It would be a real disadvantage [if I didn't have it]. I'd have to hire someone to take me to my monthly doctor appointments and/or shopping." "I do not know how I would survive without my granddaughter. She is great company and is often my legs. . . . In 5 years she will be in University and I will be 76 years old. I wonder how I will be able to maintain my apartment and independence."

As a result of changing rural demographics and the elimination of resources and services, life in rural communities becomes much more difficult, especially for older rural women who may have increasing needs for services but less ability to access them, especially at a distance. As a consequence of limited formal and informal support, several participants noted their ongoing and essential need for social support, as one participant aptly summarized: "Friendship is [important] [otherwise] nobody is going to be there to come and see you. . . ."

Health-Promotion Resources of Older Rural Women

Health-promotion resources for the women included and relied upon their independence and self-sufficiency. One woman summarized several participants' perspectives when she stated, "The isolation of a farming community is fine as long as you're self-sufficient." Inasmuch as the women were able to walk or drive to social events, health services, grocery stores, and other destinations, and thereby maintain self-sufficiency in their homes and communities, they perceived that they could maintain and promote their health. A participant noted, "If one is to have any measure of independence, one must be able to drive." Another participant wondered: "If I couldn't drive, what would happen to me? Life would not be happy. We need a car for banking, groceries, church, socializing, emergencies."

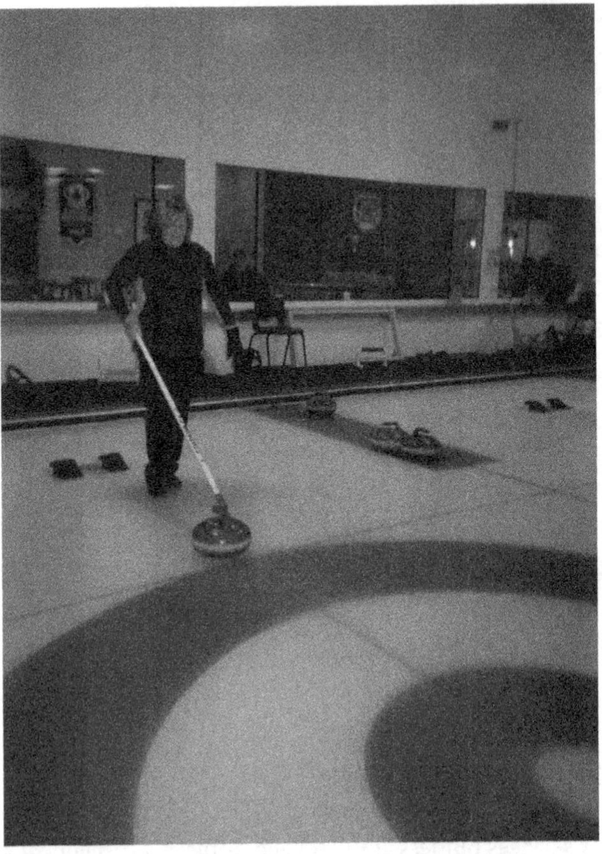

FIGURE 9.2: Stick curling

The curling rink and associated activities were identified as key resources to facilitate rural older women's health and their need to gather and socialize with others. Curling was described as a physically accessible sport for aging women. Stick curling, in which curlers use an assistive rod to deliver stones down the sheet of ice, facilitated curling for individuals with physical disabilities such as painful hips and knees (Figure 9.2). One participant noted, "with [the] stick now people are curling longer. . . . I know myself if my knees give out I would use the stick."

Social support was a key health-promotion resource for virtually all of the women in both studies. Participants noted that instrumental support was vital and offered in many ways, including assisting with travel to mutually enjoyable events, and participating together in activities such as canning, church, and other community gatherings. Curling, in particular, affirmed rural older women's abilities to be active and involved in a community sport, and also provided opportunities for their abilities, such as cooking and baking, to be profiled and valued in curling banquets and bonspiel events (Figure 9.3).

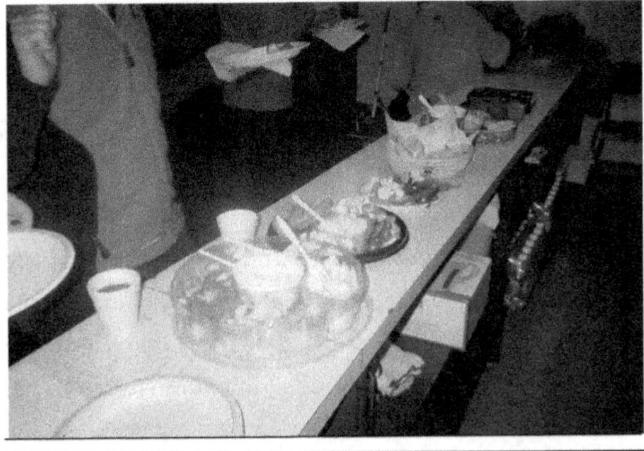

FIGURE 9.3: Food display

However, several women also noted that key rural venues, such as coffee shops, cafés, churches, and curling rinks where social interaction

Box 9.1

The Nature of Valued Rural Social Support

One woman vividly described the importance of interaction with people when she stated, "This way we interact with a person, not with a mop, not with a television, not with a computer, not with the telephone, but with an actual person, and I think for all of our well-being, it's really important."

The older women curlers also remarked on the significance of curling for social interaction. One 85-year-old woman who had recently taken up curling described why the sport was important to her social health: "It gives ya something to look forward to and as you get older, you have less and less of those things so you're caught in your house. . . . I've got . . . lots of books to read, but after a while you wanna do something, you wanna see people." Especially in the long winter months, curling provided women with something to look forward to. As these quotes indicate, the mental health and abilities of older women are significantly enhanced through the relationships they develop in rural community settings such as the curling rink. As curling is one of the few sports both available in rural settings (especially in winter) and receptive to involvement by seniors, it represents a key social and physical health resource for rural older women.

could take place, were disappearing in rural communities. Women remarked upon the financial challenges curling rinks faced due to depopulation of younger residents and loss of employment in rural areas, and lower incomes of seniors. One participant noted, "And looking to the future of the club . . . [we have] financial difficulties [and] we just aren't getting enough volunteers signing up to do the work." The erosion of social resources in many rural communities is accelerated with the closure of curling rinks. The closure of such facilities directly impacts older rural women's health because of the consequent loss of opportunities for social support as well as physical activity.

Perhaps the most valued social support noted by study participants was in assisting them to deal with or access care for health conditions. One participant noted that "the extended family is more in evidence in rural communities. . . . The senior knows that if she needs any help, it is close by." Another participant described her family's assistance in the final weeks of her husband's life so that she could "get some much-needed sleep," and her support to her current husband when he experienced a bad fall, and when travel and waiting times in distant health care settings prohibited access to care. Family and friends often drove participants to health care, and known and trusted nurses in the community were often consulted for information and to assist with care, decision-making, and access to care. One participant noted, "Nursing services [here] are excellent," and another woman stated, "B. is a registered nurse. A good friend to have when I have medical questions." In addition, neighbours often looked out for participants: "She looks after me, checks to see if my window blinds are open. We tell each other if we are going away for a few days. Other neighbours across the driveway help me and check that I am okay." The reliance on one another was evidenced by participants referring to their curling colleagues as "family." Venues such as curling rinks provided vital community places where senior women gather to stay connected with their neighbours (Figure 9.4). As a result of the fostering of this familiarity and friendship, other resources, such as transportation, advice, and support, can also be enhanced and arranged.

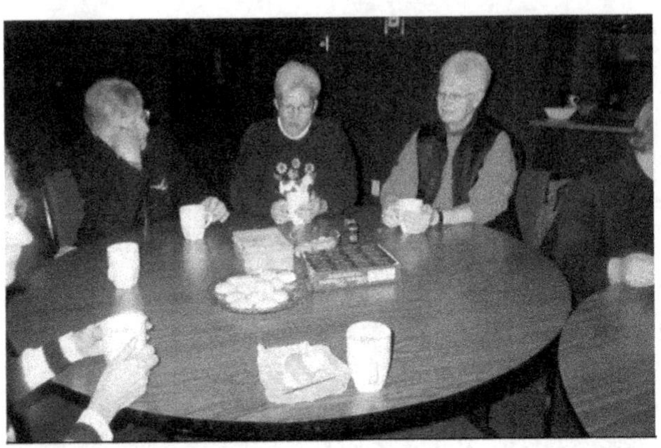

FIGURE 9.4: Rural social support

Several participants took pictures of telephones, and some women owned several types—cordless, with cords, cell phone—including answering machines; these were deemed "positive necessities of our life" in helping participants be safe and independent in their homes and vehicles.

The pride women had in their ability to be self-sustaining was evident in their narratives and pictures of beautifully kept property and full freezers and pantries. Property "becomes very personal. . . . I got this plant from somebody and I gave somebody something else . . . it's a social [thing]" and "You take great pride in it." Full pantries illustrated pride in self-sufficiency and preparedness, greater food variety and control of food choices, and opportunities to engage in enjoyable pastimes of food preservation.

In addition, full pantries helped provide affordable and diverse food options. These options are particularly important for rural older women who often have limited incomes and limited abilities to purchase off-season food and fresh fruits and vegetables, which are costly in isolated rural environments. A participant explained: "My husband and I can, preserve, and freeze [food] . . . giving us variety, [and] security for instant hospitality. There's always food for unexpected company [you can't order in, in a rural community] . . . and we give treats to shut-ins. My husband likes to put meat in the freezer and I like to bake. . . . Doing this [preserving and giving] makes us happy. It [also] saves time and helps me follow my [no red meat] diet."

Providing food at the curling rink was a source of pride and accomplishment for senior women. Women explained that they often put in significant amounts of time for food preparation for their clubs, both for social activities but also for fundraising events. One small club, for example, although with few members, successfully hosted a major curling competition. The decision to host the event was made in part to fund the club improvements but also to proudly showcase the renovated club to the greater curling community.

Senior women put in countless hours of food preparation for this event. One older woman described her involvement: "I wish I would've kept track of how many hours I actually put in. I know one day it was 13, almost 14 hours just in one day and that wasn't even including any leg work that was done ahead of time."

Utility of Photovoice for Health-Promotion Research with Older Rural Women

Participants revealed utility merits of photovoice through their comments and photos. Narratives and pictures of study participants and perspectives of the researchers revealed that photovoice is an excellent method for the conduct of health-promotion research with older rural women. First, the camera-orientation session provides an opportunity for social connection that not only facilitates open discussion in the focus group interview, but also fosters connections apart from the research. After the interview session, several women shared contact information and commented that they would get together for future social events. Thus, the method fostered the provision of rich forthright data as well as more long-term social support.

Box 9.2

Pictures and Narratives Used Together Enhance Research

One participant explained: "Pictures are worth a thousand words. If I showed you that picture, you'd say, 'What does that have to do with health?' But the reason I took that one is [goes on to verbalize what the picture means to health]. . . . The pictures help me express."

A participant noted that taking pictures helped her to see and highlight things that she would have had difficulty remembering in an interview alone. Another woman noted that knowing that the researchers would ask "why we took that picture" caused her to reflect on her life and "we just feel good that we can live in our own home, do our own thing . . . [reflect on] something we take for granted and you made us think about it." Thus, the pictures, logbook, and interview together proved affirming and enlightening in ways that either method alone would be more limited in accomplishing or could not reveal.

In addition, the use of cameras and focus group and logbook data-collection methods facilitate participant involvement in and benefit from the research. For example, a participant who initially considered dropping out of the study in the camera-orientation session ultimately took useful and informative pictures, wrote insightful comments in her logbook, and made astute comments in the focus group interview. In her logbook, she wrote, "Thank you for inviting me to be part of this study. . . . I have enjoyed it. It has made me more aware and more appreciative of living in a rural setting, its pros and cons where seniors' health is concerned."

The researchers observed that at focus group interviews the use of pictures helped some of the women to overcome reticence and forget that they felt that they could not participate or did not have anything of significance to contribute, as some had indicated in the camera-orientation session. The pictures and attendant discussion stimulated women to reflect and speak when—as indicated by their comments and participation in the camera-orientation session, or one-on-one interviews or focus group interviews without pictures—they would probably have been silent or reluctant participants. Thus, the photos acted as "intermediary artifacts" (Prosser, 2011, p. 484) that minimized lack of confidence or undervaluing of perspectives and promoted voice and participation. Clearly, the method sparks thought, fosters the provision of rich data, and serves as an empowerment tool for rural older women who often are not included, or do not include themselves, in rural research. The method also helps these women realize that they have knowledge important to their health and the health of others, and may thus assist in giving back to participants' important affirmation in terms of self-valuing, knowledge, and valuing of others.

Participants' advice to women in using photovoice in subsequent research included: "Take the camera everywhere . . . in your car . . . in your purse" to facilitate picture taking at opportune moments; "I made a list of pictures I wanted to take so that helped"; and "A digital camera would have been easier to use" for women with limited eyesight or picture-taking abilities. Nonetheless, many women took a full roll of relevant pictures. Logbooks were used for various purposes, including providing a listing of pictures, thoughts about pictures taken, or comments to the researchers. In rural settings where everyone knows everyone, the logbooks helped participants to include confidential information that might not otherwise have been offered in focus group settings. Thus, the logbooks, too, provided valuable information, particularly in this rural context.

Issues for Further Investigation

Some pictures could not be taken. For example, sometimes women forgot the camera or it was the wrong time of year. Some women would have liked to take pictures in other seasons to reveal additional health-promotion problems and resources, or at times outside of the study time frame, such as when a bonspiel was hosted at their curling rink, to reveal additional health-related opportunities or issues. Some problems, such as health and travel issues, did not occur during the period of the research, and sometimes people whose pictures participants wished to take were not available or refused to be included in pictures. This latter reason has particular relevance for older people as they are often advised to not sign papers without family present to prevent possible exploitation. This advice precluded some potential older photo subjects from signing the consent form and thus prevented their inclusion in the study. In addition, frail seniors sometimes required assistance in taking pictures, and assistants, such as family or neighbours, were not always available. Nonetheless, in spite of—and perhaps due to—the challenges and limitations noted here, additional photovoice research is clearly indicated.

Conclusions

These studies revealed that photovoice is an appropriate and effective research method for exploring and obtaining rich information about health-promotion needs and resources of older rural women. Photovoice also provided valuable information on senior rural women's contribution to and need for health resources. Study participants provided diverse, detailed, and creative pictorial and descriptive narratives, not only about health-promotion needs and resources, but also about local and systemic factors that affect these needs and resources. For example, the closure of local churches, the financial viability of small rural curling rinks, and decisions by Canada Post to eliminate rural mail delivery minimize rural older women's ability to foster and sustain both distant and local social support networks. These findings also reveal rich insights about rural culture and day-to-day ways that rural women connect to foster health. For example, mailboxes are used as conduits for the exchange of other than mail items such as magazines, baking, and personal messages, and curling rinks represent important places of acceptance, inclusion, and support. Thus, photovoice fosters understanding that could significantly affect systemic policy such as rural mail delivery and recreation, as well as assist health care providers in health promotion and social support of rural women by incorporating their priorities and ways of being into rural practices.

These studies also revealed important information about contextual and conceptual factors that affect photovoice methodology as well as rural older women's health. For example, the season in which a photovoice study is undertaken will affect the nature and conception of the questions that can be addressed and the data that can be provided. Summer pictures reveal needs and resources that differ from pictures taken during the snow, ice, and storm conditions of winter, when questions about winter sports such as curling readily lend themselves to photovoice inquiry.

In addition, the studies provided important information about sampling, financial and personal costs, and methodological issues of using photovoice in research with older rural women. Although recruitment and retention of rural samples can be challenging due to sparse populations, distance, and transportation issues, the novelty of using a camera proved attractive in recruitment and retention efforts in these studies. In addition, several participants requested the opportunity to participate in future photovoice research. Thus, this method may be important methodologically in recruiting and retaining diverse participation in rural research.

Perhaps the most significant finding of these studies was the ability of photovoice to foster empowerment of rural older women. Due to distance, rural location, the limited focus in research on older rural women's health, and the predominance of quantitative research, it is unlikely that any of the study participants had participated in formal research before. Although study participants agreed to participate, it was not assured that the women would remain in the study or that they would feel confident and comfortable to take pictures and discuss in a focus group format. However, all of the women (except for two, who withdrew due to illness or other conflicting commitments) remained in the studies after the camera-orientation session, and all were able to provide rich pictorial and narrative information. More confident expressions and postures and eagerness to discuss pictures indicated that the women gained a sense of empowerment and confidence in their participation. Thus, photovoice can be not only an effective method for accessing information, it can also foster ways of being that can help rural older women advance their health and the health of others in their communities.

Future photovoice research should expand the numbers, diversity, and locations of rural participants and sites to extend understanding and generalizability. Nonetheless, these small studies effectively generated rich data and new knowledge regarding an underserved population, under-researched settings, and effectiveness of an innovative research method for collecting meaningful data about rural women's lives. The studies also provide important insights into the value of photovoice for empowering women through a process of consciousness-raising and speaking out (Wang, 1999). Clearly, photovoice studies enrich conceptual and methodological understanding of older rural women's health-promotion needs and resources.

Acknowledgements

The authors thank Jennifer Smith, Dr. Heather Mair, Dr. Lynn Scruby, and Dr. Donna Meagher-Stewart for valuable contributions to the research and perspectives referenced in this chapter.

Note

1. Logbooks and audio tape recordings of focus group interviews were transcribed verbatim; transcripts were checked for accuracy by reviewing them with their corresponding tapes and logbooks. Each transcript was then analyzed using the process of content analysis (Patton, 2002). Line-by-line review of the transcripts revealed codes that identified key words and phrases regarding advantages (i.e., personal choice of the pictures to take) and disadvantages (i.e., forgetting about the camera) of the photovoice method; contextual factors (i.e., weather and distance); sampling issues (i.e., how to ensure diversity); financial (i.e., travel expenses) and personal costs (i.e., time to take pictures); methodological and conceptual issues (i.e., how health-promotion needs and resources are represented in photos and focus group interviews); and the nature of the data provided (i.e., pictures taken and explanations of health-promotion needs and resources). Codes were then examined for emerging themes about the appropriateness and fit of the photovoice method with

the population of older rural women, and about health-promotion needs and resources. To develop in-depth and accurate understanding, we compared themes within and across transcripts and the interview locations, as well as within the context of the pictures that were taken, those that were singled out for discussion, and those not included in the discussion. The qualitative software program NVIVO (QSR International, 2006) assisted with labelling and retrieving codes and themes during analysis.

To maintain rigour and trustworthiness: (a) focus group interviews were recorded and transcribed verbatim; (b) transcribed data were edited to accurately present recorded data; (c) participants' pictures, perspectives, and language formed the bases of the analysis; (d) transcribed and analyzed information was reviewed by two investigators to facilitate interpretive rigour; and (e) an audit trail will be achieved by keeping raw data and analytical memos for a minimum of seven years (Hall & Stevens, 1991; Lincoln & Guba, 1985; Wang & Burris, 1997).

References

Aitcheson, C. (2003). *Gender and Leisure: Social and Cultural Perspectives.* New York: Routledge.

Butler, L. M., & A. M. Xet-Mull. (2001). A Community-Based Approach to Understanding Factors Influencing TB Control and Prevention in Contra Costa County, California. Human Rights Center Summer Fellowship 2001 Final Report. Retrieved from www.hrcberkeley.org/fellowships/fellowships_selectreports.html.

Canadian Institute for Health Information. (2011). *Health Care in Canada, 2011: A Focus on Seniors and Aging.* Ottawa: Author. Retrieved from https://secure.cihi.ca/free_products/HCIC_2011_seniors_report_en.pdf.

Cerhan, J., & R. Wallace. (1993). Predictors of Decline in Social Relationships in the Rural Elderly. *American Journal of Epidemiology* 137(8): 870–880.

Clark, K., & B. Leipert. (2007). Strengthening and Sustaining Social Supports for Rural Elders. *Online Journal of Rural Nursing and Health Care* 7(1): 13–26.

Dolan, H., & D. Thien. (2008). Relations of Care: A Framework for Placing Women and Health in Rural Communities. *Canadian Review of Public Health* 99(Nov./Dec.): S38–S42.

du Plessis, V., R. Beshiri, R. Bollman, & H. Clemenson. (2001). Definitions of Rural. *Rural and Small Town Canada Analysis Bulletin* 3(3): 1–16. Cat. no. 21-006-XIE. Ottawa: Statistics Canada.

Gilmore, J. (2010). *Provincial Drop-Out Rates—Trends and Consequences* (Education Matters: Insights on Education, Learning, and Training in Canada Publication No. 7[4]). Ottawa: Statistics Canada. Retrieved from http://www.statcan.gc.ca/pub/81-004-x/2010004/article/11339-eng.htm.

Hall, J., & P. Stevens. (1991). Rigor in Feminist Research. *Advances in Nursing Science* 13(3): 16–29.

Hinck, S. (2004). The Lived Experience of Oldest-Old Rural Adults. *Qualitative Health Research* 14(6): 779–791.

Keating, N., J. Keefe, & B. Dobbs. (2001). A Good Place to Grow Old? Rural Communities and Support to Seniors. In R. Epp & D. Whitson (Eds.), *Writing off the Rural West: Globalization, Governments, and the Transformation of Rural Communities* (pp. 263–277). Edmonton: University of Alberta Press.

Leipert, B. (2013). Rural and Remote Women and Resilience: Grounded Theory and Photovoice Variations on a Theme. In C. Winters (Ed.), *Rural Nursing: Concepts, Theory, and Practice* (4th ed.; pp. 95 –117). New York: Springer.

Leipert, B., B. Leach, & W. Thurston (Eds.). (2012). *Rural Women's Health.* Toronto: University of Toronto Press.

Leipert, B., R. Plunkett, D. Meagher-Stewart, L. Scruby, H. Mair, & K. Wamsley. (2011). I Couldn't Imagine My Life Without It! Curling and Health Promotion: A Photovoice Study. *The Canadian Journal of Nursing Research* 43(1): 60–78.

Leipert, B., L. Scruby, & D. Meagher-Stewart. (under review). Sport, Health, and Rural Community: Curling and Rural Women: A National Photovoice Study. *Journal of Rural and Community Development.*

Lincoln, Y., & E. Guba. (1985). Establishing Trustworthiness. In Y. Lincoln & E. Guba (Eds.), *Naturalistic Inquiry* (pp. 289–331). New Delhi: Sage.

Mair, H. (2007). Curling in Canada: From Gathering Place to International Spectacle. *International Journal of Canadian Studies* 35: 39–60.

Mair, H. (2009). Club Life: Third Place and Shared Leisure in Rural Canada. *Leisure Sciences,* 31(5): 450–465.

Ministerial Advisory Council on Rural Health. (2002). *Rural Health in Rural Hands: Strategic Direction for Rural, Remote, Northern, and Aboriginal Communities.* Retrieved from www.phac-aspc.gc.ca/rh-sr/rural_hands-mains_rurales_e.html.

Ministry of Industry. (2006). *Women in Canada: A Gender-Based Statistical Report.* Ottawa: Statistics Canada.

Morrow, D., & K. Wamsley. (2013). Chapter 8: Gender, Body, and Sport. In D. Morrow & K. Wamsley (Eds.), *Sport in Canada* (3rd ed., pp. 179–206). Don Mills, ON: Oxford University Press.

National Advisory Council on Aging. (2002). *Writings in Gerontology: Mental Health and Aging* 18(October). Cat. no. H88-3/29-2003E. Retrieved from www.naca.ca/writings_gerontology/writ18/writ18_toc_e.htm.

Olesen, V. (2011). Feminist Qualitative Research in the Millennium's First Decade. In N. Denzin & Y. Lincoln (Eds.), *The Sage Handbook of Qualitative Research* (4th ed.; pp. 129–146). London: Sage.

Oliffe, J., J. Bottorff, M. Kelly, & M. Halpin. (2008). Analyzing Participant Produced Photographs from an Ethnographic Study of Fatherhood and Smoking. *Research in Nursing & Health* 31(5): 529–539. doi: 10.1002/nur.20269.

Patton, M. (2002). *Qualitative Research and Evaluation Methods* (3rd ed.). London: Sage.

Plunkett, R., & B. Leipert. (2013). Women's Health Promotion in the Rural Church: A Canadian Perspective. *Journal of Religion and Health* 52(3): 877–889. doi: 10.1007/s10943-011-9535-z.

Prosser, J. (2011). Visual Methodology. In N. Denzin & Y. Lincoln (Eds.), *The Sage Handbook of Qualitative Research* (4th ed., pp. 479–495). London, UK: Sage.

Pullen, C., S. Walker, & K. Fiandt. (2001). Determinants of Health-Promoting Lifestyle Behaviors in Rural Older Women. *Family and Community Health* 24(2): 49–72.

QSR International. (2006). *NVIVO 7.* Doncaster, Australia: QSR International PTY Ltd.

Rockwood, K., X. Song, C. MacKnight, H. Bergman, D. Hogan, I. McDowell, & A. Mitniski. (2005). A Global Clinical Measure of Fitness and Frailty in Elderly People. *Canadian Medical Association Journal* 173(5): 489–495.

Romanow, R. (2002). *Building on Values: The Future of Health Care in Canada.* Ottawa: Commission of the Future of Health Care in Canada.

Song, X., C. MacKnight, R. Latta, A. B. Mitnitski, & K. Rockwood. (2007). Frailty and Survival of Rural and Urban Seniors: Results from the Canadian Study of Health and Aging. *Aging Clinical and Experimental Research* 19(2):145–153. doi: 10.1007/BF03324681.

Standing Senate Committee on Agriculture and Forestry. (2006). *Understanding Freefall: The Challenge of the Rural Poor* (Interim report). Ottawa: Standing Senate Committee on Agriculture and Forestry. Retrieved from www.parl.gc.ca.

Statistics Canada. (2011). *Projected Population, by Projection Scenario, Sex, and Age Group as of July 1, Canada, Provinces, and Territories, Annual* (CANSIM table 052-0005). Ottawa: Author.

Sutherns, R., M. McPhedran, & M. Haworth-Brockman. (2004). *Rural, Remote, and Northern Women's Health: Policy and Research Directions.* Ottawa: Centres of Excellence for Women's Health.

Thomeer, M. B. (2013). Aging and Gender. In W. Cockerham (Ed.), *The Wiley Blackwell Encyclopedia of Health, Illness, Behavior, and Society* (pp. 36–42). doi: 10.1002/9781118410868.wbehibs119.

Tonts, M. (2005). Competitive Sport and Social Capital in Rural Australia. *Journal of Rural Studies* 21(2): 137–149.

Trussell, D. E., & S. M. Shaw. (2007). Daddy's Gone and He'll Be Back in October: Farm Women's Experiences of Family Leisure. *Journal of Leisure Research* 39(2): 366–387.

Turner, L., & I. Gutmanis. (2005). *Rural Health Matters: A Look at Farming in Southwest Ontario: Part 2.* London, ON: Southwest Region Health Information Partnership.

Wang, C. (1999). Photovoice: A Participatory Action Research Strategy Applied to Women's Health. *Journal of Women's Health* 8(2): 185–192.

Wang, C., & M. Burris. (1997). Photovoice: Concept, Methodology, and Use for Participatory Needs Assessment. *Health Education and Behavior* 24(3): 369–387.

Wang, C., M. Burris, & X. Ping. (1996). Chinese Village Women as Visual Anthropologists: A Participatory Approach to Reaching Policy Makers. *Social Science and Medicine* 42(10): 1391–1400.

Wang, C., W. Yi, Z. Tao, & K. Carovano. (1998). Photovoice as a Participatory Health Promotion Strategy. *Health Promotion International* 13(1): 75–86.

Ward-Griffin, C., & J. Ploeg. (1997). A Feminist Approach to Health Promotion for Older Women. *Canadian Journal on Aging* 16(2): 279–296.

Warner-Smith, P., & P. Brown. (2002). "The Town Dictates What I Do": The Leisure, Health, and Well-Being of Women in a Small Australian County Town. *Leisure Studies* 21(1): 39–56.

World Health Organization. (2014). *Health Promotion.* Retrieved from http://www.who.int/topics/health_promotion/en/.

Further Reading

Leipert, B., B. Leach, & W. Thurston. (2012). *Rural Women's Health.* Toronto: University of Toronto Press.

Ministry of Industry. (2006). *Women in Canada: A Gender-Based Statistical Report.* Ottawa: Canada: Statistics Canada.

Relevant Websites

Centre for Rural and Northern Health Research: http://www.cranhr.ca/hands.html

Public Health Agency of Canada, Aging and Seniors: http://www.phac-aspc.gc.ca/seniors-aines/index-eng.php

Statistics Canada. (2012). *Canadian Seniors: A Demographic Profile*: http://www.elections.ca/content.aspx?section=res&dir=rec/part/sen&document=index&lang=e

CHAPTER 10

The Health of Sexual Minority Women and Trans People:
An Ontario Perspective

Anna Travers

Introduction

This chapter will look at the health and well-being of sexual and gender minority women—that is, women who identify as lesbian, bisexual, and two-spirit, as well as people who identify as trans (an overarching term for transgender, transsexual, genderqueer, etc.). As I write the updated version of this chapter after seven years, I am pleased to note the increasing amount and variety of Canadian research focused on sexual and gender minority women, some small but notable improvements in access to appropriate health care services, and greater visibility of LGBT people in health-promotion initiatives.

Since the subject matter is so broad, I have chosen to discuss a few key health-related concerns and to highlight some of the more invisible and vulnerable subgroups within this population, such as bisexual women, trans people, youth, and seniors. In Canada, the research on LGBT health issues (apart from HIV) is still in an early stage of development and there are many gaps, especially in population-level data. It is not always possible, therefore, to focus on women separately from the broader LGBT population. Likewise, although I have focused on Canadian research, it is necessary to look at the broader context, particularly the United States, the United Kingdom, and Australia, to discuss trends in population health.

As the director of Rainbow Health Ontario, a knowledge translation and exchange program funded by the provincial Ministry of Health and Long-Term Care, I have had the privilege of being involved in numerous initiatives to build capacity and foster networks among health care providers, researchers, policy-makers and decision-makers in Ontario. This is the only such program in Canada that is focused broadly on LGBT health and it has allowed for the development of new knowledge networks, communities of practice, and

Knowledge Transfer and Exchange (KTE) resources (see www.rainbowhealthontario.ca). As a result, examples of innovative approaches and promising practices are drawn mainly from projects with which I am familiar.

Measuring the Prevalence of Sexual and Gender Minorities in Canada

The first question that most people ask is about the prevalence of lesbian, gay, bisexual, and transgender people in Canada. This is a very hard question to answer for a number of reasons. Firstly, people are naturally cautious about revealing a stigmatized identity on a government form or even to a family member or health care provider. We should assume, therefore, that self-reported measures regarding sexual and gender minority status will be very conservative, although by asking frequently we do give the message that this is a normal part of human diversity and therefore encourage increases in reporting (Tjepkema, 2008).

Secondly, sexual orientation and gender identity are not easy concepts to define or measure. Many epidemiologists contend that sexual orientation is made up of several different components: sexual identity, sexual behaviour, and sexual attraction. On surveys such as the Canadian Community Health Survey (CCHS), sexual-orientation questions ask only about sexual identity: "Do you identify as heterosexual, gay, lesbian or bisexual?" (Tjepkema, 2008). This narrow range of descriptors excludes, for example, "two-spirited," a term used by some Aboriginal peoples to describe both sexual orientation and gender, or "queer," a term that is commonly used by younger people.

Based on the combined 2003 and 2005 CCHS data, only 1.9 percent of adults aged between 18 and 59 self-identified as gay, lesbian, or bisexual. Within these groups the relative numbers of people identifying as gay or lesbian (homosexual) or bisexual is shown. Interestingly, more women identify as bisexual than lesbian, which points to a more fluid sense of sexuality among women (Tjepkema, 2008).

Over time, the number of people disclosing sexual minority status is gradually increasing, but the nature of the questions asked on surveys also makes a difference. For example, surveys used in the United States and other countries frequently ask about both sexual identity and same-sex sexual behaviour, and some also ask about same-sex sexual attraction (Chandra, Mosher, & Copen, 2011). Gary Gates conducted a meta-analysis of different U.S. survey tools and showed that numbers changed substantially depending on which aspect of sexuality was measured. For example, whereas 3.5 percent of Americans identified as gay, lesbian, or bisexual, 8.2 percent reported that they had engaged in same-sex sexual behaviour and 11 percent acknowledged at least some same-sex sexual attraction (Gates, 2011).

In Canada, the Ontario Health Study, a longitudinal study begun in 2010, now asks participants several questions about both sexual orientation and sexual behaviour. At the request of LGBT leaders and researchers, changes were made soon after the launch of

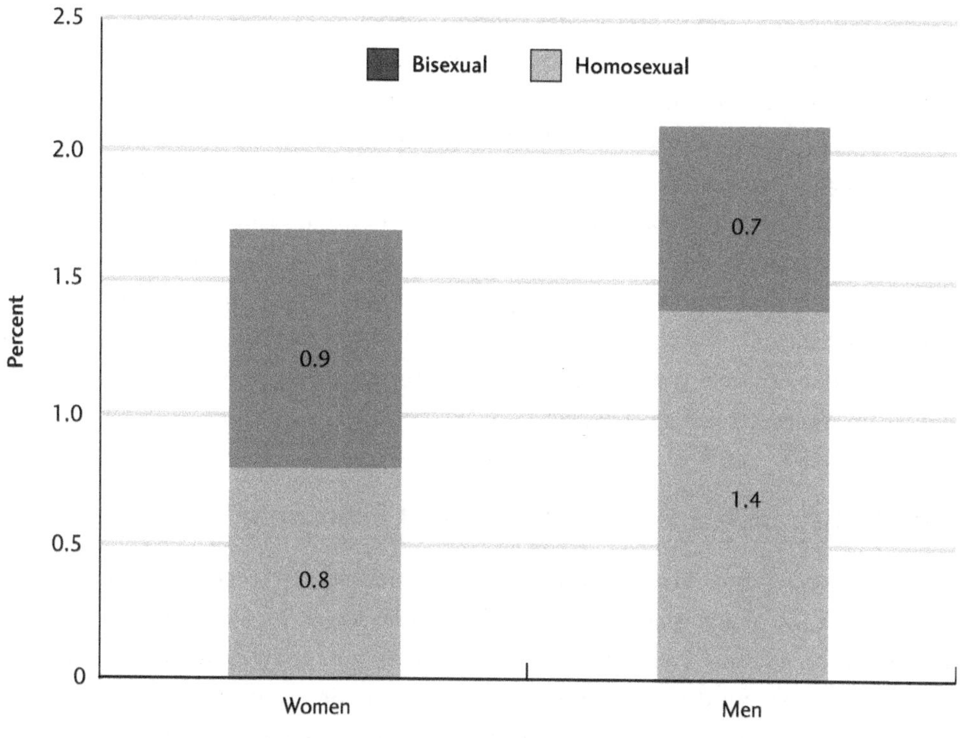

FIGURE 10.1: Percentage of Canadians identifying as homosexual or bisexual in the Canadian Community Health Survey

Source: M. Tjepkema, 2008, Health Care Use among Gay, Lesbian, and Bisexual Canadians. *Statistics Canada, Health Reports* 19(1): 53–64.

this study so that both the health questions and skip patterns embedded in the survey are inclusive of LGBT people—that is, they allow for variations in sexual partners, body parts, "gendered" medical tests and treatments, etc. Over time, this survey will provide unique, high-quality information about the health of LGBT Ontarians.

While categories describing gender—transgender or cisgender (current terminology for non-trans)—are often conflated with sexual orientation, gender is a separate spectrum of experience that describes one's internal sense of being masculine or feminine, man or woman, or some blend of both. People's internal sense of gender may or may not be aligned with their biological sex or birth-assigned gender. Canada does not collect data on the number of trans people in society, but population studies in the United States indicate that people who self-identify as trans (including transgender, transsexual, genderqueer, and some two-spirited people) are a growing population and currently comprise about one in 200 or 0.5 percent of the population (Conron, Scott, Stowell, & Landers, 2012).

In a chapter focused on women's health, the inclusion of trans people may challenge our typical ways of thinking about gender as an immutable and binary concept. The majority of trans people either begin their gender journey as female and move toward the male end of the spectrum, or begin as male and move toward the female end; others find a comfort zone somewhere in the middle or combine aspects of both (genderqueer, genderfluid). Many trans people choose to access medical treatments such as hormones and surgeries and therefore acquire some of the characteristics of the preferred gender at a physiological level, while others choose only a social transition (through clothing, presentation, name, pronoun, ID changes) but live in the world in the social role of the preferred gender. Genderqueer people may blend male and female and may also choose certain medical treatments or procedures (Scheim & Bower, 2014). Authorities such as the World Professional Association of Transgender Health now recognize the validity of a wide range of gender identities and health care choices (Coleman et al., 2011).

Health Disparities, Health Needs, and Promising Practices

Although Canada is a world leader with respect to human rights protections and progressive legislation for sexual and gender minorities, it takes far longer for these changes to trickle down to the broader policy, institutional, interpersonal, and individual levels. In Canada, there has also been little direct government policy or direction to inform LGBT citizens what they can expect from our health care system, or to provide guidance to health care providers at the federal or provincial levels (Mulé et al., 2009; Daley, 2005). This is in contrast to other English-speaking countries where governments have taken a much more active role in tackling health disparities affecting sexual and gender minorities and in setting standards to achieve greater equity in health (U.S. Department of Health and Human Services, 2013; U.K. Government, 2011a; Australian Government, 2012).

In Canada, it has been very much left to individual champions—scholars, activist groups, progressive organizations, and service providers—to lead the way in identifying research priorities and developing culturally and clinically competent services for LGBT people. Despite the existence of many innovative and valuable initiatives, the lack of any overarching policy framework reinforces a culture of invisibility and silence at the institutional level and makes it harder to work toward common goals (Makadon, 2011; Institute of Medicine, 2011). The diagram below, created by the author, uses an ecological framework to show the impact of discrimination, silence, and invisibility surrounding sexual and gender minority people, and the way that these processes reinforce one another in different domains of life.

Academic studies and community surveys alike document significant inequities in the health and well-being of sexual and gender minority communities in North America (GLMA, 2001; Institute of Medicine, 2011; Tjepkema, 2008; Bauer, Jairam, & Baidoobonso, 2010). In Canada's 2003 and 2005 Community Health Surveys, Statistics Canada data showed that among individuals aged 18–59, 21.8 percent of homosexuals and bisexuals reported that they had an unmet health care need—nearly twice the proportion of heterosexuals

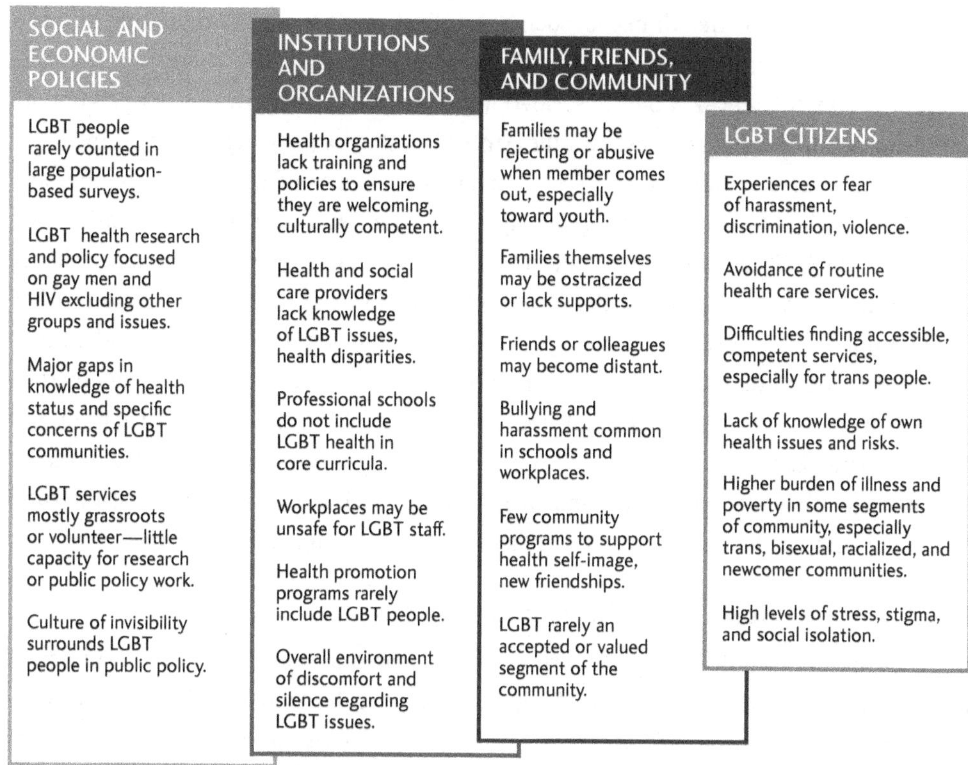

FIGURE 10.2: A social-ecological model showing multi-level barriers to LGBT health and wellness

Source: Adapted from Dahlberg and Krug's (2002) model of violence for the World Health Organization. L. L. Dahlberg & E. G. Krug, 2002, Violence—A Global Public Health Problem, in E. G. Krug, L. L. Dahlberg, J. A. Mercy, A. B. Zwi, & R. Lozano (Eds.), *World Report on Violence and Health* (Geneva: World Health Organization), pp. 1–56.

(12.7 percent). In addition, homosexual and bisexual people were more likely than heterosexuals to find life stressful (Tjepkema, 2008). The Trans Pulse Study, which provided population-level data for trans people in Ontario, showed that among trans people, unmet health needs and stress-related concerns were far higher than among cisgender people (Scanlon, Travers, Coleman, Bauer, & Boyce, 2010; Bauer, Pyne, Francino, & Hammond, 2013; Rotondi et al., 2011).

It is often assumed that HIV is the only health issue of relevance to LGBT communities; indeed, the number of research articles on HIV is twice the number on all other health conditions combined (Snyder, 2011). But HIV is not the *only* issue affecting LGBT people, especially queer and trans women. The most prevalent health disparities across the entire LGBT population are related to mental health and substance-use problems (McCabe et al., 2010; Meyer, 2003; Tjepkema, 2008), and tobacco is actually responsible for more deaths among sexual and gender minority communities than HIV (Offen, Smith, & Malone, 2008).

There are also specific health needs, such as medical care for gender transition and services related to becoming a parent, which may be different for LGBT communities. These disparities and differences will be described in more detail together with examples of both problematic and helpful responses on the part of health care providers and systems.

In health service delivery, there are certainly instances of overt homophobia and transphobia, which are expressed in rejecting and hostile behaviours (Rosario, Schrimshaw, & Hunter, 2009; Grant et al., 2011) but more commonly LGBT people experience silence and invisibility when engaging with health and social service providers (Makadon, 2011). This reinforces the sense that being open about sexual orientation or gender identity is not a good idea. In their efforts not to cause offence, health care providers frequently miss important cues and conversations that would build trust, elicit important information, and facilitate better care. In addition, LGBT people frequently censor themselves due to shame or the expectation of disapproval; some avoid care as much as possible (Steele, Tinmouth, & Lu, 2006; Bauer, Scheim, Deutsch, & Massarella, 2014; Rotondi et al., 2013).

Mental Health, Substance Abuse, and Tobacco

LGBT people as a whole are significantly overrepresented in reported rates of depression, anxiety, suicidality, and substance use (Boehmer, Xiaopeng, Linkletter, & Clark, 2014; Bauer, Pyne, Francino, & Hammond, 2013). This is related to the stress of stigma, discrimination, and anticipated harassment or violence rather than being an innate characteristic of LGBT people. Mental illness has a particular negative resonance for queer people because during the twentieth century when psychological paradigms gained dominance over religious/moral paradigms, LGBT individuals were regarded as both sexually deviant and mentally unstable. Many were sent to mental hospitals for treatment, including for psychoanalysis and electroshock (American Psychiatric Association, 2000). A significant number of professionals, as well as some community members themselves, still believe that LGBT people are emotionally unstable or damaged in some way.

Ilan Meyer is credited with developing the Minority Stress Model to explain the chronic psychological strain resulting from stigma and expectations of rejection and discrimination, decisions about disclosure of sexual identity, and the internalization of homophobia that LGBT people face in a heterosexist society (Meyer, 2003). Ongoing stress, especially when associated with social isolation, affects internal psychological processes such as mood and cognitive beliefs resulting in anxiety, depression, and suicidality as well as the use of external coping/numbing mechanisms such as alcohol, drugs, or tobacco (Hatzenbuehler, Nolen-Hoeksma, & Dovidio, 2009). Not surprisingly, the effects of several types of societal marginalization, such as being both lesbian *and* from a racialized group, or being bisexual *and* disabled can lead to cumulative levels of stress with greater psychological impacts (McLaughlin, Hatzenbuehler, & Keyes, 2010; Ryan, Brotman, Baradaran, & Lee, 2008; Steele, Tinmouth, & Lu, 2006). Transphobia at all levels has a similar detrimental effect on mental health and has been directly linked to depression in trans people (Rotondi et al., 2011).

Of course, many LGBT people and members of other minoritized groups demonstrate robust mental health and resilience despite being targeted or constrained by discriminatory acts or systems. This is partially attributable to individual factors, but the literature shows that resilience and self-efficacy flourish in environments where there are others who openly share their experiences, where there is social support, and where groups can mobilize against their marginalized status (Hatzenbuehler, Nolen-Hoeksma, & Dovidio, 2009).

Current evidence from the United States shows that lesbian and bisexual women not only consume more alcohol than their heterosexual counterparts but that they continue to drink at higher levels in their senior years (Ritter, Matthew-Simmons, & Carragher, 2012). Similarly, the data from the United States and Australia on substance use indicate that lesbian and bisexual women have higher rates of substance use, with bisexual women's use of cannabis being especially marked (Bauer, Jairam, & Baidoobonso, 2010; Wilsnack et al., 2008). In Canada, studies on high school students in British Columbia show that LGB students were more likely than their straight peers to report using substances and that lesbian and bisexual youth were the heaviest users of "club" drugs and had high rates of binge drinking (Lampinen, McGhee, & Martin, 2006; Saewyc et al., 2007).

When it comes to tobacco use, a 2007 study conducted in Toronto (Clarke & Coughlin, 2012) showed that people who self-identify as LGBTQ are twice as likely to smoke tobacco as the city's general population—36 percent compared with 18 percent. A sample size of over 3,000 enabled a robust breakdown of subgroups within the LGBTQ population and revealed that the highest smoking rates were among bisexual people. Compared with adults in the survey, youth reported very high smoking rates with 50 percent of those under 15 and 57 percent of those aged 15–19 being current smokers. Young women smoked the most of all.

In 2013, a qualitative study conducted by Toronto Public Health, Rainbow Health Ontario, and others explored the drivers behind the high rates of smoking among LGBT youth and invited youth themselves to produce "Why You Puffin'?" a photovoice book to share personal and social links between smoking and LGBTQ identities (Toronto Public Health and Partners, 2014). For this population, as well as adult smokers, quitting programs need to be tailored to the audience and must include stress management and mutual support strategies that respond to the specific causes of distress (Rosario, Schrimshaw, & Hunter, 2009; Lombardi, 2007).

Specialized programs that provide mental health support or treatment for substance or tobacco use are rare and found only in major cities. Most people will have access only to generic or mainstream programs, but workers in these programs rarely receive professional education or ongoing training in how to serve these communities competently (Makadon, Mayer, Potter, & Goldhammer, 2008; GLMA, 2001). It would be ideal if more focused content on LGBT health were integrated into professional education programs. A study of medical schools in the United States and Canada showed that the LGBT-related education averaged just over five hours over the students' entire medical education (Obedin-Maliver et al., 2011).

Physical and Sexual Health

Discussing intimate health issues can be hard for anyone. For a lesbian or bisexual woman, anxiety about a health care visit may be heightened or relieved by the clues she picks up from the environment: the graphics and brochures on display; the way she is addressed; and the forms that are used to collect information. For trans people the stress of disclosure is even greater and there may be great apprehension about discussions and procedures related to the chest/breast and genital areas. Intake forms that request a range of demographic information, including questions about sexual orientation and gender identity, are not only good for service planning and evaluation, they also signal that the organization expects diversity and is ready to provide competent services. In 2013 in Toronto, planning and funding bodies such as the Toronto Central Local Health Integration Network (LHIN) started to require hospitals to gather eight categories of demographic information, including sexual orientation and gender identity, and this expectation will later extend to the community sector as well. Figure 10.3 shows part of the intake form used for all clients at Toronto's Sherbourne Health Centre, a primary health care centre that specializes in care for homeless and newcomer communities as well as LGBT clients and which is the home base for Rainbow Health Ontario.

Lesbian and bisexual women and their health care providers typically lack information about their need for Pap tests and other sexual health screenings and tests. As a result, some conditions are not diagnosed until they are more advanced and less amenable to treatment. (Mravcak, 2006). Doctors and nurses who are unfamiliar with LGBT people may avoid asking questions out of embarrassment or fear of offending the client, but providers need to know how to make it easy for clients to disclose their sexual orientation and/or gender identity. Beyond this they must also ask detailed, non-judgmental questions about sexual behaviours and partners in order to screen appropriately for sexually transmitted infections or provide effective sexual health education (Power, McNair, & Carr, 2009; Sanchez, Hailpern, Lowe, & Calderon, 2007).

In addition to health promotion that is provided in the clinical setting, Canada relies on major charitable organizations to provide vital information and disease-specific health-promotion strategies to the public. Examples include the Canadian Cancer Society, the Alzheimer Society, the Heart and Stroke Association, the Lung Association, and a host of others. To date, few have undertaken campaigns focused on LGBT people even though this is warranted in terms of risk factors, the prevalence of certain health conditions, and the need to be audience-specific in order to be effective. In Canada, we are starting to see a change in this trend as charitable associations begin to partner with LGBT groups to address specific public health concerns.

✓ Can we contact you at home? ❑ Yes ❑ No
✓ Can we leave private message if necessary? ❑ Yes ❑ No
✓ Can we use your preferred name in correspondence? ❑ Yes ❑ No

Gender:		**Sexual Orientation:**	
❑ Female	❑ Male	❑ Heterosexual (straight)	❑ Gay
❑ Intersexed	❑ Two Spirit	❑ Lesbian	❑ Bisexual
❑ Transgender	❑ Genderqueer	❑ Two-Spirit	❑ Queer
❑ Prefer not to answer	❑ Do not know	❑ Pansexual	❑ Prefer not to answer
❑ Other ____________		❑ Do not know	❑ Other ____________
		❑ Not Applicable	

Do you have concerns related to your sexual orientation?
❑ Not at all ❑ A little ❑ Somewhat ❑ A lot ❑ Prefer not to answer

Are you currently sexually active? ❑ Yes ❑ No ❑ Prefer not to answer

Do you practice safe sex? ❑ Yes ❑ No ❑ Prefer not to answer

Are you currently in a relationship? ❑ Yes ❑ No ❑ Prefer not to answer

Is/Are your partner(s):
❑ Female ❑ Male ❑ Intersexed ❑ Transgender ❑ Two Spirit ❑ Other ______________
Were your previous partner(s):
❑ Female ❑ Male ❑ Intersexed ❑ Transgender ❑ Two Spirit ❑ Other ______________

FIGURE 10.3: Excerpt from the intake form used at Sherbourne Health Centre, Toronto, Ontario, 2014

In 2013, the Canadian Cancer Society developed the Get Screened campaign in partnership with Rainbow Health Ontario and community volunteers. Special graphics and posters were created resembling well-known film posters, but with same-sex couples replacing straight couples. The Get Screened campaign has been featured at dozens of LGBT events and directs audiences to a specialized website (Canadian Cancer Society, 2014). The text on the website says:

> Did you know that we have higher risk factors for colon and breast cancer, and studies show that we are less likely to go to the doctor because of actual or feared mistreatment due to homophobia? And that some health care providers believe that we don't need to get checked out for cervical cancer, even though we do?

Another feature of the campaign involves a partnership with trainers at Rainbow Health Ontario, which has resulted in hundreds of medical imaging technologists learning appropriate language and terminology and how to work respectfully with trans people whose bodies may not conform to their gender presentation. This campaign is an example of the way mainstream organizations can reach out to LGBT people at risk with appropriate, inclusive messaging and services.

Children and Families

Members of Canada's gender and sexual minorities are frequently parents or wish to form their own families through donor insemination, adoption, surrogacy, and co-parenting arrangements. They need reliable information and services to support them in deciding how they will become parents and how to raise children in a culture that does not always recognize or legitimize families that fall outside the heterosexual, cisgender, nuclear family norm (Chan, Raboy, & Patterson, 2008). For a queer woman, being a parent frequently means she is assumed to be heterosexual and her female partner is often left out of the picture altogether. In the case of a parent who transitions, there is a common myth that the children would be better off without contact with the parent altogether. Thus, trans people are often pressured to give up their rights and sever contact with their children (Pyne, 2012).

Whether in the fertility clinic, the obstetrician's office, the hospital, daycare, school, or neighbourhood, queer and trans families continually have to explain themselves, educate others, and insist on their rights (Ross, Steele, & Epstein, 2006). Children in these families are exposed to frequent homophobic comments in the schoolyard; they too must continually decide when and where it is safe to come out (Epstein, 2004; Bos & Van Balen, 2008). Despite these challenges, the literature indicates that children raised in LGB families show a robust sense of self-esteem and are more empathic than other children (Murray & McClintock, 2005).

Many helpful resources have been created to inform and educate service providers, policy-makers, and community members about the needs of LGBT families. Table 10.1 shows just some of the ways that organizations can change their language to become more welcoming and inclusive.

In Toronto, the LGBTQ Parenting Network is a unique program that serves sexual and gender minority families by providing family-planning courses, parent education, and family-oriented social events. The Network also reaches a broader audience through its website and social media to disseminate policy briefs, research studies, guidebooks, and posters.

Instead of:	Use:	Comment
Are you married?	Do you have a spouse or domestic partner?	Does not assume sexual orientation or gender of sexual partners.
Boyfriend/girlfriend	Partner	As above.
Are you the mother/father?	Are you the parent or guardian?	More inclusive of different types of families.
Who is the real father/mother?	Who is the biological father/ mother?	Describes the genetic parent and is useful if genetic information is needed.

TABLE 10.1: Examples of Inclusive Language

Source: S. Mravcak, 2006, Primary Care for Lesbian and Bisexual Women, *American Family Physician* 74:2. Adapted with permission from M. Laret, 2004, *Inclusive Language Policy* (San Francisco, CA: University of San Francisco Medical Center).

Youth

"Coming out"—the recognition of a queer or trans identity—now takes place earlier in life as a result of greater public awareness and media coverage, typically in early to mid-adolescence. The 2011 Climate Survey of over 4,000 Canadian high school students showed that 70 percent of LGBT students are exposed daily to homophobic/transphobic comments. They also report high rates of verbal, physical, and sexual harassment (Taylor & Peter, 2011).

These experiences in turn are linked to higher levels of anxiety and depression, increased drug and alcohol use, early school leaving, and homelessness (Abramovic, 2012; Boehmer et al., 2014). A Canadian study estimated that the risk of suicide among LGB youth is 14 times higher than for their heterosexual peers (Benibgui, 2011). Among trans people, 43 percent reported ever having attempted suicide attempt and of these, two-thirds were under 20 when they made their first suicide attempt (Bauer et al., 2013).

Supports for families and adolescents that normalize, even celebrate, the existence of LGBT people, as well as enforcement of anti-bullying policies and gay–straight alliances in schools are proven ways to create safety and to keep young people connected to their families and peers (Ryan, Russell, Huebner et al., 2010). In many communities in Ontario, increasing numbers of agency or community-initiated programs have been established to provide information, support, and safe spaces for LGBT youth. One of the largest and most comprehensive is Supporting Our Youth at Sherbourne Health Centre in Toronto.

> Supporting Our Youth (SOY) is an exciting, dynamic community development program designed to improve the lives of lesbian, gay, bisexual, transsexual and transgendered youth in Toronto through the active involvement of youth and adult communities. We work to create healthy arts, culture and recreational spaces for young people; to provide supportive housing and employment opportunities; and to increase youth access to adult mentoring and support. (Supporting Our Youth, 2014)

This program serves hundreds of diverse LGBT youth every week including newcomers and refugees, black queer youth, homeless and street involved youth, and trans youth. SOY has grown and evolved since 1998 and has served as a model for programs internationally (see Lepischak, 2004).

Trans People

Trans people are coming out younger and in greater numbers than ever before (Scheim & Bauer, 2014). Sadly, they lag far behind LGB communities with regard to basic human rights, experiences of discrimination and violence, and access to health care. Ninety-eight percent of trans people who participated in the Trans Pulse Study had experienced transphobia, including being beaten up, told they weren't normal, dismissed from work, and excluded from family events (Marcellin, Scheim, Bauer, & Redman, 2013).

In health care, trans people who are seeking gender change through hormone treatment are frequently told that their needs are beyond the family physician's scope of practice. This creates a kind of Catch-22 since hormone treatment is now considered within the scope of primary health care by the World Professional Association of Transgender Health (Coleman et al., 2011), but there are so few physicians or nurses who have received training in this area and, understandably, they lack knowledge and confidence in providing this kind of service. This means that large numbers of trans people are unable to access care and many wait years to find a doctor who will prescribe hormones. Others end up purchasing hormones on the Internet or from friends, but then have no access to medical follow-up to establish the correct dosage, be monitored for dangerous side effects, or receive education and support (Rotondi et al., 2013).

The Trans Pulse Project provided an analysis of the key factors that contributed to suicidality. The findings show that once people have decided on a medical transition, being unable to access care can have very detrimental effects on their mental health, leading to a significant spike in suicide levels (Bauer et al., 2013). Thus, as much as physicians worry that hormonal transition carries risks, there are also very real risks in denying access to hormones.

To address the serious gaps in services for trans people in Ontario, Rainbow Health Ontario received special funds from the Ontario Ministry of Health in 2011 to build communities of practice in trans care across the province. Regional groups of interdisciplinary providers from primary and community agencies receive intensive training over four days to learn to deliver health care and support to trans people. They also work across sectors and agencies to design respectful, comprehensive services that meet their communities' needs. Between 2011 and 2014, over 2,000 professionals were trained and trans health services were initiated in over 10 localities across Ontario (Rainbow Health Ontario, 2014).

Not all trans people want sex-reassignment surgery (SRS) (also known as gender-confirmation surgery), but for some it is critical to their sense of body integrity and ability to move forward with their lives (Scheim & Bauer, 2014). While many of the procedures that are part of gender-confirmation surgery are now covered under public health insurance in most Canadian provinces, gaining approval for government funding usually involves a long wait to be seen in a gender identity clinic, and the only approved surgical facility for SRS in Canada is in Montreal. Thus, the majority of trans people in Canada have to travel outside their home province or even out of the country to have their surgeries (Centre for Addiction and Mental Health, 2014).

The health of trans people is very dependent on the social environment, but is also highly dependent on the availability of appropriate health care services. Services in Canada and other countries are still inadequate, waiting lists are often years long, and trans people are still often mistreated in health and social service settings (Marcellin et al., 2013; Grant et al., 2011).

Bisexual Communities

To many people, it comes as a surprise to learn that the health status of bisexual people is generally worse than that of their lesbian or gay counterparts (Tjepkema, 2008). One might assume that bisexual people face fewer barriers than lesbian or gay people, but the opposite is the case and there is additional discrimination and greater social isolation for bisexual people. Poorer mental health and quality-of-life scores reflect the fact that bisexual people encounter prejudice from both straight and queer communities, are often labelled as indecisive or immature, and made to feel unwelcome by both groups (Ross, Dobinson, & Eady, 2010).

Bisexual women report poorer mental and physical health and higher rates of disability than bisexual men (Tjepkema, 2008, Boehmer et al., 2014). They are less likely to have a regular family doctor and also report negative experiences with health care providers, including judgment or dismissiveness toward their bisexual identity, and invasive or inappropriate questions related to their sexuality (Koh & Ross, 2006; Steele, Tinmouth, & Lu, 2006).

A new cohort of Canadian researchers is beginning to expand our knowledge of bisexual health by exploring the specific factors behind higher levels of alcohol and drug use, increased levels of anxiety and depression, and experiences of physical violence and sexual assault. Many of these studies include initiatives to raise the visibility and legitimacy of bisexual communities. Rainbow Health Ontario is a partner with the Centre for Addiction and Mental Health in This Is Our Community: The Bisexuality Anti-stigma Campaign, a poster campaign designed to promote awareness of bisexual identities and the research study that seeks to understand their mental health issues (www.rainbowhealthontario.ca/resources).

Seniors

In long-term care and other seniors' settings, service providers often have little awareness that there are sexual or gender minority people among their patients or residents. They often feel that this is a private issue that concerns sexual behaviour only (Brotman et al., 2007). In reality, open discussion of sexual orientation and gender identity may also open up dialogue about the partner of a resident or the one she has lost; the quality of her relationships with her biological family members (many LGBT people have been rejected by their families or have strained relationships with them); and the importance of her friends as her chosen family (de Vries & Megathlin, 2009). Understanding sexual orientation and gender identity in the context of the older people's lives offers a rich history of residents' social and cultural history and the ways that they have coped and adapted.

Many seniors avoid using services such as home care, day programs, and long-term care because they feel they must choose between the social isolation of the closet and the risk of ridicule or rough treatment (Chamberland, Heffernan, & Paquin, 2004; Brotman et al., 2007). For trans people, the prospect of being cared for by untrained and perhaps transphobic staff can be terrifying. Placement in the highly gendered spaces of residential care is the first challenge; being entirely dependent on others for bathing, toileting, dressing, and grooming is the second. Many trans seniors will have been denied medical transition services or may have only had access to certain ones, perhaps hormones, but not surgeries. Others may have chosen a social transition only. Without clear policies, staff training, and an explicit commitment to serve trans seniors, they are highly vulnerable to being forced into the "wrong gender," being ridiculed, not receiving appropriate care, or being assaulted by other residents or staff (Marcellin et al., 2013; Grant et al., 2011)

In Toronto, a LGBT Diversity Task Force was inaugurated in late 2006 by the municipal government to assist city-operated long-term care facilities to develop respectful, competent care for LGBT seniors. Policies were developed that applied to all city-run homes, and three adopted explicit programming and events that were focused on the interests of LGBT residents. A tool kit was published in 2008 (City of Toronto, 2008). At the time of writing this chapter, this is believed to be the only such initiative in Canada. With a large cohort of seniors beginning to require home care, long-term care, and other services, there has been little preparation in the sector for the significant influx of elderly LGBT people who will form part of this group.

Gaps in Research and Public Health Policy

Understandably, significant research and policy resources have been targeted toward HIV/AIDS prevention and care and this has led to the development of some exceptional models of community-based research and services. At the same time, other critical issues have not received enough focus to give us accurate information about the health status, health care needs, and health-related experiences of our sexual and gender minority communities, especially queer women and trans people.

With no dedicated programs of LGBT research except in the area of HIV, Canadian academic researchers find it challenging to obtain funding through current government granting streams such as the Canadian Institutes of Health Research. Despite this, a growing number of younger researchers are building their careers and contributing to our knowledge and understanding of Canada's diverse sexual and gender minorities. Women are prominent among these researchers, as are some young trans scholars.

Canada has gained worldwide attention for its progressive legislation concerning sexual and gender minorities. This, in turn, has created a climate where LGBT people increasingly expect to be acknowledged as legitimate citizens within a proudly diverse society. However, compared with other jurisdictions, our governments and regulatory bodies have taken a laissez-faire approach to health and social services regarding lesbian, gay, bisexual, and trans populations. In Australia, the United States, and the United Kingdom, high-level government policies have been enacted that are driving initiatives at the research, policy, and practice levels. Australia has recently produced government policy statements on aging

(Australian Government, 2012), and on LGBT people and social inclusion (South Australian Strategy for the Inclusion of Lesbian, Gay, Bisexual, Transgender, Intersex, and Queer People 2014–2016, 2013). In the United Kingdom, following the passage of the 2010 Equality Act, there are now nationally sponsored action plans on minority sexual orientation and gender identity communities that are set up to coordinate policies across multiple government departments and to set targets and deadlines for action (U.K. Government, 2011b). In the United States, the national department of Health and Human Services has developed a series of initiatives on issues ranging from youth bullying, to improving care for LGBT seniors, to funding a national LGBT Health Education Centre to improve professional education (U.S. HHS, 2013).

In Canada, it is mainly individual organizations and advocacy groups that are leading the way, albeit with a certain amount of government funding. As a result, the development of more targeted services and more responsive health-promotion initiatives for LGBT people is taking place in a more haphazard way (if at all), and there is no overall tracking or coordination of these efforts. In Ontario, the existence of Rainbow Health Ontario,which is supported by the Ontario Ministry of Health and Long-Term Care, means that at least in Ontario, there is a dedicated knowledge hub for LGBT health from which training, best practices, a biennial conference, print resources, and research and policy-related activities can be accessed and coordinated.

Conclusion

In conclusion, there are signs of progress in the breadth of research being carried out on LGBT health issues and in a growing awareness and responsiveness on the part of service providers, especially at the community level. In the absence of significant national or provincial government efforts to provide leadership and coordination, however, it will be challenging to sustain widespread, consistent improvements in the health of sexual and gender minority populations and this is especially true when it comes to lesbian and bisexual women and trans people since gay men's health is monitored much more systematically through existing HIV-related initiatives. Progressive government policies with clear goals and timelines are needed to encourage planning bodies, health delivery systems, professional education institutions, and research institutes to deliver a higher standard of care for this and for all marginalized communities.

References

Abramovic, I.A. (2012). No Safe Place to Go: LGBTQ Youth Homelessness in Canada: Reviewing the Literature. *Canadian Journal of Family & Youth* 4(1): 29–51.

American Psychiatric Association. (2000). *Therapies Focused on Attempts to Change Sexual Orientation (Conversion and Reparative Therapies).* Arlington, VA.: Author. Retrieved from www.psychiatry.org/advocacy--newsroom/position-statements.

Australian Government. (2012). *National Lesbian, Gay, Bisexual, Transgender, and Intersex (LGBTI) Ageing and Aged Care Strategy.* Department of Health and Ageing.

Bauer, G. R., J. Jairam, & S. Baidoobonso. (2010). Sexual Health, Risk Behaviours, and Substance Use in Heterosexual Women with Female Sex Partners: 2002 U.S. National Survey of Family Growth. *Sexually Transmitted Diseases* 37(9): 531–537.

Bauer, G. R., J. Pyne, M. Francino, & R. Hammond. (2013). La suicidabilité parmi les personnes trans en Ontario: Implications en travail social et en justice sociale [Suicidality among Trans People in Ontario: Implications for Social Work and Social Justice]. *Service Social* 59(1): 35–62. doi:10.7202=1017478ar.

Bauer, G. R., A. I. Scheim, M. B. Deutsch, & C. Massarella. (2014). Reported Emergency Department Avoidance, Use, and Experiences of Transgender Persons in Ontario, Canada: Results from a Respondent-Driven Sampling Survey. *Annals of Emergency Medicine* 63(6): 713–720.

Benibgui, M. (2011). *Mental Health Challenges and Resilience in Lesbian, Gay, and Bisexual Young Adults: Biological and Psychological Internalization of Minority Stress and Victimization* (doctoral dissertation). Concordia University, Montreal.

Boehmer, U., M. Xiaopeng, C. Linkletter, & M. Clark. (2014). Health Conditions in Younger, Middle, and Older Ages: Are There Differences by Sexual Orientation? *LGBT Health* 2(00), Mary Ann Liebert, Inc. doi: 10.1089/lgbt.2013.0033.

Bos, H. M. W., & F. Van Balen. (2008). Children in Planned Lesbian Families: Stigmatization, Psychological Adjustment, and Protective Factors. *Culture, Health & Sexuality* 10(3): 221–236.

Brotman S., B. Ryan, S. Collins, L. Chamberland, R. Cormier, D. Julien, E. Mayer, A. Peterkin, & B. Richard. (2007). Coming out to Care. *The Gerontologist* 47(4): 490–503.

Canadian Cancer Society. (2014). *Get Screened Campaign.* Retrieved from http://convio.cancer.ca/site/.

Centre for Addiction and Mental Health (CAMH). (2014). *Gender Identity Clinic Guidelines.* Retrieved from www.camh.ca/en/hospital/care_program_and_services/hospital_services/Pages/gid/ guide_to_camh.aspx.

Chamberland, L., D. Heffernan, & J. Paquin. (2004). *The Adaptation of Residential Services for Aging Lesbians in an Equal Rights Environment.* Montreal: Université du Québec à Montréal.

Chan, R., B. Raboy, & C. Patterson. (2008). Psychosocial Adjustment among Children Conceived Via Donor Insemination by Lesbian and Heterosexual Mothers. *Child Development* 69(2): 443–457.

Chandra, A., W. D. Mosher, & C. Copen. (2011). Sexual Behavior, Sexual Attraction, and Sexual Identity in the United States: Data from the 2006–2008 National Survey of Family Growth. *National Health Statistics Report.* Washington, DC.

City of Toronto. (2008). *LGBT Toolkit for Creating Culturally Competent Care for Lesbian, Gay, Bisexual, and Transgender Persons.* Retrieved from www1.toronto.ca/city_of_toronto/long-term_care_homes__services/files/pdf/lgbt_toolkit_2008.pdf.

Clarke, M., & R. Coughlin. (2012). Prevalence of Smoking among the Lesbian, Gay, Bisexual,

Transsexual, Transgender, and Queer (LGBTTQ) Subpopulations in Toronto—The Toronto Rainbow Tobacco Survey (TRTS). *Canadian Journal of Public Health* 103(2): 132–136.

Coleman, E., W. Bockting, M. Botzer, P. Cohen-Kettenis, G. DeCuypere, J. Feldman, & K. Zucker. (2011). Standards of Care for the Health of Transsexual, Transgender, and Gender-Nonconforming People, Version 7. *International Journal of Transgenderism* 13(4):165–232. doi: 10.1080/15532739.2011.700873.

Conron, K. J., G. Scott, G. S. Stowell, & S. J. Landers. (2012). Transgender Health in Massachusetts: Results from a Household Probability Sample of Adults. *American Journal of Public Health* 102(1):118–122. doi:10.2105=AJPH.2011.300315.

Dahlberg, L. L., & E. G. Krug. (2002). Violence—A Global Public Health Problem. In E. G. Krug, L. L. Dahlberg, J. A. Mercy, A. B. Zwi, & R. Lozano (Eds.), *World Report on Violence and Health* (pp. 1–56). Geneva: World Health Organization.

Daley, A. (2005). Lesbian and Gay Health Issues: OUTside of the Health Policy Arena. *Critical Social Policy* 26(4): 794–816.

de Vries, B., & D. Megathlin. (2009). The Meaning of Friendship for Gay Men and Lesbians in the Second Half of Life. *Journal of GLBT Family Studies* 5(1): 82–98.

Epstein, R. (2004). Our Kids in the Hall: Lesbian Families Negotiate the Public School System. In A. O'Reilly (Ed.), *Mother Outlaws: Theories and Practices of Empowered Mothering* (pp. 145–154). Toronto: Women's Press.

Gates, G. (2011). *How Many People Are Lesbian, Gay, Bisexual, and Transgender?* Los Angeles: Williams Institute, UCLA. Retrieved from http://williamsinstitute.law.ucla.edu/wp-content/uploads/Gates-How-Many-People-LGBT-Apr-2011.pdf.

Gay and Lesbian Medical Association (GLMA). (2001). *Healthy People 2010 Companion Document for LGBT Health.* Washington, DC: Gay and Lesbian Medical Association.

Grant, J. M., L. A. Mottet, J. Tanis, J. Harrison, J. L. Herman, & M. Keisling. (2011). *Injustice at Every Turn: A Report of the National Transgender Discrimination Survey.* Washington, DC: National Center for Transgender Equality and National Gay and Lesbian Task Force.

Hatzenbuehler, M., S. Nolen-Hoeksma, & J. Dovidio. (2009). How Does Sexual Minority Stigma "Get under the Skin"? A Psychological Mediation Framework. *Psychological Bulletin* 135(5): 707–730. doi: 10.1037/a0016441.

Institute of Medicine. (2011). *The Health of Lesbian, Gay, Bisexual, and Transgender People: Building a Foundation for Better Understanding.* Washington, DC: The National Academies Press. Retrieved from www.nap.edu/catalog.php?record_id = 13128.

Koh, A. S., & L. K. Ross. (2006). Mental Health Issues: A Comparison of Lesbian, Bisexual, and Heterosexual Women. *Journal of Homosexuality* 51(1), 33–57.

Lampinen, T. M., D. McGhee, & I. Martin. (2006). Increased Risk of "Club" Drug Use among Gay and Bisexual High Schools Students in British Columbia. *Journal of Adolescent Health* 38(4): 458–461.

Lepischak, B. (2004). Building Community for Toronto's Lesbian, Gay, Bisexual, Transsexual, and Transgender Youth. *Journal of Gay & Lesbian Social Services* 16(3–4): 81–98.

Lombardi, E. (2007). Substance Use Treatment Experiences of Transgender/Transsexual Men and Women. *Journal of LGBT Health Research* 3(2): 37–47.

Makadon, H. J. (2011). Ending LGBT Invisibility in Health Care: The First Step in Ensuring Equitable Care. *Cleveland Clinical Journal of Medicine* 78(4): 220–224.

Makadon, H. J., K. H. Mayer, J. Potter, & H. Goldhammer. (2008). *Fenway Guide to Lesbian, Gay, Bisexual, and Transgender Health.* Philadelphia: American College of Physicians Press.

Marcellin, R., A. Scheim, G. Bauer, & N. Redman. (2013). Experiences of Transphobia among Trans Ontarians. *Trans PULSE e-Bulletin* 3(2). Retrieved from http://www.transpulseproject.ca.

McCabe, S. E., W. B. Bostwick, T. L. Hughes, B. T. West, & C. J. Boyd. (2010). The Relationship between Discrimination and Substance Use Disorders among Lesbian, Gay, and Bisexual Adults in the United States. *American Journal of Public Health* 100(10): 1946–1952.

McLaughlin, K., M. Hatzenbuehler, & K. Keyes. (2010). Responses to Discrimination and Psychiatric Disorders among Black, Hispanic, Female, and Lesbian, Gay, and Bisexual Individuals. *American Journal of Public Health* 100(8): 1477–1484.

Meyer, I. (2003). Prejudice, Social Stress, and Mental Health in Lesbian, Gay, and Bisexual Populations: Conceptual Issues and Research Evidence. *Psychological Bulletin* 129(5): 674–697.

Mravcak, S. (2006). Primary Care for Lesbian and Bisexual Women. *American Family Physician* 74: 2.

Mulé, N., L. Ross, B. Deeprose, B. Jackson, A. Daley, A. Travers, & D. Moore. (2009). Promoting LGBT Health and Wellbeing through Inclusive Policy Development. *International Journal for Equity in Health* 8(18).

Murray, P., & K. McClintock. (2005). Children of the Closet. *Journal of Homosexuality* 49(1): 77–95.

Obedin-Maliver, J., E. S. Goldsmith, L. Stewart, W. White, E. Tran, S. Brenman, M. Wells, D. M. Fetterman, G. Garcia, & M. R. Lunn. (2011). Lesbian, Gay, Bisexual, and Transgender-Related Content in Undergraduate Medical Education. *Journal of the American Medical Association* 306(9): 971–977.

Offen, N., E. A. Smith, & R. E. Malone. (2008). Is Tobacco a Gay Issue? Interviews with Leaders of the Lesbian, Gay, Bisexual, and Transgender Community. *Culture, Health, and Sexuality* 10(2): 143–157.

Power, J., R. McNair, & S. Carr. (2009). Absent Sexual Scripts: Lesbian and Bisexual Women's Knowledge, Attitudes, and Action Regarding Safer Sex and Sexual Health Information. *Culture, Health, and Sexuality* 11(1): 67–81.

Pyne, J. (2012). *Transforming Family: Trans Parents and Their Struggles, Strategies, and Strengths.* Toronto: LGBTQ Parenting Network, Sherbourne Health Centre. Retrieved from http://www.lgbtqparentingnetwork.ca/socialchange/TransformingFamilyReport.cfm.

Rainbow Health Ontario. (2014). *Productivity Report to the Ontario Ministry of Health and Long-Term Care, Toronto* (unpublished).

Ritter, A., F. Matthew-Simmons, & N. Carragher. (2012). Monograph No. 23: *Prevalence of and Interventions for Mental Health and Alcohol and Other Drug Problems amongst the Gay, Lesbian, Bisexual, and Transgender Community: A Review of the Literature.* DPMP Monograph Series. Sydney: National Drug and Alcohol Research Centre. Retrieved from http://ndarc.med.unsw.edu.au/resource/23-prevalence-and-interventions-mental-health-and-alcohol-and-other-drug-problems-amongst.

Rosario, M., E. Schrimshaw, & J. Hunter. (2009). Disclosure of Sexual Orientation and Subsequent Substance Use and Abuse among Lesbian, Gay, and Bisexual Youths: Critical Role of Disclosure Reactions. *Psychology of Addictive Behaviour* 23(1): 175–184.

Ross, L., C. Dobinson, & A. Eady. (2010). Perceived Determinants of Mental Health for Bisexual

People: A Qualitative Examination. *American Journal of Public Health* 100(3): 496–502. doi: 10.2105/AJPH.2008.156307.

Ross, L., L. Steele, & R. Epstein. (2006). Service Use and Gaps in Services for Lesbian and Bisexual Women during Donor Insemination, Pregnancy, and the Postpartum Period. *Journal of Obstetrics and Gynaecology Canada* 28(5): 505–511.

Rotondi, N., G. Bauer, K. Scanlon, M. Kaay, R. Travers, & A. Travers. (2013). Non-prescribed Hormone Use and Self-Performed Surgeries: "Do-It-Yourself" Transitions in Transgender Communities in Ontario, Canada. *American Journal of Public Health* 103(10): 1830–1836.

Rotondi, N., G. Bauer, R. Travers, A. Travers, K. Scanlon, & M. Kaay. (2011). Depression in Male-to-Female Transgender Ontarians. *Canadian Journal of Community Mental Health* 30(2): 113–133.

Ryan, B., S. Brotman, A. Baradaran, & E. Lee. (2008). The Colour of Queer Health Care: Experiences of Multiple Oppression in the Lives of Queer People of Colour in Canada. In S. Brotman & J. Lévy (Eds.), *Intersections: Cultures, sexualités et genres* (pp. 307–317). Québec: Presses de l'Université du Québec.

Ryan, C., S. T. Russell, D. Huebner, R. Diaz, & J. Sanchez. (2010). Family Acceptance in Adolescence and the Health of LGBT Young Adults. *Journal of Child and Adolescent Psychiatric Nursing* 23(4): 205–213.

Saewyc, E., C. Poon, N. Wang, Y. Homma, A. Smith, & the McCreary Centre Society. (2007). *Not Yet Equal: The Health of Lesbian, Gay, & Bisexual Youth in BC.* Vancouver: McCreary Centre Society.

Sanchez, J., S. Hailpern, C. Lowe, & Y. Calderon. (2007). Factors Associated with Emergency Department Utilization by Urban Lesbian, Gay, and Bisexual Individuals. *Journal of Community Health: The Publication for Health Promotion and Disease Prevention* 32(2): 149–156.

Scanlon, K., R. Travers, T. Coleman, G. Bauer, & M. Boyce. (2010). Ontario's Trans Communities and Suicide: Transphobia Is Bad for Our Health. *Trans PULSE E-Bulletin.* Retrieved from http://www.transpulseproject.ca.

Scheim, A., & G. Bauer. (2014). Sex and Gender Diversity among Transgender Persons in Ontario, Canada: Results from a Respondent-Driven Sampling Survey. *The Journal of Sex Research* 52(1). doi:10.1080/00224499.2014.893553.

Snyder, J. E. (2011). Trend Analysis of Medical Publications about LGBT Persons: 1950–2007. *Journal of Homosexuality* 58(2): 164–188.

South Australian Strategy for the Inclusion of Lesbian, Gay, Bisexual, Transgender, Intersex, and Queer People 2014–2016. (2013). Department for Communities and Social Inclusion. Retrieved from www.sa.gov.au/__data/assets/pdf_file/0007/59470/DCSI-608-PCD-LGBTIQ-Strategy-2014-Booklet_WEB.pdf.

Steele, L. S., J. M. Tinmouth, & A. Lu. (2006). Regular Health Care Use by Lesbians: A Path Analysis of Predictive Factors. *Family Practice* 23(6): 631–636.

Supporting Our Youth, a program of Sherbourne Health Centre. Retrieved from www.soytoronto.org.

Taylor, C., & T. Peter. (2011). *Every Class in Every School: The First National Climate Survey on Homophobia, Biphobia, and Transphobia in Canadian Schools.* Final Report. Toronto: Egale Canada Human Rights Trust.

Tjepkema, M. (2008). Health Care Use among Gay, Lesbian, and Bisexual Canadians. *Statistics Canada, Health Reports* 19(1) (March): 53–64.

Toronto Public Health and Partners. (2014). Why You Puffin'? Photovoice Project. Retrieved from www.rainbowhealthontario,ca/resources/whyyoupuffin.

U.K. Government. (2011a). *Supporting Pages to the Equality Act 2010.* Retrieved from www.gov.uk/government/policies/creating-a-fairer-and-more-equal-society/supporting-pages/promoting-and-protecting-the-rights-of-lesbian-gay-bisexual-and-transgender-people.

U.K. Government. (2011b). *Working for Lesbian, Gay, Bisexual, and Transgender Equality: Moving Forward.* Retrieved from www.gov.uk/government/uploads/system/uploads/attachment_ data/file/206347/lgbt-action-plan.pdf.

U.S. Department of Health and Human Services (U.S. HHS). (2013). *HHS LGBT Issues Coordinating Committee 2013 Report.* Retrieved from www.hhs.gov/secretary/about/lgbthealth_objectives_2013.html.

Wilsnack, S., T. Hughes, P. Johnson, B. Bostwick, L. Szalacha, P. Benson, F. Aranda, & K. Kinnison. (2008). Drinking and Drinking-Related Problems among Heterosexual and Sexual Minority Women. *Journal of Studies on Alcohol and Drugs* 69(January): 129–139.

Further Reading

Epstein, R. (2012). *Welcoming and Celebrating Sexual Orientation and Gender Diversity in Families, from Preconception to Preschool.* Toronto: Best Start Resource Centre/Health Nexus. Retrieved from www.beststart@healthnexus.ca.

Peterkin, A., & C. Risdon. (2003). *Caring for Lesbian and Gay People: A Clinical Guide.* Toronto: University of Toronto Press.

Relevant Websites

The LGBTQ Parenting Network (a program of Sherbourne Health Centre): www.LGBTQparentingnetwork.ca

Rainbow Health Ontario (a program of Sherbourne Health Centre): www.rainbowhealthontario.ca

The Trans PULSE Project: www.transpulseproject.ca

CHAPTER 11

Girls' Perspectives on Girls' Groups

Nancy Poole, Christina Talbot, Jennifer Bernier, Cheryl van Daalen-Smith, Tatiana Fraser, and Bilkis Vissandjée

Introduction

In 1977, an article by Carol Gilligan in the *Harvard Educational Review* illuminated the role of gender and power inequities in the way that girls and boys view morality and put to rest a model of moral development that deemed girls to be morally inferior to boys. In her research, she found that men are more likely to consider the rules and rights of others and make a moral judgment ("lens of justice"), while women are more likely to consider relationships and responsibilities to others and seek moral understanding ("lens of care") (Gilligan, 1977). This knowledge of women's and girls' relational orientation is a key component of girl- and women-centred care (BCCEWH, 1997; Hills & Mullet, 2002; VCH, 2009). Since that time, while the fields of women's studies and women's health have grown, as a field, girlhood studies remains less developed and girls' health understudied. Yet worldwide, there is a recognized need for girl-centred programming in order to improve girls' health (Austrian & Ghati, 2010). This chapter considers an emerging model for girls' health promotion, and its relationship to conceptions of women-centred health care.

Girls' sense of health and well-being is intertwined with their everyday experience of life (Larsson, Sundler, & Ekebergh, 2012). Patterns of behaviour that affect health are set down in adolescence and influenced by culture, race, gender, sex, ethnicity, age, and class (Temin & Levin, 2009; Woods, 2009). These influences and intersections affect girls' agency and thereby their sense of belonging, self-efficacy, and well-being. In the case of physical activity, girls are opting out of physical education at school when it is not compulsory because girl-centred models that promote fun, friendship, and participation are not present (van Daalen, 2005). Beyond evaluative school models, we know that cultural norms may affect how girls feel about dressing in sports clothes or participating in co-ed spaces. Socially constructed ideas of femininity may cause girls to feel that physical activity makes them appear less feminine or will change their body shape (Wallace & Wilchins, 2013). Girls living in a rural setting may not have access to team sports or exercise facilities. Girls living in poverty may not have the time or money to participate in physical activities as they may need to care for family members or take a job. Similarly, girls who are disabled, lesbian, or transgendered, or otherwise socially marginalized, may be discouraged or prohibited from participating in physical activities that support health.

Understanding these critical intersections of girls' health matters because they co-determine the social, educational, and political direction of girls' lives. In developing countries, the lack of private and clean sanitation facilities in schools means that girls drop out or cannot go to school during menstruation, consequently limiting their opportunities for a better life (Khau, 2011). Seventy percent of those living in poverty worldwide are women and girls (Woods, 2009). In developed countries, black girls "have unique race and gendered experiences of discrimination," resulting in weakened immune systems and, consequently, diminished health and well-being (Wallace & Wilchins, 2013). Rates of HIV and STDs are increasing among Latina girls, and in recent years they have had the highest rate of teen pregnancies among all ethnic groups in the United States (Gumbrian & DiFulvio, 2011). And while most discussion about women's and girls' health focuses on reproductive health, tobacco use among girls is rising in developing countries, and chronic diseases associated with social determinants of health, like diabetes, cardiovascular disease, and cancer, are the leading causes of mortality of women worldwide (Davidson et al., 2011; Pederson, Haworth-Brockman, Clow, Isfeld, & Liwander, 2013; Temin & Levin, 2009). The researchers involved in the study described in this article were concerned about these and related trends in girls' health such as the rise in risky drinking found in school surveys in British Columbia and Ontario (McCreary Centre Society, 2009; Paglia-Boak, Mann, Adlaf, & Rehm, 2009). We sought to understand approaches to health promotion for girls that took into consideration the determinants of girls' health, and drew on principles from women-centred approaches such as empowerment and self-determination.

Even though there is concern for the health of girls, according to Caron (2011), their perspectives and involvement in policy, programs, and research are rarely solicited. She asserts that girls need to become "part of us" rather than "women to be." Listening to girls and soliciting their perspectives in the decision-making processes that affect their lives develops their self-esteem and sense of worth, which, in turn, supports their "political health"—a sense of being a valued citizen and worthy of participating in political processes and deliberations (Caron, 2011). Political health, as she describes it, is the mandate of girls' empowerment groups and what sets them apart from traditional girls' groups. We undertook this research project to gather those perspectives of girls in empowerment groups across Canada and to further our understanding of girl-centred health promotion.

Principles of Girl- and Women-Centred Approaches

Women-centred approaches to health care, health promotion, and disease prevention have been developed in the context of primary care, substance use, mental health, and violence against women, to name a few, and each incorporates its own nuances. Overall, women-centred approaches have been expressed through principles: among these are safety, self-determination, connection with others, and empowerment. Safety includes not only physical safety, but also cultural, spiritual, and emotional, so that respecting the diversity of community, socio-economic status, sexual identity, religious beliefs, and life experiences—including the likelihood of violence in women's lives—are key to providing a safe environment for women and girls (BCCEWH, 1997; Hills & Mullet, 2002; VCH, 2009). Self-determination supports the participation of women in their own care by building collaborative environments where women can define their problems and goals based on their unique concerns. Connection with others respects women's relational orientation toward interaction, communication, and values of providing care and support to others, and seeks to strengthen relationships among women. All of the principles are intertwined with the empowerment of girls and women—confirming and supporting their agency to make choices, take action in their lives, and learn from and with each other (BCCEWH, 1997; Hills & Mullet, 2002; VCH, 2009).

Amaro, Covington, and others have integrated these principles into gender-specific models of prevention of substance use and support related to trauma for girls (Amaro, Blake, Schwartz, & Flinchbaugh, 2001; Covington, 2004). Amaro notes that prevention programs designed to reach at-risk adolescents in general address neither the risk factors for girls, nor the consequences of them. For example, girls' rate of sexual abuse significantly increases between the ages of 14 and 18 years; girls are also more likely than boys to experience more severe health problems from drinking. Further girls' relational orientation makes them more vulnerable to the influence of others, likely to put their needs below the needs of others, or to not speak their minds in order to maintain harmony in relationships (Amaro et al., 2001; Brown, 2001; Gilligan, 1977). Consequently, prevention and health-promotion models that seek to reinforce protective factors for girls must explore gender and power inequities, foster self-determination, and build on girls' relational orientation by strengthening key health-promoting relationships (Amaro et al., 2001).

Girls' Group Models

The Girls Action Foundation is a Canadian organization that facilitates a national network and provides resources and training to girls' programs across the country. Leadership skills, media literacy, sexual health, and violence prevention are fostered through all-girls spaces, along with encouragement for girls to be agents of change in their own social networks. Girls

Action programs employ a unique multi-faceted framework, each facet drawn from critical social theory and applied to the realm of girls, thus creating empowerment programs that address individual, relational, and systemic issues in girls' lives and communities.

Groups affiliated with the Girls Action Foundation, like models developed in the United States, build on girl-centred approaches. In the United States, Lyn Mikel Brown and LeCroy and Daley have incorporated these principles into support and empowerment groups with the aim of building resiliency and mitigating risks for girls. Through the organization Hardy Girls, Healthy Women, girls can participate in groups that encourage them to speak up and take action with a strong emphasis on building healthy relationships with other girls (Brown, 2001). The Go Grrrls program employs a curriculum developed to follow critical developmental tasks for girls, like developing healthy peer relationships and body image, understanding sexuality, and building skills in decision-making and future planning (LeCroy, 2004).

The Canadian Girls Action Foundation model is built upon a framework of five principles: Popular Education, Integrated Feminist Analysis, Transformational Change, Critically Asset-Based, and Organic Formation (Girls Action Foundation, 2009). In relation to the women- and girl-centred approaches described above we can see parallels and distinctions with these Girls Action Foundation principles. *Popular education* puts girls at the centre of their own learning and connected to others with common issues. It is an anti-oppression approach that validates the individual experiences within a group and, through empowerment and critical reflection, supports collective action. *An integrated feminist analysis framework* involves identifying systemic issues in girls' lives, seeing where they intersect, and understanding the power structures that support them (Girls Action Foundation, 2009). According to de Finney, Loiselle, and Dean (2011), girls-only groups and spaces are not in and of themselves transformative—it is this critical gender analysis of intersecting relations of race, class, and sexuality that makes transformational change possible. It is by way of this critical analysis, coupled with assessing personal and community strengths, that a *critical asset-based dynamic* is created: girls recognize the barriers that they face, as well as the assets they have and then take action, thereby expanding their own knowledge and skills. Through an organic process of learning, reflecting, researching, acting, and evaluating, the aim is to remain relevant to girls' lives (Girls Action Foundation, 2009), just as the involvement of women in their health care is part of women-centred care.

All-girl groups that promote girls' health and empowerment, like those associated with the Girls Action Foundation, have not received a great deal of research attention. The existing research on gender-responsive prevention programming for girls have found girls' groups to be effective because they address specific risk factors for adolescent girls, including body dissatisfaction, low self-esteem, cigarette and alcohol use, depression, influence of media and pop culture, socio-culturally based pressures, and experiences of trauma and violence (Amaro et al., 2001; LeCroy & Mann, 2008). Emerging frameworks for girls' health promotion, such as that advocated by the VALIDITY project team at the Centre for Addiction and Mental Health in Ontario (Validity ♀ Team CAMH, 2009), promote a move from issue-specific interventions toward health-determinant-oriented approaches that address interconnected factors and socio-cultural conditions that affect girls' health. Indeed, our scan of academic and grey literature in girl-specific health promotion found nine promising approaches common to groups in a range of girls' health issues, including: skill-building, girl-centred, girl-driven (participatory), enhancing social connections, building self-esteem, including multiple components, culturally safe, strengths-based, and empowerment oriented (Poole et al., 2012). In this article we focus on how girls see these approaches in practice.

Gathering Girls' Perspectives

Our research team had noted concerning trends in girls' health, such as the rise in risky alcohol drinking by girls. We partnered with the Girls Action Foundation to study how/if girls' empowerment groups were addressing these issues, and what girls saw as helpful when learning about and making decisions about their health. We were interested to know how/if what the girls saw as helpful fit with the promising approaches arising from the literature and with principles of girl/women-centred care.

The Girls' Group Settings

The girls' groups linked to the Girls Action Foundation are located in multiple settings, in schools, and in communities across Canada. Some groups have a specific mandate to bring together girls with shared experiences such as cultural identity or experiences of trauma. Other groups bring together girls who live in the same rural region, while some have specific mandates such as artistic endeavours, sciences and technology, or promotion of physical activity. The non-prescriptive, organic nature of Girls Action Foundation supports local, contextualized work in these multiple settings.

What Girls' Groups Offer

Girls Action Foundation has developed the *Amplify Toolkit* for facilitators, which describes their role as "learners" rather than "leaders," and provides information for organizing groups as well as a "workshop" curriculum. Facilitators create and organize the group, make it emotionally and physically safe, and use workshop ideas from the tool kit or create their own using an activity template. As girls explore topics of interest, express themselves, and build on their problem-solving skills, the facilitators provide guidance, information, and opportunities (Girls Action Foundation, 2009). Groups usually have an age range, but often girls who have previously been in a group act as peer mentors to the younger girls. In this study we gathered perspectives from nine groups in five provinces.

The Study Participants

Between November 2011 and February 2012, we gathered the perspectives of participants in girls' groups through focus groups, and of former participants through individual interviews. A question was also posted online on the "Kickaction" blog on the website of the Girls Action Foundation. The Girls Action Foundation worked with the research team to engage a convenience sample of girls' groups, including both rural and urban groups wherever possible, within five provinces (Nova Scotia, Quebec, Ontario, Manitoba, and British Columbia) to participate in the study. We sought to reach girls aged 13 to 15 years, currently participating in groups, as well as older girls who had participated in these groups when they were of that age range. (We also interviewed girls' group program facilitators; however, facilitators' perspectives are not reported on here.) Once the group facilitators identified interest in their group as a site for the study, researchers working in each of the five provinces handled the study recruitment, enrolment, and data collection for local sites. Interviews and focus groups were digitally recorded with participants' permission. All participants were given an honorarium.

Nine focus groups of girls aged 13 to 15 were conducted across Canada and seven individual interviews with girls aged 16 to 18 were conducted in four of the five provinces. The key characteristics of each focus group are described below:

- Nova Scotia
  - school-based group—girls identified as Caucasian and Hispanic/Caucasian
  - school-based group—girls identified as Caucasian

- Ontario
  - community-based group—girls identified as Somali
  - community-based group for newcomers—girls largely of South Asian descent

- Manitoba
  - group focus on sexual exploitation—girls identified as Aboriginal

- British Columbia
  - community-based group in rural area—girls identified as Caucasian or of mixed race
  - school-based group to train older girls to mentor younger girls coming into high school—girls identified as Caucasian

- Quebec
  - school-based group—girls identified as Caucasian or of mixed race
  - school-based group—girls identified as Caucasian or of mixed race

In order to compare what girls get from girls' empowerment groups with known promising practices for age- and gender-specific health promotion as identified in our literature search, we asked girls questions such as: What kinds of topics did you discuss, and activities or actions have you done as a group? Has the group helped you with choices about things like smoking, drinking, and having sex? Have you had any discussion or activity or learning in the group about healthy and unhealthy relationships or body image? In this chapter we focus on three key topics and principles identified by the girls on the contributions of girls' empowerment groups to enhance self-esteem and in turn girl identity and healthy body image; to create a safe space and in turn physical, emotional, and cultural safety; and to develop critical thinking skills.

Self Esteem

Self-esteem was most often mentioned by the girls as a benefit of participation in the groups:

> But if you have confidence you'll be like "yeah, whatsoever. I am who I am," right. So it more depends on confident and being in this group I would say everyone has developed more confidence, so if we have confident we won't care about, like we would care about our, usually like how we look, but we won't care about people, what they think or what they say to us.

> I think the best part is . . . I think it helps you build more confidence in yourself. It helps you make strong self-esteem. It brings your self-esteem up and you just feel that you can talk about things once you know the people [in the group] and you . . . can call them your friends, right. Because if you don't know them as well, like not very much, then you just feel shy talking to them. But once you know them you just feel more comfortable.

> I guess they weren't like "No, this is wrong, this is wrong." They were just, it was more like "How do you value yourself?" and that's kind of where we started was, you have to value yourself, other people devalue . . . you, and then make better decisions, and are we to really focus on us caring about ourselves and like building our confidence, which is something I think that was really good for us, and that's what just what we stuck on.

Girls also reported that the groups increased their self-acceptance, and gave them the confidence to resist social pressures to engage in risky health behaviours such as drinking and smoking:

> I love it because you could just be yourself; it's amazing!
>
> It helps us to feel that we're not alone too. Like if I have an issue and like someone else might have an issue and like we talk about it and we feel more like, okay, like you don't feel that bad. . . .
>
> But I think it did help like make our choices like about those things [alcohol, drugs, tobacco, sex], because from the girls' group we felt confident about ourselves. So, we didn't feel like, you know, there was a need to like, you know, fit in. There was no need to, you know, do things to make, you know, make yourself feel confident, like you know, to have sex or . . . to smoke with people just to fit in. Like you don't have that urge, because you know, you're already confident about yourself. Like this group helped you to be, you know, it just helped you to be confident about ourselves, so I think it did help in that aspect.
>
> Yeah . . . to own your own body, to love your body, to have that big piece on self-esteem too, to present that piece as well as you're presenting safe sex as well.

Girls mentioned how body image is closely linked with self-esteem and how important the group discussions of body image were:

> Like before I wouldn't wear like, because regarding the self-esteem and body image thing. Like before I wouldn't wear certain clothes because I felt they made me look fat, and I didn't look like the girls in the magazines and I didn't look all pretty like that. And now I can, I feel like I can wear whatever I want, especially to [name of group], and it's like, ahh.
>
> Like if some people like me like that's good; the ones that they don't, I don't really care because like they're not worth it, and I don't know, I guess that's how the girls' group helped me, like seeing like you don't really need to impress people, you just, yeah, just make friends and they won't care what you do with your body or anything, they won't care. And . . . the ones that don't matter, yeah, don't, it doesn't matter!
>
> Body issues are probably the number one thing that gets talked about in most of the girls' groups around here.

The body image issue most often cited by girls was the pressure to be thin. In addition, the culturally specific practice of "shadism" and skin bleaching was discussed as a body-image issue. Some girls mentioned learning during groups about media portrayal of girls and women and the pressure to be thin, and felt this was a valuable discussion point.

Safe Space

Girls in all focus groups discussed the benefits of participating in a girls-only space. Girls felt that the girls-only format of groups enabled them to create bonds with other girls, and experience a sense of empowerment with being a girl:

> [This] group just makes me feel more like powerful for being a girl.
>
> Where I used to live there used to be a lot of, I guess girls were kind of put down more, and when I came here and I found out that there was a girls' group it kind of made me feel more important as a girl because I know how girls used to be discriminated against and we used to not be able to do anything, and now it kind of feels good.
>
> It's alright to, to be around girls. Like you know, having you have that trust issue and how to, how to cope with each other and just how to have fun being with other girls.

Girls also mentioned that they felt more comfortable and less judgment from participating in girls-only, rather than co-ed groups. Participants noted how they could freely share what they were experiencing as girls, suggesting that the groups provided a space for them to relax, develop their voice, and feel comfortable with the way they look:

> Like with girls it's just like we just chill and we can talk about like almost anything you know, and you just feel more comfortable.
>
> It was people that I already grew up [with] and I already knew, and no boys, so I was more comfortable in coming in a t-shirt and just being okay.
>
> I, there's a lot of judgement between women when men are around, and there's still a lot of judgement when men aren't around. But if you're in a place that's like "Yeah, this is a girls' group" people seem to put away their judgement and just be real and be there for you know, the hour or some.

The safe environment created by the girls' groups gave the girls the ability to talk about any issue relevant in their lives. Trust and confidentiality were key:

> With girls it's just like we just chill and we can talk about like almost anything you know, and you just feel more comfortable.
>
> It's really nice to have like a safe place to go and just be able to talk about whatever you want and like know that it's completely confidential.

> It's very helpful and you can like pretty much just talk about whatever the heck you want to and without being judged, and just, you can, don't have to be afraid of anything like leaving here.

> I like the people in it because they actually feel like they like care about everybody, not just they're here to only care about themselves. They feel like—like I feel like I can trust them and stuff without them going off and telling people what has been said in group.

> What I was going to say, this is a very, like I said, like a gazillion times before, it's so safe and everyone feels so welcome, and it's just a, it's a very healthy place. So just girls can come together and talk about the things they don't feel comfortable talking to with anyone else, because they're at the same age group, maybe that's why. So they feel like, you know, whatever is going through with me might be going through with someone else. So they feel a bit safer and easier to discuss the same problem with others.

> Everyone acts different, because it's a safe environment and so I find everyone there is themselves. Like some of my friends outside of [name of girls' group] they kind of act like they have walls up, but in here it seems like they've taken them down.

> I feel welcomed here, like it's a place where I feel safe.

By having a safe space to talk, girls' self-expression and self-disclosure increased, which challenged their notions of being different from others:

> Just made it feel like it's more supportive, like I wasn't, I didn't feel like, oh yeah, I'm the only one that feels like this. Just, I don't know, it felt good to know that somebody else deals with that same thing, or something really similar.

Some girls revealed that participating in the girls' group helped them to find their voice and place as a new immigrant to Canada. Native language programming was viewed as important for discussing problems. Some girls spoke about the unique pressures girls from specific ethnocultural groups encounter, including family rules and pressures, which create an additional hurdle as girls integrate to be "Canadians."

> I'm going to add that the importance of girls' group is going to be like the cultural specific, the understanding. Like you can go to any girls' group . . . but if they don't understand the cultural background you come from, it's going to be hard to get your information.

> Joining a girl group does have something to do with—of like it being all females, because it gives you that sense of like sisterhood, which a lot of [named ethnic group] girls are lacking.

> I've been to a lot of girl groups and stuff but it's just like there's only so much you can share when you know this person doesn't speak your language. There's only, sometimes you can only express yourself in your language.

> That is like so important, so it's like I always felt like I went to a girls' group if they weren't culturally specifically, I only shared this much to get whatever I needed, but if it's a total package you can be like okay, so at home you know this, because our parents are like this, you know this, because the cultural is like this, but this is, it's like you can add that, because that's the complexity we come with, because we always have to look at things from the cultural perspective, the religious perspective and then from your own family and your language, and then where do you stand? So it's like every time you're in a girl group somebody has to be aware of that, because you can give me advice but if it violates the culture, what happens?

Critical Thinking

The groups introduced girls to different perspectives, supported reflection on their own beliefs and values, and helped them integrate different world views:

> I think like when, when we started being part of girl groups and when I started being part of girl groups it was just the fact that you hear different perspectives, and sometimes you see a girl who is strong and "I'm not going to do it!" and you see that in that girl and you're like, wow, you know, it's amazing to see that. And then you wonder why she's like that and then you try it and you know, it's just seeing different perspectives was good enough to be like, okay, everybody doesn't think that way. I'm not the only one that thinks that way. And then after a while I might be in a comfortable place where I can share where I'm at.

> And you get to see like other people's point of view too.

> [The girls' groups were] helpful in many ways because we learn from other people's experiences and we get to like talk about things and learn more.

> And so it's, I find it really interesting to hear other people's experiences and you know, depending on their experiences I'm sure it does have some effect on you know, my decisions in the moment, like "Oh, but so and so said this, and maybe that's not okay."

> Like I always think of other people's point of view.

Girls also talked about how the groups had supported them in working through various issues they have experienced such as peer pressure, bullying, abuse, grief, and suicide. In one group, the participants had recently dealt with the suicides of peers, and spoke about how the group was helpful in dealing with grief:

> Yeah, I have to agree with everyone. Just getting a fuller understanding of just suicide, grief and loss and all that definitely helped, and also gave you like, I don't know, what you call it, maybe school skills, or just like life skills that you can like use like outside of group, and like to help other people.

Older girls described analyzing media messages and images of beauty and being aware that what they see in the media is different from reality. Media literacy was almost always talked about within the context of body image and acceptance. Becoming media literate was helpful for older girls and considered important by the peer facilitators, but they still acknowledged that the messages are strong and some struggle to maintain a positive body image:

> I was thinking about this the other day and I was wondering what would happen if we, like just for like maybe 24 hours, 48 hours, swapped everyone on TV and every like, in all of the media sources, same names, same such, but change their appearances a bit to be, you know, like bigger or not so air-brushed and have a, have like weird moles and like every once in a while they get a rash and, [laughs] you know . . . like just have like them be human for 24 hours and see what happens to the world.

Engaging in activities during girls' groups allowed girls to think about different issues and how they might respond to certain situations so they are prepared if/when they happen, such as having sexual relationships and smoking.

> So you're not faced like, you know, like whoa, like what do I do and then you just do something that you're not thinking properly. So you already think about it before and then you think about it again when you're faced with it.

> . . . like knowing that there's all sort of problems and knowing different ways to figure it out, like being able to fix it besides like just trying to figure it out on your own.

> So these girls' groups, I feel like these girl groups can help because at the end of the day no one can help you make your decision, you know. Your decision is your decision. But at least you'll know that there's two sides.

> But I think we're learning a lot and I think I'm going to get a lot out of it, like for experience for when I'm older and stuff.

> ... listening to women talk honestly about drug use, alcohol use and sex, it gives you a good idea of where people are at, and not that you, not that it makes you feel like you have to match them, but you know, that way you know where most people stand on those sort of issues, which can, if you're struggling with finding that place for yourself, can really help you, I think.

> Yeah, like ... well if they didn't have the girls' group you wouldn't know what's right or wrong, you would probably just, just go with it, and with the girls' group you're like "We talked about this," and like the situation that they are in, and how they made the choice, and then yeah, it'd be like much different.

> Like knowing that there's all sort of problems and knowing different ways to figure it out, like being able to fix it besides like just trying to figure it out on your own.

> I think girls' groups are important because it helps us, it helps girls open their minds to different opportunities out there for them, whether it's career-wise, whether it's you know, you know, it helps them build their personalities, it helps them learn relationship problems, issues, how to help them in I would say in almost every aspect of their life, so.

As such the girls participating in girls' empowerment groups eloquently expressed the benefits of girls' empowerment groups in fostering self-esteem, providing vital safe spaces for co-learning, discussion, and action, as well as opportunity to critically consider health and socio-cultural complexities, and make decisions for facing the challenges and opportunities presented.

Listening to Girls: What Girls Valued

The perspectives of girls are not always sought or considered when designing and implementing programs for them. Yet a program focused on reducing violence against girls found that by simply asking girls the season of the year, times of day, and daily situations where girls felt vulnerable made safety planning more effective (Bruce, 2011). This study with Girls Action Foundation provided an opportunity to listen to girls and to validate them as experts in their own lives, a central component of popular education as well as of women- and girl-centred care.

A theme that emerged from the girls' reflections on their experiences with girls' groups was that the groups provided a "refuge"—a space away from their daily stressors. The groups provided both physical and psychological space. Of course, within the groups themselves, there were dynamics and power struggles. In fact, providing an environment where girls can "experience conflict, embody difference and grapple with problems" is essential to empowering girls (Brown, 2013). With the presence of the facilitators and peer mentors, and a focus on empowerment, the girls explained that they were able to open up and relax. For in the groups, the girls told us there was less judgment. They told us that they came to realize that they weren't alone, weren't at fault, and maybe—just maybe—weren't entirely inadequate.

Developing and maintaining relationships that are genuine in which girls can identify and express their beliefs, needs, and desires—emphasizing "being real" over "sounding good"—correlates to positive self-esteem in girls (Tolman, Impett, Tracy, & Michael, 2006). Girls felt that the opportunity to build friendships with other girls, and share what they are going through, was helpful in improving their self-esteem. Girls reported that the group increased their self-respect and self-acceptance, helped them overcome shyness, and gave them the confidence to resist peer pressure.

Many girls reported that they valued the experience of having a safe and confidential space to share their experiences with other girls. Some girls mentioned how the groups allowed girls to share both similar and different experiences and opinions in a safe and non-judgmental space. Many girls talked about how groups provided a safe space to discuss issues that are normally avoided or regarded as taboo, and provided an opportunity for girls to gather reliable information. For example, popular topics girls felt were valuable to discuss or were interested in discussing more included sexuality, sex, substance use, suicide, and eating disorders.

Girls felt less restricted in girls' groups: they felt freer in what they said, how they said it, what they wore, and what they believed. They felt more open to be themselves, and to speak openly about what was going on in their lives. This was the glue that held groups together: they were afforded the opportunity to talk to others who were facing *similar struggles* in a climate of safety, acceptance, and respect.

Still, girls' groups are not meant to be a place for girls to bond because of their suffering, but a place where they can come to understand their personal experiences within a systemic context and act to make changes in their lives (Brown, 2001). Some girls revealed that participating in the girls' group helped them to find their voice as new immigrants to Canada. They spoke about the unique pressures that specific ethnocultural groups of girls encounter, including family rules and pressures, and suggested that these groups are helpful for minority groups to experience a sense of sisterhood with their peers. Several girls mentioned the need for girls' groups to be either culturally relevant, or to include facilitators who are aware of specific cultural differences and issues. They made it clear that a one-size-fits-all approach is not workable to create space for discussion of the complex realities girls are navigating.

Preparing, Not "Fixing," Girls

Girls talked about their lives within the context of the "bigger picture." They talked about how they wanted to live their lives, as well as the influence of the media and its messages. Deciphering messages in the media is a particularly important skill now that "girl power" has become a brand and a marketing tool (Klein, 2000). Some girls said they felt more independent because of the skills they had learned in the groups. As girls learn skills in these girls' groups, they are encouraged to take action in their lives. Actions fall on a continuum from personal actions, such as refocusing negative self-talk, to global action to change inequitable policies. This is the ethos of Girls Action Foundation's model. An empowerment model that incorporates principles and practices from strength-based, popular education, and civic engagement approaches is upstream work where the focus is not centred on learning coping skills, or teaching girls to make "better choices," or to have a "healthy lifestyle." It is about mobilizing girls and young women to come together for social change—to name and eliminate systemic racism, sexism, heterosexism, classism, ableism, and other forms of power imbalances that lead to inequities so that *safety* might no longer be the key reason girls seek refuge in girls' groups.

Girl-Centred Support: Lessons for Women-Centred Care?

The girls who participated in this study describe how important girls' group spaces are in supporting their self-esteem, helping them to recognize and resist peer and socio-cultural pressure, develop and strengthen critical thinking skills, as well as to build or strengthen connections with other girls (as peers and mentors). This challenges narrowly focused health-issue approaches, which do not address the context of girls' lives and the broader determinants of girls' health. As such this study has allowed us to think about the importance of linking emerging findings about promising practices in health promotion with empowerment-oriented models and frameworks for promoting health.

Although group sessions were not limited to specific health risks or topics, the focus on empowering girls enhances the protective factors associated with health risks such as substance use, unhealthy relationships, unhealthy weight, and physical inactivity and related health concerns for youth. By providing a safe, non-judgmental space where girls can create connections with peers, mentors, and facilitators, and work through the problems and concerns they are encountering, girls expressed that they felt more confident and had more skills to make decisions about their health and deal with other challenges in life.

Overall, girls' groups have built on and extended effective practices in promoting healthy living and girl- and women-centred care while simultaneously addressing the social and political issues that their members face. The emphasis of girls' groups on skill-building, strengthening of social connections, and empowerment provides girls with the opportunities to learn about issues that are relevant to them, apply the tools they acquire into practice with the support of others, and provide a foundation for further exploration of concepts of healthy living. This girl-centred approach extends the application of principles of women-centred care and could prompt a revisiting of role of empowerment groups in women's lives as well.

Acknowledgements

This study was the result of a partnership among researchers at the British Columbia Centre of Excellence for Women's Health, the Girls Action Foundation, the Atlantic Centre of Excellence for Women's Health, the Prairie Women's Health Centre of Excellence, York University, and the Université de Montréal. This study was made possible through a financial contribution from the Women's Health Contribution program of Health Canada. The views expressed herein do not necessarily represent the views of Health Canada.

References

Amaro, H., S. M. Blake, P. M. Schwartz, & L. J. Flinchbaugh. (2001). Developing Theory-Based Substance Abuse Prevention Programs for Young Adolescent Girls. *Journal of Early Adolescence* 21(3): 256–293.

Austrian, K., & D. Ghati. (2010). *Girl Centered Program Design: A Toolkit to Develop, Strengthen and Expand Adolescent Girls' Programs.* New York: Population Council.

BCCEWH. (1997). *Key Aspects of Women-Centred Care.* Vancouver: Author.

Brown, L. M. (2001). *Cultivating Hardiness Zones for Adolescent Girls.* In the *Girls' Health Summit.* Retrieved from http://web.colby.edu/ed332/files/2010/08/HardinessZones.pdf.

Brown, L. M. (2013, February 4). *Beyond Mean Girls: Futures without Violence.* Slide presentation.

Bruce, J. (2011). *Violence against Adolescent Girls: A Fundamental Challenge to Meaningful Equality.* New York: Population Council.

Caron, C. (2011). Getting Girls and Teens into the Vocabulary of Citizenship. *Girlhood Studies* 4(2): 70–91.

Covington, S. S. (2004). *Voices: A Program for Self-Discovery and Empowerment for Girls.* Facilitator Guide. Carson City, NV: The Change Companies.

Davidson, P. M., S. J. McGrath, A. I. Meleis, P. Stern, M. DiGiacomo, T. Dharmendra, & R. Correa-de-Araujo. (2011). The Health of Women and Girls Determines the Health and Well-being of Our Modern World: A White Paper from the International Council on Women's Health Issues. *Health Care for Women International* 32(10): 870–886.

de Finney, S., E. Loiselle, & M. Dean. (2011). Bottom of the Food Chain: The Minoritization of Girls in Child and Youth Care. In A. Pense & J. White (Eds.), *Child and Youth Care: Critical Perspectives on Pedagogy, Practice, and Policy* (pp. 70–94). Vancouver: University of British Columbia Press.

Gilligan, C. (1977). In a Different Voice: Women's Conceptions of Self and Morality. *Harvard Educational Review* 47(4): 481–517.

Girls Action Foundation. (2009). *Amplify. Designing Spaces and Programs for Girls.* A tool kit. Montreal: Girls Action Foundation http://girlsactionfoundation.ca/en/amplify-toolkit.

Gumbrian, A. C., & G. T. DiFulvio. (2011). Girls in the World: Digital Storytelling as a Feminist Public Health Approach. *Girlhood Studies* 4(2): 28–48.

Hills, M., & J. Mullet. (2002). Women-Centred Care: Working Collaboratively to Develop Gender Inclusive Health Policy. *Health Care for Women International* 23(1): 84–97.

Khau, M. (2011). Growing Up a Girl in a Developing Country: Challenges for the Female Body in Education. *Girlhood Studies* 4(2): 130–147. doi: 10.3167/ghs.2011.040209.

Klein, N. (2000). *No Logo: Taking Aim at the Brand Bullies*. Toronto: Vintage Canada.

Larsson, M., A. Sundler, & M. Ekebergh. (2012). Beyond Self-Rated Health: The Adolescent Girl's Lived Experience of Health in Sweden. *The Journal of School of Nursing* 29(1): 71–79.

LeCroy, C. W. (2004). Evaluation of an Empowerment Program for Early Adolescent Girls. *Adolescence* 39(155): 427–441.

LeCroy, C. W., & J. E. Mann. (2008). *Handbook of Prevention and Intervention Programs for Adolescent Girls*. Hoboken, NJ: John Wiley & Sons.

McCreary Centre Society. (2009). *A Picture of Health: Regional Reports*. Vancouver: McCreary Centre Society.

Paglia-Boak, A., R. E. Mann, E. M. Adlaf, & J. Rehm. (2009). *Drug Use among Ontario Students, 1977–2009: OSDUHS Highlights*. CAMH Research Document Series no. 28. Toronto: Centre for Addiction and Mental Health.

Pederson, A., M. J. Haworth-Brockman, B. Clow, H. Isfeld, & A. Liwander. (2013). *Rethinking Women and Healthy Living in Canada*. Vancouver: British Columbia Centre of Excellence for Women's Health.

Poole, N., C. Talbot, T. Fraser, J. Bernier, C. van Daalen-Smith, B. Vissandjee, & S. Thakur. (2012). *"I Love It Because You Could Just Be Yourself": A Study of Girls' Perspectives on Girls' Groups and Healthy Living*. Retrieved from http://promotinghealthinwomen.ca/wordpress/wp-content/uploads/2012/08/I-love-it-because-you-could-just-be-yourself-Full-Report.pdf.

Temin, M., & R. Levin. (2009). *Start with a Girl: A New Agenda for Global Health*. Washington, DC: Center for Global Development.

Tolman, D. L., E. A. Impett, A. J. Tracy, & A. Michael. (2006). Looking Good, Sounding Good: Femininity Ideology and Adolescent Girls' Mental Health. *Psychology of Women Quarterly* 30(1): 85–95.

Validity ♀ Team CAMH. (2009). *Girls Talk: An Anti-Stigma Program for Young Women to Promote Understanding of and Awareness about Depression*. Facilitator's manual. Toronto: Centre for Addiction and Mental Health. Retrieved from http://www.camh.net/Publications/Resources_for_Professionals/Validity/girl_talk.html.

van Daalen, C. (2005). Girls' Experiences in Physical Education: Competition, Evaluation, and Degradation. *The Journal of School Nursing* 21(2): 115–121. doi: 10.1177/10598405050210020901.

VCH. (2009). *A Framework for Women-Centred Health*. Vancouver: Vancouver Coastal Health Women's Health Committee.

Wallace, S., & R. Wilchins. (2013). *Gender Norms: A Key to Improving Health and Wellness among Black Women and Girls*. Retrieved from http://www.truechild.org/Images/Interior/findtools/heinz%20report.pdf.

Woods, N. F. (2009). A Global Imperative: Development, Safety, and Health from Girl Child to Woman. *Health Care for Women International* 30(3): 195–214.

Further Reading

British Columbia Centre of Excellence for Women's Health. (2011). *Your Rights in Research: A Guide for Girls*. Retrieved from http://www.coalescing-vc.org/virtualLearning/section3/documents/YourRightsinResearch17Nov2011.pdf.

British Columbia Centre of Excellence for Women's Health and Girls Action Foundation. (2012). *Girls' Perspectives on Girls' Groups and Health Living: Research Summary*. Retrieved from http://girlsactionfoundation.ca/en/girls-perspectives-on-girls-groups-and-healthy-living.

Gonneau, G., & N. Poole. (2012). *Preventing Heavy Alcohol Use among Girls & Young Women: Practical Tools & Resources for Practitioners & Girls' Programmers*. Vancouver: British Columbia Centre of Excellence for Women's Health. Retrieved from http://www.coalescing-vc.org/virtualLearning/section3/documents/BCCEWH_Preventing_Heavy_Alcohol_Use_Among_Girls_Young_Women_Practical_Tools_Resources_for_Pr.pdf.

Greaves, L., N. Jategaonkar, & L. McCullough. (2007). Research Highlight: Smoking and Disordered Eating among Adolescent Girls: Investigating the Links. Excerpted from N. Poole, L. Greaves, & Centre for Addiction and Mental Health (Eds.), *Highs & Lows: Canadian Perspectives on Women and Substance Use*. Retrieved from http://knowledgex.camh.net/amhspecialists/specialized_treatment/smoking/women_treatment/Documents/smoking_disordered_eating_highs_lows.pdf.

Greaves, L., A. Pederson, & N. Poole (Eds.). (2014). *Making It Better: Gender-Transformative Health Promotion*. Toronto: Women's Press.

Student Drug Use Surveys Working Group. (2013). *The Value of Student Alcohol and Drug Use Surveys*. Ottawa: Canadian Centre on Substance Abuse. Retrieved from http://www.mcs.bc.ca/pdf/Value_of_SDUS.pdf.

Manuals and Facilitator Guides for Girls' Groups and Programs

Examples of manuals and guides from five different organizations that use a girl-centred approach to health promotion, including addressing substance use and related risk factors:

Bell-Gadsby, C., N. Clark, & S. Hunt. (2006). *It's A Girl Thang! A Manual on Creating Girls Groups*. Vancouver: McCreary Youth Foundation. Retrieved from http://www.mcs.bc.ca/pdf/its_a_girl_thang.pdf.

Centre for Addiction and Mental Health. (2009). *Girls Talk Program: Facilitator's Manual*. Retrieved from https://knowledgex.camh.net/amhspecialists/resources_families/Documents/Girls_Talk.pdf.

Crooks, C.V., D. Chiodo, & D. Thomas. (2009). Engaging and Empowering Aboriginal Youth: A Toolkit for Service Providers. Retrieved from http://master.fnbc.info/sites/default/files/resource-files/Engaging%20and%20Empowering%20Aboriginal%20Youth%20-%20Toolkit%20for%20Service%20Providers_0.pdf.

Girls Action Foundation. (2009). *Amplify: Designing Spaces and Programs for Girls Toolkit*. Retrieved from http://girlsactionfoundation.ca/files/Amplify_2010_LR_0.pdf.

Promundo, Instituto PAPAI, Salud y Género, & ECOS. (2013). *Program H/M/D: A Toolkit for Action: Engaging Youth to Achieve Gender Equity*. Rio de Janeiro/Washington, DC: Promundo. Retrieved from http://www.promundo.org.br/en/publications-for-youth/.

Relevant Websites

Canadian Women's Foundation: http://www.canadianwomen.org/
Centre for Addiction and Mental Health (Canada): http://www.camh.ca/en/hospital/Pages/home.aspx
Centre for Addictions Research of BC, University of Victoria: http://www.carbc.ca/
The Center on Alcohol Marketing and Youth (U.S.): http://www.camy.org/
Coalescing on Women and Substance Use: Young Women, Alcohol, and Other Substance Use: http://coalescing-vc.org/virtualLearning/section3/default.htm
Girls Action Foundation: http://girlsactionfoundation.ca/en
The Girl Effect: http://www.girleffect.org/
Girl Talk (U.S.): https://grltlk.wordpress.com/
Hardy Girls, Healthy Women (U.S.): http://www.hghw.org/
Jean Kilbourne: http://www.jeankilbourne.com/
National Roundtable on Girls, Women, and Alcohol: http://girlswomenalcohol.org/
One Circle Foundation: https://onecirclefoundation.org/
Population Council: http://www.popcouncil.org/

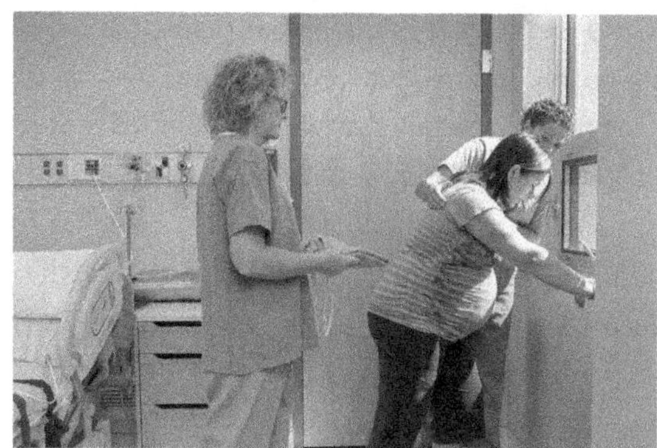

Gendering Care Work

No book on health and care would be complete without a discussion of the health care labour force. Simply put, without providers there is no care. The discussion of care work is particularly important in a book on women's health, given that women account for the overwhelming majority of paid providers and of those who are responsible for unpaid personal care. Section Three examines women's paid and unpaid work and how such work affects the lives and, in turn, the health status of women.

The section begins with Chapter 12 providing an overview of the division of labour in the Canadian system of health and social care, using a feminist political economy approach informed by the literature on the determinants of health. Kate Laxer, a post-doctoral fellow working on the development of a large, accessible database on gender and work, offers a statistical picture of who does what kind of work where, demonstrating that inside and outside institutions, care work is women's work. She pays particular attention to the aging of this labour force, identifying the issues this raises for women's health now and in the future. In the following chapter, Pat Armstrong, a sociologist and a former Canadian Health Services Research Foundation and Canadian Institutes of Health Research Chair in Health Services and Nursing Research, explores the extent and impact of women's growing unpaid health care work. Like Laxer, she uses a feminist political economy approach to understand the forces that shape this growing labour force. She argues that the failure to recognize such work as both skilled and essential to care threatens the health of not only these providers but also of those who need care. With unpaid care accounting for the overwhelming majority of the labour provided, she contends that the nature and extent of unpaid labour is an indicator of equity.

Chapter 14, by Linda Silas and Carol Reichert, is about women's struggles for recognition and support as health care providers. In this case, the story is about nurses and the story is told by a nurse who is president of the Canadian Federation of Nurses' Unions and by a policy and research specialist working with nurses' unions. Both are involved in policy on a daily basis. This chapter makes it clear why nurses need unions and how unions protect patients as well as providers. In Chapter 15, midwife Wendy Katherine takes up another struggle—for midwives to gain and keep recognition as valuable members of the health care team. Built on notions of health promotion and supportive care, Ontario midwives like Wendy Katherine have worked hard to ensure that midwifery protects women and their families in ways that follow feminist principles.

This section begins with an overview of the paid labour force before moving on to consider the nature and conditions of work for the two largest components in the health care workforce—namely, unpaid care providers and nurses. In the case of unpaid health care work, the argument focuses on the need for collective strategies while in the case of nurses, the emphasis is on how collective strategies have worked and how such actions continue to be necessary. The most obvious changes have happened in midwifery and medicine. Both demonstrate the effectiveness of collective action. Feminists' successful demands to remove quotas on admission to medical school have been critical to the female majority in medical schools today (Armstrong, 2012). And midwifes have become not only legal but also funded by the state in multiple jurisdictions as a result of women's collective struggles for recognition (MacDonald & Bourgeault, 2009). There are other occupational groups that deserve focused attention and these occupations, too, call out for a gender analysis of the sort provided here.

These chapters raise multiple questions, including:

1. Who should be counted as a health care worker?
2. Who can and should provide care in the home?
3. Should health care workers such as nurses and midwives be involved in policy?
4. Should there be a compulsory retirement age for health care workers?

References

Armstrong, P. (2012). Women's Work in Health Care. In P. Armstrong, B. Clow, K. Grant et al. (Eds.), *Thinking Women: Reforming Care* (pp. 167–192). Toronto: Women's Press.

MacDonald, M., & I. L. Bourgeault. (2009). The Ontario Midwifery Model of Care. In R. Davis-Floyd, L. Barclay, & J. Tritten (Eds.), *Birth Models That Work* (pp. 89–117). Berkeley: University of California Press.

CHAPTER 12

Who Counts in Care?
Gender, Power, and Aging Populations

Katherine Laxer

Introduction

Populations are aging, including the workforces in care, with implications for the organization and financing of care work. This chapter charts the workforce in care, including those typically excluded from analysis such as personal care providers and support workers. It examines the shifting industrial and occupational division of labour in care in Canada with an examination of who does what care work and where, and how this is evolving in the Canadian system of health and social care. The evidence suggests that the evolving divisions of labour in care reflect gendered work intensification and deskilling and is demonstrated by increasing numbers of providers with fewer credentialed skills replacing the work of more expensive professionalized occupation groups. This chapter also asks how the paid care workforce is both racialized and aging and how this demonstrates inequitable segregations in care that have long existed in Canada. By mapping all occupation groups in health and social care and by comparing across the sub-industries of care over time, this chapter establishes that the industrial division of labour in care is shifting dramatically in Canada. These shifts are related to neo-liberal changes in health and social care as well as to gender.

Counting is one means through which the critical relationship between working conditions and the conditions of care can be assessed. Counting is also a means to reveal structurally embedded exploitation, unfairness, and discrimination. Through an exploration of how statistical data on care work are assembled, this chapter employs a feminist political economy framework to unveil the varied ways the data reflect neo-liberal priorities. The framing of care is also influenced by medical notions of care and by the failure to account for gender. These blind spots in measuring care work point to the limits to statistical infrastructure for adequately measuring workforces for providing a basis to address the continuing supply of labour as the population ages. Finally, evidence from the data suggests that the public not-for-profit sector and unionization are critical shelters for the providers in care, most of whom are women.

Working conditions, skill levels, pay, and benefits for the labour force in some areas of care are largely invisible given that much of the data are not provided evenly by sub-industry in health and social care. The main emphasis of health workforce planning is on mapping the availability of physicians, nursing professionals, and various associate professionals, leaving out half of those who work for pay in health and social care and all of those who provide unpaid care (Armstrong, Armstrong, & Scott-Dixon, 2008; Armstrong, Chapter 13 in this book). This chapter aims to contribute to emerging discussions on health and social care, gender, and aging populations by mapping a broad spectrum of workers in care while using this exercise to raise larger empirical and theoretical questions about data collection and about the conditions of work in this sector.

Box 12.1

Data Sources

The ensuing analysis relies upon my calculations based on statistical data from the Gender and Work Database (GWD) and the Comparative Perspectives on Precarious Employment Database (CPD). The GWD data featured in this chapter is drawn from the Statistics Canada Survey of Labour and Income Dynamics. The surveys used in the CPD are: the Statistics Canada Survey of Labour and Income Dynamics, the Statistics Canada Labour Force Survey, the United States Current Population Survey, and the European Union Labour Force Survey. The source surveys within the GWD and CPD include principal and reliable sources of data that are regularly drawn upon for labour force analysis. Please see "Relevant Websites" below for information on accessing the GWD and CPD.

Feminist Political Economy

This chapter fits within a long tradition in sociology of understanding data as socially constructed, reflecting values as much as facts. Throughout, this chapter applies the lens of feminist political economy to evaluate and interpret the data in these contexts. This theoretical framework places the dynamics of gender, race, and class centre-stage and allows for the analysis of care relationships as they unfold in the everyday and across several levels, including the local, national, and international. A core legacy of feminist political economy is the connecting of production and reproduction, seeking to demonstrate that much of what is defined as productive in conventional economic terms is possible only through caring for people through paid and unpaid labour. Assuming data are not simple reflections of objective reality, this theoretical framework encourages explorations of whose interests are served and whose are not by how work is counted and categorized.

Intersectional analysis is increasingly adopted through feminist political economy scholarship and has helped demonstrate the interrelationships among citizenship statuses, migration, race, ethnicity, and social reproduction and production in high-income countries (Vosko, 2002). Applied research on care providers demonstrates the racialized segregations and inequities in care work and how these are distinct from the segregations and inequities faced by non-racialized groups in society (Das Gupta, 2009; Duffy, 2011).

In the process of challenging both dominant political economy and silences within feminist political economy related to marginalized social locations, feminist political economists have confronted the categories in statistical data and exposed many of the embedded assumptions (Vosko, 2006, 2014; Armstrong et al., 2007). For example, scholars have pointed to the absence of data on unpaid work, on non-standard forms of employment (Vosko, 2006), and on the gender-blindness of occupational health measures (Messing, 1998; Le Jeune, 2009). This scholarship has encouraged researchers across many disciplines of the social sciences to acknowledge the economic and social significance of unpaid work performed mostly by women, particularly in caregiving roles. Further, it has pointed to ongoing segregations of women and other marginalized groups into less secure forms of employment with high risks of ill health.

This dominant approach of mapping health and social care workforces understands health care in terms of medical procedures, diagnoses, and pharmaceutical intervention, but not in terms of much of the direct attention involved in care such as bathing, feeding, changing, cleaning, and coordinating teams of care (Armstrong, Armstrong, & Scott-Dixon, 2008). Of course, much care for aging populations includes *social care*, often left out of a medical model framework, and, in health and social care, much of the labour falls into these other areas and is not defined as skilled (Armstrong, 2013). To understand and map care work in many areas, the realities can best be captured with a concept of care that is both material and relational, including medical and social aspects of care.

Insights from feminist political economists have contributed to a conceptualization of care that focuses on the relational aspects of health care work, which are particularly invisible and are learned abilities rather than innate to women. Relational care work involves emotional labour such as sensitivity, patience, interpersonal skills, and adaptive learning, among other qualities. These skills are particularly invisible and are typically depicted as personality traits rather than acquired competencies (Armstrong, 2013; Hochschild, 2000). The reframing of concepts of care and of understandings of skills through the lens of feminist political economy offers the capacity to interpret differences in work organization and the quality of care, particularly in how this lens allows for more sophisticated and critical understandings of care and skill. Feminist political economy provides the foundation for alternate conceptualizations centrally related to the field of care—concepts of what constitutes work, what shapes health and well-being, what skills are required for appropriate care, and how care work is gendered, contributing to inequality, marginalization, and invisibility.

Neo-liberalism and Austerity

The role of the state in providing for care is changing to reflect the expansion of neo-liberalism across high-income states, and in recent years, the spread of austerity measures. As an approach to governing, neo-liberalism is not an accident but reflects specific interests that have over the last couple decades been able to guide policy in many countries (Harvey, 2007). Steered by the notion that human well-being is best served by enhancing the individual freedom to pursue unbridled entrepreneurship in a context of free trade and free markets, those encouraging neo-liberal shifts aim to protect and enhance the rights of individuals to private property, reduced taxation, and increased profit through so-called efficiencies and innovations (Harvey, 2007; Braedley & Luxton, 2010). Neo-liberal interests have gained tremendous strength since the 1980s when governments in the United States and the United Kingdom, under Reagan and Thatcher respectively, began to implement far-reaching changes to public and welfare state programs.

In Canada, similar changes took place under various federal and provincial governments, most notably beginning with the Mulroney Progressive Conservative government in the late 1980s and the Harris government in Ontario in the 1990s (McBride & Shields, 1997; Sears, 1999). Neo-liberalism has gained more strength in recent years in Canada under the federal Conservative government led by Harper, who since 2006 has implemented far-reaching changes to health and social care programs, along with changes to how the activities of Canadians are accounted for in national statistics. Among some of the early reforms made by the Harper government were the elimination of plans for a national childcare strategy that was replaced with the somewhat trivial Universal Child Care Benefit (Bezanson, 2010), the cuts to numerous women's programs and organizations, and the changes to unemployment insurance.

The impacts of neo-liberal reforms for care and for women workers are numerous. Over the last few decades these changes have included the privatization and contracting out of support services, the use of private sector managerial practices and managed competition, increased private and for-profit care, and the shifting of care out of institutions into community and home settings. All of these changes have contributed to the casualization of employment relationships, deskilling, and the intensification of care work (Armstrong & Armstrong, 2010), so that many workers are less likely to have job security and more likely to have their work defined as unskilled despite undertaking more demanding and complicated tasks.

Privatization, in particular, has been found to increase the precariousness experienced by support workers who have been contracted out (Armstrong & Laxer, 2011), some to multinational corporations. The underlying political and commercial interests represented by trade agreements, such as the North American Free Trade Agreement (NAFTA), depict these aspects of globalization as unavoidable while supporting health delivery that is increasingly private and for-profit.

Despite the spread of privatized care and neo-liberal approaches to governing, there are jurisdictional differences in health and social care delivery models. For example, there are differences in how care is valued in different provinces in Canada and across countries. Liberal welfare states such as Canada differ from Scandinavian social democratic states in how care is framed with most Canadian jurisdictions framing some types of care as a private responsibility, whereas Sweden frames a broader range of care services as a universal right. Nevertheless, the framing of care is shifting across high-income countries, so that countries like Sweden are pressured to adopt the values and practices typical of neo-liberalism.

The value placed on care influences delivery. The delivery of care in the market and informal sectors coincides with a restructuring of collective values pertaining to the rights and choices of individuals. Choices of individuals and families are deeply rooted in circumstances and wider context, including the availability of social supports and financial resources as well as ideas about gender. Indeed, choice cannot be separated from material and social circumstances. Choice is challenging to define for individuals grappling with complicated conditions, including illness, limited resources, along with hidden or overt assumptions about gender. There are grim consequences for conceiving of choice as boundless when it comes to appropriate care. Individuals often have very narrow choices if they lack social reinforcement such as family members—often women—who are available to provide attention, economic resources, and support.

Box 12.2

Who Has Choice?

Choice as a concept in care is reserved for recipients of care with no coinciding notion of choice for the majority of those providing the care, undermining both recipients and providers who are less able to engage in more suitable relational care. As Smele and Seeley (2013) point out, both formal and informal care providers—most of whom are women—are excluded from the choice-making narrative in health and social care policy. Choice is difficult to measure, but it is critical to consider since providers need a degree of autonomy in order to respond appropriately in varied and complicated situations of care. Existing research suggests that some workers in care have more choices than others (e.g., Daly & Szebehely, 2012).

The Shifting Division of Labour, Work Intensification, and Deskilling

Health and social care in Canada takes place across all sectors, including the public, private, for-profit, and not-for-profit sectors. The primary objective of Canadian health policy is "to protect, promote and restore the physical and mental well-being of residents of Canada and to facilitate reasonable access to health services without financial or other barriers" (Health Canada, 2014). The Canada Health Care Act covers insured health services, which are: "hospital services provided to in-patients or out-patients, if the services are medically necessary for the purpose of maintaining health, preventing disease or diagnosing or treating an injury, illness, or disability; and medically required physician services rendered by medical practitioners" (Health Canada, 2014). Provinces and territories may also offer additional benefits funded and delivered on their own terms and conditions, such as prescription drugs, dental care, optometric, chiropractic, and ambulance services. Universal access to hospital and doctor care has been particularly important for women, given that women use the system more than men and are less likely to have resources to pay for care. Conversely, the gaps in universal care have an especially negative impact on women and on particular groups of women.

Box 12.3

The Hidden Rise of For-Profit Care

The only sub-industry in health and social care in Canada that is entirely publicly funded is the hospital industry and almost all hospitals are not-for-profit. There is considerable variation in the ownership of other services. However, mapping ownership and delivery models is limited by the classification of public and private sector used by Statistics Canada labour force surveys. Statistics Canada labour force surveys define the public sector as including institutions and services that are part of government and/or publicly owned. The private sector is defined as including all institutions and businesses outside government services, whether for-profit or not-for-profit, as well as private households. The most significant limitation to the sector variable is the lack of data on the not-for-profit and for-profit sectors, as well as on public-private partnerships in hospitals that blur the lines between public and private. This omission is quite consequential in Ontario, where for example, there has been a considerable rise in provincial government funding for-profit long-term residential care.

There are four sub-industries in health and social care in Canada: ambulatory, hospital, nursing and residential, and social assistance (Minister of Industry, 2012). Ambulatory services comprise physician, dentist, and other health practitioner offices along with out-patient care, diagnostic laboratories, and medical home care. The hospital sub-industry includes general medical and surgical hospitals, psychiatric and substance-abuse hospitals, and specialty hospitals. Nursing and residential care includes nursing care facilities; "residential developmental handicap, mental health and substance abuse facilities" (Minister of Industry, 2012, p. 59); community care facilities for the elderly; and other residential care facilities. Finally, social assistance (not to be confused with welfare) includes individual and family services; community food and housing, and emergency and other relief services; vocational rehabilitation services; and child daycare services (Minister of Industry, 2012). Non-medical home care is classified within social assistance and includes services for older people and people with disabilities.

The size of the workforce in each of the sub-industries of health and social care (Figure 12.1) points to the significance of the measurable paid health and social care work in the Canadian economy.

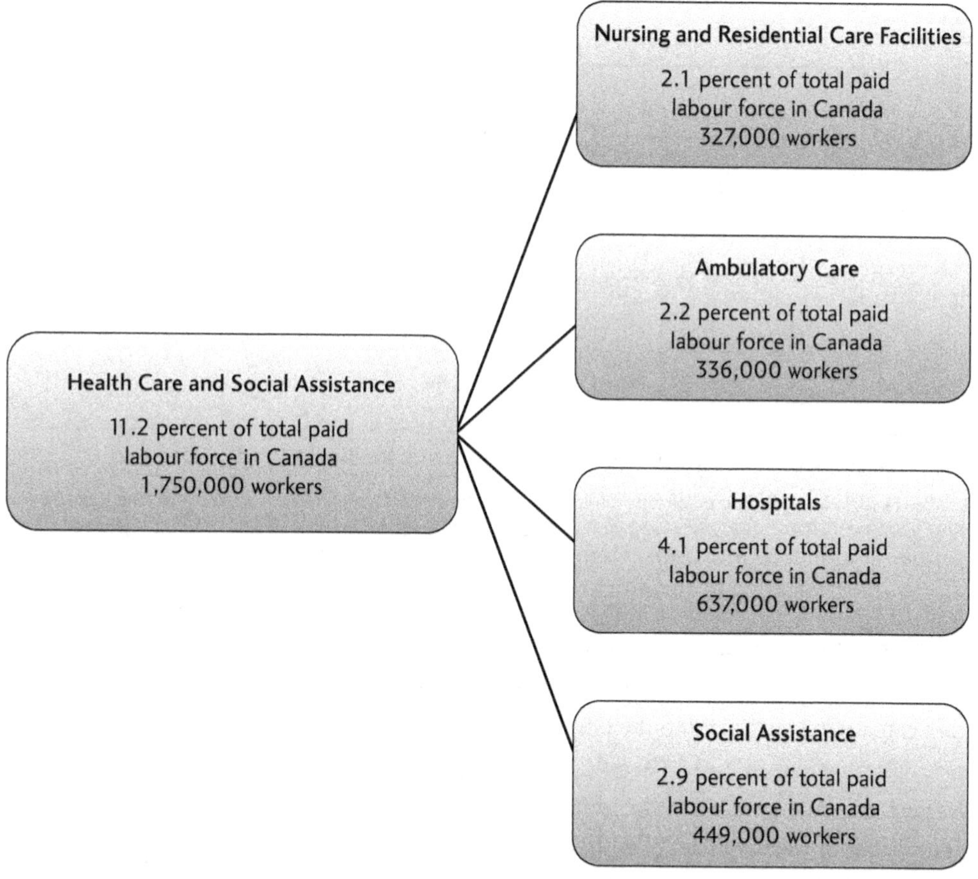

FIGURE 12.1: Canada's industries of health and social care, 2009

Source: Health industry and occupation by full-time and part-time employment, class of worker, and caregiving absence 1993–2009 (HC SLID G-3). Gender and Work Database, York University. Retrieved from http://www.genderwork.ca/gwd. Data from Statistics Canada Survey of Labour and Income Dynamics, 1993–2009.

The health and social care industry has seen considerable changes over the last couple of decades. Most significantly, the division of labour across the four sub-industries is changing with critical implications for both care providers and recipients of care. Figure 12.2 shows the growth in numbers of the paid labour force in each of ambulatory, hospitals, nursing and residential care, and social assistance between 1993 and 2009. Evident is the dramatic rise of social assistance, where non-medical home care is classified. Between 1993 and 2009, the labour force in social assistance grew by more than 200,000 workers, considerably outpacing the growth in each of the other sub-industries.

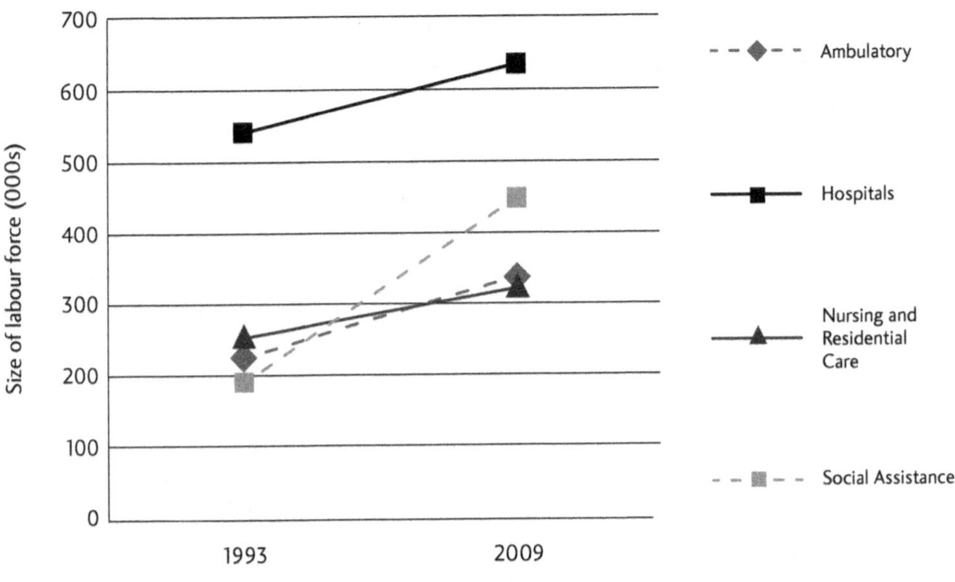

FIGURE 12.2: Growth of the paid labour force in sub-industries of care

Source: Health industry and occupation by full-time and part-time employment, class of worker, and caregiving absence 1993–2009 (HC SLID G-3). Gender and Work Database, York University. Retrieved from http://www.genderwork.ca/gwd. Data from Statistics Canada Survey of Labour and Income Dynamics, 1993–2009.

Ambulatory care has also grown more than the average across all the sub-industries, though its growth hardly compares to that of social assistance. This growth in ambulatory care can also be attributed to the emphasis in the last two decades on home care. Hospital care has grown by only 14.5 percent, the smallest growth of the four sub-industries in care. As Figure 12.3 demonstrates, the varied rate of growth of the sub-industries has led to a realignment of the relative sizes of each. In 1993, 44 percent of health care and social assistance took place in hospitals, but by 2009, only 36.4 percent of care is hospital care. Meanwhile, in 1993, 15.9 percent of all care was social assistance care. However, by 2009, the latter sub-industry comprised 25.7 percent of all of health care and social assistance. In sum, the last two decades in Canada have seen a dramatic shift in the direction of care work, and the paid labour force in both medical and non-medical home care has grown considerably.

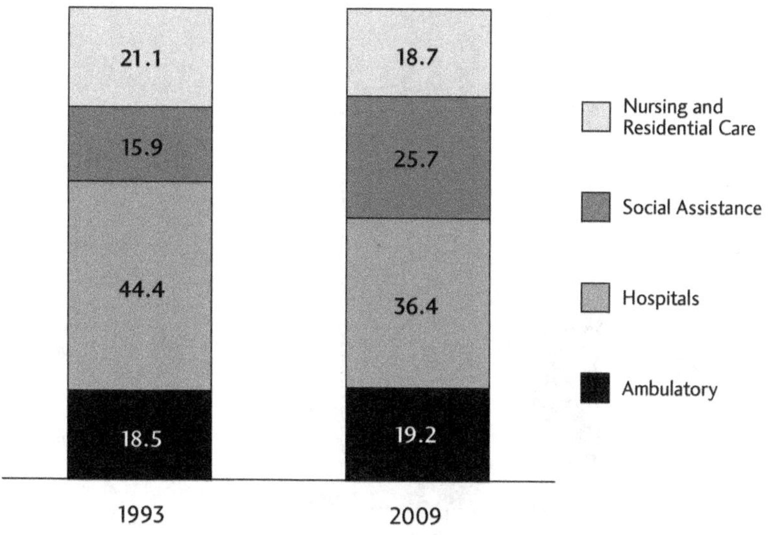

FIGURE 12.3: Change in relative size of sub-industries in care (percent)

Source: Health industry and occupation by full-time and part-time employment, class of worker, and caregiving absence, 1993–2009 (HC SLID G-3). Gender and Work Database, York University. Retrieved from http://www.genderwork.ca/gwd. Data from Statistics Canada Survey of Labour and Income Dynamics, 1993–2009.

Each of the sub-industries in health care and social assistance in Canada has a distinct configuration of care providers (Figure 12.4). Professionals are concentrated in ambulatory services, nurses are concentrated in hospitals, workers in assisting occupations (such as personal support workers) are primarily in nursing and residential care, and support workers are in social assistance. Hence, the most highly trained, highly paid workers are in the ambulatory and hospital sub-industries where they provide the most specialized care to patients with more acute needs—care typically defined within the medical model. Those with the least formal training are in nursing and residential care and social assistance. At the same time, acuity levels are rising, with more people with heavy care needs living outside hospitals.

The growth of home care and the shrinking of hospitals also corresponds with the push to marketize, privatize, and turn a profit from care, all approaches to care delivery that are guided by neo-liberal values. Governments are shifting funding from hospital care to less expensive contexts where more care can be provided privately, in the market, and for-profit. In this way, governments are key contributors to both work intensification and deskilling in health and social care, particularly in some jurisdictions such as Ontario, where hospital care is being substituted with less costly care in nursing and residential facilities and in home care. Both of the latter two areas of care are unprotected by the Canada Health Care Act and have faced the increased implementation of neo-liberal measures such as managed competition and outright privatization.

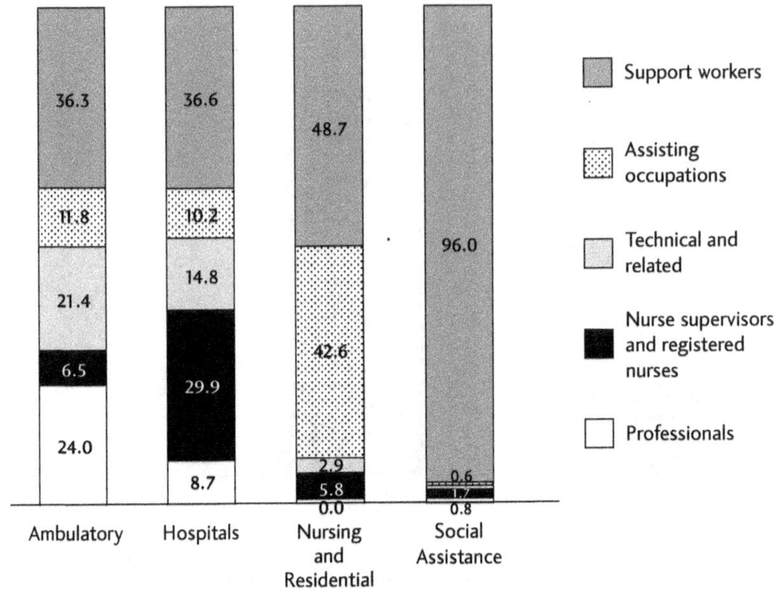

FIGURE 12.4: Occupational division of labour by sub-industry in care, 2009 (percent)

Source: Health industry and occupation by full-time and part-time employment, class of worker, and caregiving absence, 1993–2009 (HC SLID G-3). Gender and Work Database, York University. Retrieved from http://www.genderwork.ca/gwd. Data from Statistics Canada Survey of Labour and Income Dynamics, 1993–2009.

Box 12.4

Silences in the Data

The division of labour is in part obscured by the contracting out of support services in health and social care in Canada over the last decade, since it is likely some workers are no longer classified within the industry of health care and social assistance (Armstrong & Laxer, 2011). Also absent in the data are the unpaid providers in these settings, including volunteers and family members who provide care, along with unpaid hours performed by paid employees (Baines, 2004). Further, personal companions and other informal providers who are often hired privately within facilities to supplement care cannot be mapped using Canadian labour force data. There is growing evidence that informal care providers are critical workers who augment the insufficient care found in some health and social care contexts (Armstrong & Braedley, 2013).

The distinction between medical and social care, along with the exclusion of those who provide social care from labour force planning, is unjustifiable in the wake of neo-liberal health care reforms. By relocating patients with higher acuity levels into family homes and long-term care facilities, a parallel shift in the labour done in these contexts has occurred to accommodate interventions commonly defined to be medical, often by care providers who have not typically done this sort of work, nor have necessarily been trained formally to provide this level of care. As Struthers (2013) points out, this shift has not involved a change in the definition of the work of care in these contexts. As a result, providers typically defined as unskilled, including family members, are frequently performing medical tasks such as inserting feeding tubes and intravenous drips, giving injections, and operating medical equipment, including ventilators (Struthers, 2013, p. 167).

This movement of work into family homes, and often into the realm of the unpaid work done mostly by women for the care of their family, is related to how workers are valued and compensated for their contributions to care within a neo-liberal framing. As a result, the work is defined as social and/or custodial and is seen as part of the normal daily work that women are accustomed to provide in the home. So, even though health care needs are intensifying, the working conditions, pay, and narrow authority of workers mirror gendered beliefs about the unskilled nature of the work (Armstrong & Braedley, 2013) while also reflecting neo-liberal changes that prioritize the search for profit.

Gendered, Racialized, and Aging Workforces

Given the feminized nature of caring professions and occupations, it is not surprising that the largest share of providers in care, both paid and unpaid, are women. In Canada, over 80 percent of paid workers in health and social care are women. Care has long had a feminized nature and the gendered division of labour shows larger shares of men in professional occupations associated historically with more status, more power, higher pay, and superior working conditions. In the last few decades women have moved into these professional roles in medicine (Riska, 2008) at the same time as they have fought to professionalize occupations like nursing (Clark & Clark, 2003; Armstrong & Silas, 2009) and midwifery (Bourgeault, 2006).

It is striking how men's occupational concentrations differ from those for women in health and social care. Among men working in ambulatory care, for example, 48.9 percent are professionals as compared to only 11.4 percent of women in that sub-industry. These are highly paid jobs, as are management occupations, where 8.6 percent of men in nursing and residential care are employed as compared to only 3.6 percent of women.

Canadian data reveal that women from racialized groups and immigrant populations from non-dominant ethnic communities have disproportionately large concentrations among the providers of care in the lower paid areas of health and social care. The racialization of the labour force is entrenched in historical patterns of exploitation in care. Especially precarious women, whether due to their citizenship status (Bakan & Stasiulis, 1997) and/or their lack of economic and social resources, end up in the kinds of care work that few others are willing to take on (Duffy, 2011). Furthermore, credentials attained in other countries may not be recognized in Canada while it is assumed that women are naturally capable of providing care (Armstrong, 2013). Women from racialized groups are often pressured into care work, releasing privileged women from the burden of providing care (Braedley, 2013; Glenn, 2010; Das Gupta, 2009; Duffy, 2011). This inequitable segregation in care work, including concentrations of disproportionate shares of immigrants and ethnic minorities, reflects continuities in inequalities between people from different classes and social locations (Duffy, 2011).

Box 12.5

"Global Care Chains"

Many workers in care from racialized backgrounds or minority ethnic groups are migrant workers caught up in global care chains (Yeates, 2012), leaving their own countries to provide low-paid care in wealthier countries. Not only does this out-migration create a deficit of care providers in the countries of origin, it suggests that all women are capable and innately skilled to provide care, regardless of where they come from or their personal backgrounds. This then reinforces notions that social care work is unskilled or low skilled and that it is deserving of low pay (Armstrong, 2013, p. 106). Care delivery models adopted by governments influence the degree to which migrant workforces are drawn upon (Lethbridge, 2010; Twomey, 2013), but these workers are often invisible in the data since migrant workers are very difficult to trace using available statistics.

The labour force in health and social care is aging. Table 12.1 demonstrates the growth in shares of providers between the ages of 45 and 64 years of age from 1997 to 2011 in four high-income countries, including Canada. Table 12.2 shows a growth in the labour force of providers over the age of 65 in the same four countries. The growth of the workforce past age 65 is particularly striking. The only country among the four that already had notable shares of workers past age 65 in 1997 is the United States, a country with fewer public benefits, including health insurance and pension coverage. However, workers in Canada, the United Kingdom, and Sweden may be feeling pressures to continue working that are related to a reduction in pension and health coverage (Townson, 2006; Gruber & Wise, 2007). Furthermore, there has been an end to mandatory retirement in many jurisdictions and it is predicted that workers will work longer, despite current variations in mandatory retirement (European Commission, 2009). A further explanation of a growth in the size of the workforce among older groups is the demand for labour in health and social care in each of these countries. And yet, the reasons physicians work past age 65 are likely very different from the reasons nurses and assisting providers continue working, choices that are related to gender and class.

	Canada		United States		United Kingdom		Sweden	
	1997	2011	1997	2011	1997	2011	1997	2011
Managers	42.5	58.7	42.0	53.9	44.7	55.4	59.8	60.8
Physicians and other professionals	30.8	39.8	34.5	43.4	32.1	35.1	36.4	47.0
Nursing professionals	39.5	46.6	32.5	43.1	29.6	44.5	45.9	48.1
Associate professionals	25.0	34.6	28.4	42.8	33.0	43.5	39.2	58.2
Assisting occupations	35.2	43.9	25.6	34.0	32.4	38.4	36.5	44.3
Support providers	36.3	48.7	31.8	41.8	44.9	49.4	48.8	52.8

TABLE 12.1: Shares of Older Workers in Care on the Rise across High-Income Countries

Source: Education by detailed HSC occupation, Canada, United States, and EU countries, 1983-2011 (HSC DE-1). Comparative Perspectives on Precarious Employment Database York University. Retrieved from http://www.genderwork.ca/cpd.

	Canada		United States		United Kingdom		Sweden	
	1997	2011	1997	2011	1997	2011	1997	2011
Managers	2.7	2.5	2.3	4.4	0.8	2.4	0.0	2.9
Physicians and other professionals	4.0	6.5	4.5	7.7	2.8	3.0	11.9	3.7
Nursing professionals	0.2	2.7	2.3	3.6	0.8	1.6	0.0	1.3
Associate professionals	0.6	1.7	1.2	2.5	1.2	2.4	0.6	2.6
Assisting occupations	1.0	2.4	2.9	4.6	0.6	2.2	0.3	1.3
Support providers	0.9	3.3	3.3	5.3	1.7	3.7	0.0	1.7

TABLE 12.2: Working Past the Age of 65 Years

Source: Education by detailed HSC occupation, Canada, United States, and EU countries, 1983-2011 (HSC DE-1). Comparative Perspectives on Precarious Employment Database, York University. Retrieved from http://www.genderwork.ca/cpd.

Despite the aging of the labour force, it is unlikely that this is a factor in the high injury and absenteeism rates in some areas of care such as long-term residential care, particularly among workers in assisting occupations (Armstrong & Laxer, 2012). For example, absenteeism is almost twice as high for workers in assisting occupations in health and social care in Canada than for any other group of worker in health care (Daboussy & Uppal, 2012). However, similar rates of absenteeism and injury are not observed in other contexts such as Sweden, suggesting that work organization and working conditions are more likely explanations for the high rates in Canada (Armstrong & Laxer, 2012).

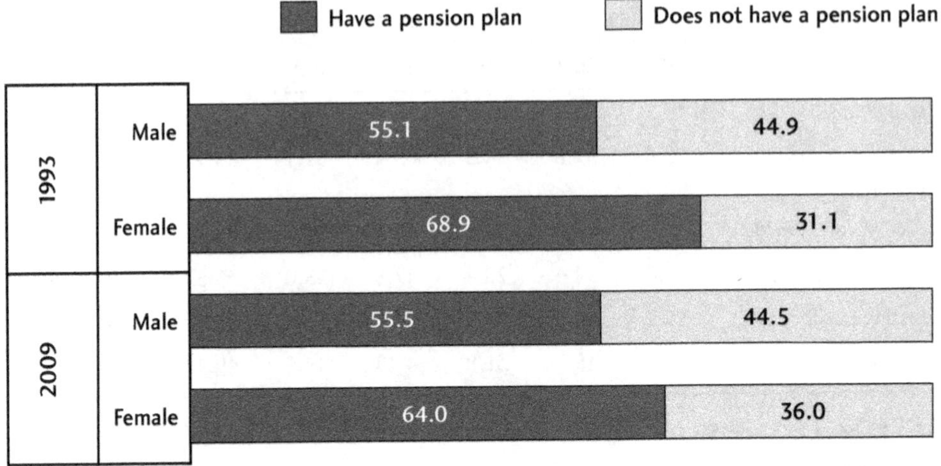

FIGURE 12.5: Pension coverage rising for men in care but not for women (percent)

Source: Health industry and occupation by pension plan coverage, union coverage, and form of employment, 1993–2009 (HC SLID A-3). Gender and Work Database, York University. Retrieved from http://www.genderwork.ca/gwd. Data from Statistics Canada Survey of Labour and Income Dynamics, 1993–2009.

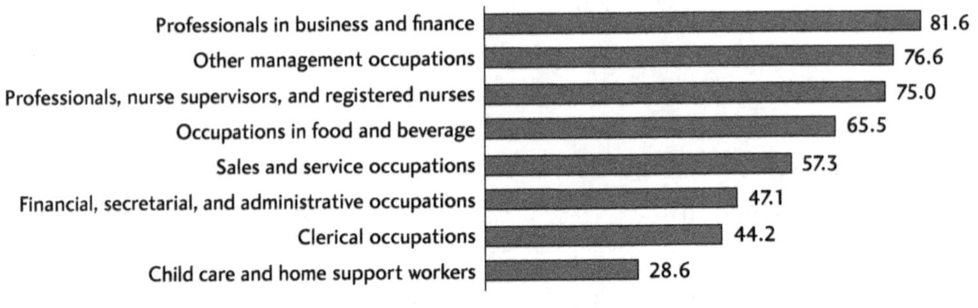

FIGURE 12.6: Pension coverage in health and social care, 2009 (percent)

Source: Pension plan by work and demographic variables (PE SLID E-1). Gender and Work Database, York University. Retrieved from http://www.genderwork.ca/gwd. Data from Statistics Canada Survey of Labour and Income Dynamics, 1993–2009.

Box 12.6

The "Choice" to Work Part-Time

The most commonly reported reason for working part-time among providers in assisting occupations such as personal care workers is "going to school." Meanwhile, among professionals in health and social care, the most common reason reported is "did not want full-time work," followed by "caring for own children." A significant reason reported among nurses is "semi-retired." Each of these reasons reflects the gendered nature of part-time work, but the data on assisting providers suggest that part-time work arrangements help accommodate additional training and education, perhaps as a means to leave precarious employment. These findings on part-time employment are consistent with other research on part-time employment in other industries and the reasons why workers end up in this form of employment (Duffy & Pupo, 1992; Duffy, Glenday, & Pupo, 2007). Further, these data are consistent with research on the "choice" to work part-time in order to accommodate other commitments outside work, revealing for example, gendered expectations about household responsibilities and caregiving (O'Reilly et al., 2009; Vosko & Zukewich, 2006).

Precarious Care

Precariousness is a defining aspect of many care workers' working conditions. Research in recent years has pointed to the unique characteristics of precarious employment for health and social care workers (see, for example, Armstrong & Armstrong, 2009). Generally, precarious employment has come to be associated with employment insecurity, less protection from regulations, low income and benefit coverage, diminished control and autonomy—particularly among non-unionized and non-professional workforces—and high risks of ill health (Vosko, 2006, 2014). Health and safety risks are of particular concern among health and social care workers in general, but especially among workers in assisting occupations such as personal care work where rates of absenteeism are very high relative to all other workers in Canada (Daboussy & Uppal, 2012).

Unique to work in these occupations are the disproportionate shares of workers employed in atypical scheduling, particularly on-call and split shifts. New managerial practices, including the increases to on-call scheduling, intensify the impact of these atypical schedules by allowing for even less choice and control among workers (Armstrong & Armstrong, 2009). These arrangements are risky to care providers, particularly for women, given that such schedules are disruptive to unpaid care commitments outside of paid employment (Armstrong & Armstrong, 2009) and to their personal health (Geiger-Brown et al., 2004; Wong, McLeod, & Demers, 2011).

Workers in assisting occupations such as those working in nursing homes are also more likely to experience violence from residents, much of which is embedded in, and a reflection of, structural aspects of care (Banerjee et al., 2012). Care providers have little recourse to address these hazards, especially if they are not unionized, and though employment standards may regulate protection against some unsafe working conditions and provide the appearance of protection, enforcement of existing standards is often lacking or weak (Vosko & Thomas, 2014). Often, workers will continue to go to work when sick or injured, referred to as *presenteeism*, creating additional hazards within workplaces that are largely invisible, such as the risk of

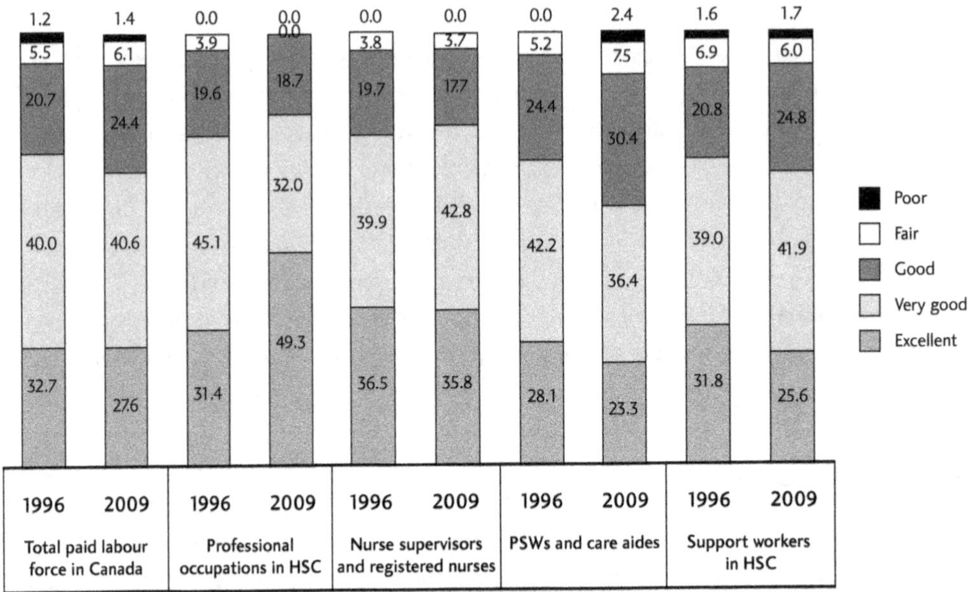

FIGURE 12.7: Self-reported health status improving for some workers but not for others in health and social care (percent)

Source: Health industry by health status, shifts, and tenure, Canada, 1993–2009 (HC SLID F-1). Gender and Work Database, York University. Retrieved from http://www.genderwork.ca/gwd. Data from Statistics Canada Survey of Labour and Income Dynamics, 1993–2009.

becoming further infected or infecting others. Hazards are particularly invisible because of the gendered normalization and individualization of injury and illness, which assume women's work is safe (Campbell, 2013), demonstrating as other scholars have that gender affects how risk is defined and measured (e.g., Le Jeune, 2009; Messing, 1998; Messing, Neis, & Dumais, 1995).

A consideration of the self-reported health status among occupation groups (Figure 12.7) shows that working conditions, including atypical scheduling, may be influencing the health of paid care workers. Notable is the larger share of professionals reporting excellent health (49.3 percent) relative to all other occupation groups. Also notable is the increase in shares of workers in only some occupations reporting fair or poor health over the time period of 1996–2009. The data on self-reported health status are striking and suggest there is a possible negative effect on health experienced by some providers more than others, which may be related to the type of work they do and their working conditions.

These union coverage differences reflect different historical labour movement organizing initiatives in health and social care, which initially focused on unionizing workers in hospitals and nursing occupations. The larger establishment sizes typical of most hospitals were more practical for organizing campaigns as workers were centralized and easily coordinated. This is also true for some nursing and residential care facilities, which can have large workplace sizes, and can be seen as more appropriate settings within which to undertake

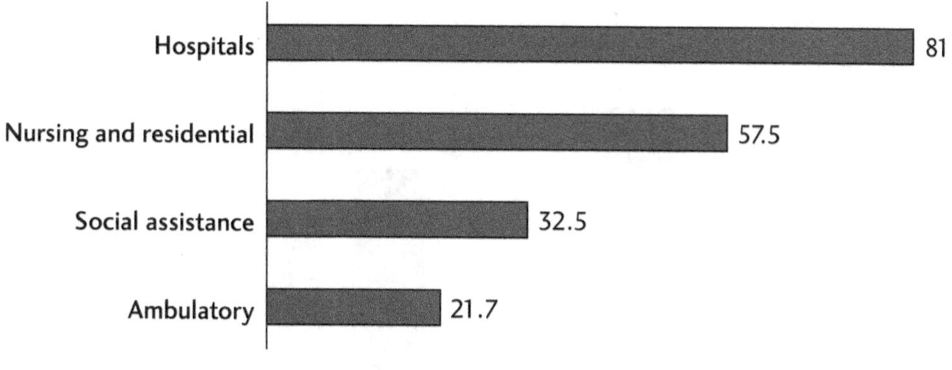

FIGURE 12.8: Union coverage, 2009 (percent)

Source: Health industry and occupation by pension plan coverage, union coverage, and form of employment, 1993–2009 (HC SLID A-3). Gender and Work Database, York University. Retrieved from http://www.genderwork.ca/gwd. Data from Statistics Canada Survey of Labour and Income Dynamics, 1993–2009.

union-organizing campaigns. Workers in ambulatory and social assistance, however, tend to be much more dispersed and therefore much more challenging to coordinate (Cranford, 2005). Factors such as workplace size have been demonstrated to present challenges to union organizing. Unions began to target women workers for organizing in the 1970s as women were moving in large numbers into paid employment, particularly in the public sector. In the last decade, unions less associated historically with both health and social care and women workers have begun focusing on organizing workplaces with large numbers of women workers. For example, the Canadian Auto Workers, now UNIFOR, has moved into organizing in health and social care settings.

Despite developments in union organizing and the union advantage many workers have in terms of pay, benefits, and other protections (Jackson, 2003; Anderson et al., 2006), data show that providers in the same occupation groups are less likely in nursing and residential care to be unionized than their counterparts in hospitals (Figure 12.9). This factor is no doubt linked to the shifting of care from hospitals to nursing and residential care facilities as a means to reduce costs for labour. These union advantages are often seen as impediments to management and government who, guided by neo-liberal ideals, seek to save on care costs by reducing the expenditures on workers. The union wage advantage for workers in health and social care in Canada is apparent in Table 12.3.

There can be little doubt that workers employed in for-profit settings in health and social care generally earn less in some jobs where profit is an economic priority guiding management. Indeed, in for-profit settings, so-called efficiencies and reductions to labour wages may be implemented not so much to reduce economic pressure on governments, but to yield a greater return for owners and shareholders. Data on the public and private sectors (despite limitations to definition of sector noted in Box 12.3) reveal differences in benefits coverage and wages for providers, demonstrating that some providers have a

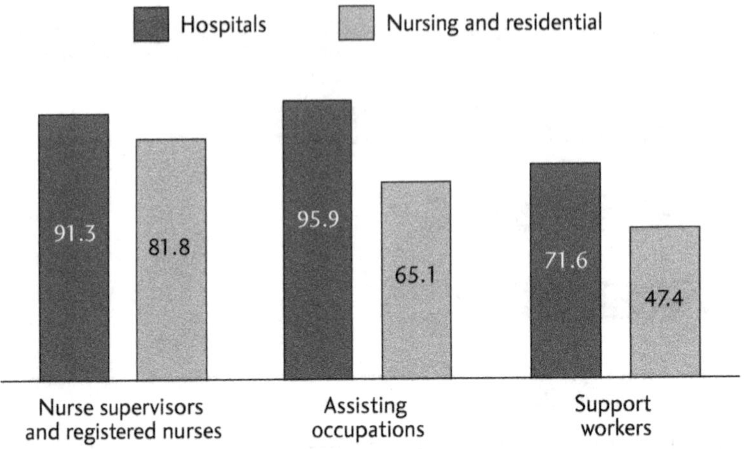

FIGURE 12.9: Union coverage by select occupations, 2009 (percent)

Source: Health industry and occupation by pension plan coverage, union coverage, and form of employment, 1993–2009 (HC SLID A-3). Gender and Work Database, York University. Retrieved from http://www.genderwork.ca/gwd. Data from Statistics Canada Survey of Labour and Income Dynamics, 1993–2009.

	Covered by a Union	Not Covered by a Union	Wage Gap
Total all health care industries	25.45	22.10	3.35
Ambulatory	28.94	23.90	5.04
Hospitals	27.49	35.16	-7.67
Nursing and residential care	20.41	16.74	3.67
Social assistance	22.97	17.98	4.99

TABLE 12.3: Average Hourly Wages by Union Coverage, 2009

Source: Health industry by establishment size, firm size, union coverage, and hourly wage, Canada and provinces, 1993–2009 (HC SLID F-2). Gender and Work Database, York University. Retrieved from http://www.genderwork.ca/gwd. Data from Statistics Canada Survey of Labour and Income Dynamics, 1993–2009.

significant public sector advantage. Put another way, some providers are more seriously affected by privatization, and earlier research has demonstrated this to be particularly true for support and ancillary providers (Armstrong & Laxer, 2011).

Not surprisingly, nurse supervisors and registered nurses in nursing and residential care have the highest wages relative to the other occupation groups in these facilities (Table 12.4). The lowest average hourly wage is for providers in assisting occupations employed in the private sector at only $16.65 in 2009. The most striking observation, however, is how much larger the wage gap is between workers in the public and private sectors for providers in the assisting occupations (such as personal support workers) and support occupations (such as cleaners and food service workers) as compared to providers in the professional nursing group (Table 12.4). Furthermore, the gap between the highest and lowest earners is larger in the private sector than in the public sector—a relative difference in earnings that has been shown to influence the self-worth and health and well-being of workers (Marmot & Wilkinson, 2001; Wilkinson & Pickett, 2009).

	Average Total ($)	Public Sector ($)	Private Sector ($)	Wage Gap ($)	Wage Gap (%)
Nurse supervisors and registered nurses	29.26	29.92	28.80	1.12	3.7
Technical and related occupations in health	21.55	22.49	21.18	1.31	5.8
Assisting occupations in support of health services	17.28	18.67	16.65	2.02	10.8
All other occupations	18.50	21.10	16.87	4.23	20.0

TABLE 12.4: Average Hourly Wages by Sector in Nursing and Residential Care, 2009

Source: Health industry and occupation by sector, employment form, and hourly wage, 1993–2009 (HC SLID B-3). Gender and Work Database, York University. Retrieved from http://www.genderwork.ca/gwd. Data from Statistics Canada Survey of Labour and Income Dynamics, 1993–2009.

Conclusion

Reflecting the medical model, the dominant approach to mapping workers in health and social care focuses on physicians, nurses, other professionals, and associate professionals. Key sources of statistical data on labour forces in care maintain this dominant focus. While there has been a move by organizations such as the Organisation for Economic Co-operation and Development to collect more data on other providers, including those in informal and personal care, these data are problematic in many ways and hardly account for their complete contribution to care.

In Canada, there has been a significant realignment in the sub-industries of health and social care. The sub-industry called social assistance has grown dramatically over the last two decades as a consequence of the push toward more home care. Meanwhile, hospital care has shrunk in relative size. There has also been a shift to more personal responsibility, defined as choice, and more individual payment. While the care workforce is gendered, racialized, and aging, some workers are doing better in some contexts than in others. Workers in care who are unionized have an advantage over those who are not. Similarly, providers in the public sector have an advantage over their private sector counterparts and this is especially true for workers in assisting and support occupations. Throughout recent changes, however, care work is still women's work and some care work is more likely performed by those from racialized populations.

References

Anderson, J., J. Beaton, & K. Laxer. (2006). The Union Dimension: Mitigating Precarious Employment? In L. Vosko (Ed.), *Precarious Employment: Understanding Labour Market Insecurity in Canada* (pp. 301–317). Montreal & Kingston: McGill-Queen's University Press.

Armstrong, P. (2013). Skills for Care. In P. Armstrong & S. Braedley (Eds.), *Troubling Care: Critical Perspectives on Research and Practices* (pp. 101–112). Toronto: Canadian Scholars' Press Inc.

Armstrong, P., & H. Armstrong. (2009). Precarious Employment in the Health-Care Sector. In L. Vosko, M. MacDonald, & M. Campbell (Eds.), *Gender and the Contours of Precarious Employment* (pp. 256–270). New York: Routledge Press.

Armstrong, P., & H. Armstrong. (2010). *Wasting Away: The Undermining of Canadian Health Care.* Wynford Project Edition. Toronto: Oxford University Press.

Armstrong, P., H. Armstrong, & K. Laxer. (2007). Doubtful Data: Why Paradigms Matter in Counting the Health Care Labour Force. In W. Clement & V. Shalla (Eds.), *Work and Labour in Tumultuous Times* (pp. 326–348). Montreal & Kingston: McGill-Queen's University Press.

Armstrong, P., H. Armstrong, & K. Scott-Dixon. (2008). *Critical to Care: The Invisible Women in Health Services.* Toronto: University of Toronto Press.

Armstrong, P., & S. Braedley (Eds.). (2013). *Troubling Care: Critical Perspectives on Research and Practices.* Toronto: Canadian Scholars' Press Inc.

Armstrong, P., & K. Laxer. (2011). Precarious Work, Privatization, and the Health Care Industry: The Case of Ancillary Workers. In V. Shalla (Ed)., *Working in a Global Era: Canadian Perspectives* (2nd ed.). Toronto: Canadian Scholars' Press Inc.

Armstrong, P., & K. Laxer. (2012). *Demanding Labour: An Aging Health Care Labour Force.* Proceedings from 2012 RC19 Annual Conference, Oslo, Norway.

Armstrong, P., & L. Silas. (2009). Taking Power, Making Change: Nurses' Unions in Canada. In M. McIntyre & C. McDonald (Eds.), *Realities of Canadian Nursing: Professional, Practice, and Power Issues* (3rd ed., pp. 316–336). Philadelphia: Lippincott Williams and Wilkins.

Baines, D. (2004). Caring for Nothing: Work Organization and Unwaged Labour in Social Services. *Work, Employment and Society* 18(2): 267–295.

Bakan, A. B., & D. Stasiulis. (1997). Foreign Domestic Worker Policy in Canada and the Social Boundaries of Modern Citizenship. In A. B. Bakan & D. Stasiuli (Eds.), *Not One of the Family: Foreign Domestic Workers in Canada* (pp. 29–52). Toronto: University of Toronto Press.

Banerjee, A., T. Daly, P. Armstrong, M. Szebehely, H. Armstrong, & S. Lafrance. (2012). Structural Violence in Long-Term, Residential Care for Older People: Comparing Canada and Scandinavia. *Social Science & Medicine* 74(3): 390–398.

Bezanson, K. (2010). "Child Care Delivered through the Mailbox": Social Reproduction, Choice, and Neoliberalism in a Theo-Conservative Canada. In S. Braedley & M. Luxton (Eds.), *Neoliberalism and Everyday Life* (pp. 90–112). Montreal & Kingston: McGill-Queen's University Press.

Bourgeault, I. L. (2006). *Push! The Struggle to Integrate Midwifery in Ontario.* Montreal & Kingston: McGill-Queen's University Press.

Braedley, S. (2013). A Gender Politics of Long-Term Residential Care: Towards an Analysis. In P. Armstrong & S. Braedley (Eds.), *Troubling Care: Critical Perspectives on Research and Practices* (pp. 59–70). Toronto: Canadian Scholars' Press Inc.

Braedley, S., & M. Luxton. (2010). *Neoliberalism and Everyday Life*. Montreal & Kingston: McGill-Queen's University Press.

Campbell, A. (2013). Work Organization, Care, and Occupational Health and Safety. In P. Armstrong & S. Braedley (Eds.), *Troubling Care: Critical Perspectives on Research and Practices* (pp. 89–100). Toronto: Canadian Scholars' Press Inc.

Clark, P. F., & D. A. Clark. (2003). Challenges Facing Nurses' Associations and Unions: A Global Perspective. *International Labour Review* 142(1): 29–47.

Cranford, C. (2005). From Precarious Workers to Unionized Employees and Back Again? The Challenges of Organizing Personal Care Workers in Ontario. In C. Cranford, J. Fudge, E. Tucker, & L. Vosko (Eds.), *Self-Employed Workers Organize* (pp. 96–135). Montreal: McGill-Queen's University Press.

Daboussy, M., & S. Uppal. (2012). Work Absences in 2011. *Perspectives on Labour and Income* 24(2). Catalogue no. 75-001-XIE. Ottawa: Statistics Canada.

Daly, T., & M. Szebehely. (2012). Unheard Voices, Unmapped Terrain: Care Work in Long-Term Residential Care for Older People in Canada and Sweden. *International Journal of Social Welfare* 21(2): 139–148.

Das Gupta, T. (2009). *Real Nurses and Others: Racism in Nursing*. Halifax: Fernwood Press.

Duffy, A., D. Glenday, & N. Pupo. (2007). Seniors in the Part-Time Labour Force: Issues of Choice and Power. *International Journal of Canadian Studies* 18(1998):133–152.

Duffy, A., & N. Pupo. (1992). Part-Time Paradox: Connecting Gender, Work, and Family. Toronto: McClelland & Stewart.

Duffy, M. (2011). *Making Care Count: A Century of Gender, Race, and Paid Care Work*. New Brunswick, NJ: Rutgers University Press.

European Commission. (2009). *European Economy No. 2/2009, The 2009 Ageing Report: Economic and Budgetary Projections for the EU-27 Member States (2008–2060)*. Luxembourg: Office for Official Publications of the European Communities.

Geiger-Brown, J., C. Muntaner, J. Lipscomb, & A. Trinkoff. (2004). Demanding Work Schedules and Mental Health in Nursing Assistants Working in Nursing Homes. *Work Stress* 18(4): 292–304.

Gender and Work Database (GWD). (2014). *Health Care Multidimensional Tables*. Data from Survey of Labour and Income Dynamics 1993–2009, York University. Retrieved from http://www.genderwork.ca.

Glenn, E. N. (2010). *Forced to Care: Coercion and Caregiving in America*. Cambridge, MA: Harvard University Press.

Gruber, J., & D. Wise. (2007). *Social Security Programs and Retirement around the World: Fiscal Implications of Reform*. Chicago: NBER Books, National Bureau of Economic Research, Inc.

Harvey, D. (2007). *A Brief History of Neoliberalism*. Oxford: Oxford University Press.

Health Canada. (2014). Homepage. Retrieved from http://www.hc-sc.gc.ca/.

Hochschild, A. (2000). Global Care Chains and Emotional Surplus Value. In T. Giddens & W. Hutton (Eds.), *On the Edge: Globalization and the New Millennium* (pp. 130–146). London: Sage Publishers.

Jackson, A. (2003). *In Solidarity: The Union Advantage*. Research paper no. 27. Ottawa: Canadian Labour Congress.

Le Jeune, G. (2009). Ungendering Women's Health: Information Systems and Occupational Health Indicators. In E. Balka, E. Green, & F. Henwood (Eds.), *Gender, Health, and Information Technology in Context*. Hampshire: Palgrave Macmillan.

Lethbridge, J. (2010). *Care Services for Older People in Europe: Challenges for Labour*. London: Public Services International Research Unit, University of Greenwich.

Marmot, M., & R. G. Wilkinson. (2001). Psychosocial and Material Pathways in the Relation between Income and Health: A Response to Lynch et al. *BMJ* 322(7296): 1233–1236.

McBride, S., & J. Shields. (1997). *Dismantling a Nation: The Transition to Corporate Rule in Canada* (2nd ed.). Toronto: Fernwood Publishing.

Messing, K. (1998). *One-Eyed Science: Occupational Health and Women Workers*. Philadelphia: Temple University Press.

Messing, K., B. Neis, & L. Dumais. (1995). *Invisible: Issues in Women's Occupational Health*. Charlottetown, PE: Gynergy Books.

Minister of Industry. (2012). *North American Industrial Classification System (NAICS) Canada*. Catalogue no. 12-501-X. Ottawa: Statistics Canada.

O'Reilly, J., J. Macinnes, T. Nazio, & J. M. Rochie. (2009). The United Kingdom: From Flexible Employment to Vulnerable Workers. In L. Vosko, M. MacDonald, & I. Campbell (Eds.), *Gender and the Contours of Precarious Employment* (pp. 108–126). New York & London: Routledge.

Riska, E. (2008). The Feminization Thesis: Discourses on Gender and Medicine. *Nordic Journal of Feminist and Gender Research* 16(1): 3–18.

Sears, A. (1999). The "Lean" State and Capitalist Restructuring: Towards a Theoretical Account. *Studies in Political Economy* 59(1999): 91–114.

Smele, S., & M. Seeley. (2013). Balancing the Tensions in Resident-Centred Care. In P. Armstrong & S. Braedley (Eds.), *Troubling Care: Critical Perspectives on Research and Practices* (pp. 143–154). Toronto: Canadian Scholars' Press Inc.

Struthers, J. (2013). Historical Perspective on Care and the Welfare State: The Rise, Retreat, Return, and Reframing of a Key Concept. In P. Armstrong & S. Braedley (Eds.), *Troubling Care: Critical Perspectives on Research and Practices* (pp. 159–170). Toronto: Canadian Scholars' Press Inc.

Townson, M. (2006). *Growing Older, Working Longer: The New Face of Retirement*. Ottawa: Canadian Centre for Policy Alternatives.

Twomey, A. (2013). Aging in Welfare States in Austere Times: Long-Term Care Reform in Japan. In P. Armstrong & S. Braedley (Eds.), *Troubling Care: Critical Perspectives on Research and Practices* (pp. 9–16). Toronto: Canadian Scholars' Press Inc.

Vosko, L. F. (2002). The Pasts (and Futures) of Feminist Political Economy in Canada: Reviving the Debate. *Studies in Political Economy* 68(2002): 55–83.

Vosko, L. F. (2006). Precarious Employment: Towards an Improved Understanding of Labour Market Insecurity. In L. F. Vosko (Ed)., *Precarious Employment: Understanding Labour Market Insecurity in Canada* (pp. 3–42). Montreal & Kingston: McGill-Queen's University Press.

Vosko, L. F. (2014). Introduction. *Comparative Perspectives on Precarious Employment Database, York University*. Retrieved from http://www.genderwork.ca/cpd/?page_id=2.

Vosko, L. F., & M. Thomas. (2014). Confronting the Employment Standards Enforcement Gap: Exploring the Potential for Union Engagement with Employment Law in Ontario, Canada. *Journal of Industrial Relations* 56(5): 631–652.

Vosko, L. F., & N. Zukewich. (2006). Precarious by Choice? Gender and Self-Employment. In L. F. Vosko (Ed.), *Precarious Employment: Understanding Labour Market Insecurity in Canada* (pp. 67–89). Montreal & Kingston: McGill-Queen's University Press.

Wilkinson, R., & K. Pickett. (2009). *The Spirit Level: Why More Equal Societies Almost Always Do Better.* London: Penguin Books.

Wong, I. S., C. B. McLeod, & P. A. Demers. (2011). Shift Work Trends and Risk of Work Injury among Canadian Workers. *Scandinavian Journal of Work, Environment and Health* 37(1): 54–61.

Yeates, N. (2012). Global Care Chains: A State-of-the-Art Review and Future Directions in Care Transnationalization Research. *Global Network* 12(2): 135–154.

Further Reading

Armstrong, P., Armstrong, H., & Scott-Dixon, K. (2008). *Critical to Care: The Invisible Women in Health Services.* Toronto: University of Toronto Press.

Armstrong, P., & K. Laxer. (2011). Precarious Work, Privatization, and the Health Care Industry: The Case of Ancillary Workers. In V. Shalla (Ed.), *Working in a Global Era: Canadian Perspectives* (2nd ed., pp. 115–140). Toronto: Canadian Scholars' Press Inc.

Armstrong, P., K. Laxer, & H. Armstrong. (2014). *The Conceptual Guide to the Health Care Module.* Gender and Work Database, York University. Retrieved from http://www.genderwork.ca/gwd/ ?page_id=20.

Briskin, L. (2013). In the Public Interest: Nurses on Strike. In S. Ross & L. Savage (Eds.), *Public Sector Unions in the Age of Austerity.* Halifax: Fernwood Press.

Canadian Institute for Health Information. (2013). *Canada's Health Care Providers: 1997–2011.* Ottawa: Author.

Das Gupta, T. (2009). *Real Nurses and Others: Racism in Nursing.* Halifax: Fernwood Press.

Duffy, M. (2011). *Making Care Count: A Century of Gender, Race, and Paid Care Work.* New Brunswick, NJ: Rutgers University Press.

Laxer, K., & P. Armstrong. (2014). *The Conceptual Guide to the Health and Social Care Module.* Comparative Perspectives on Precarious Employment Database, York University. Retrieved from http://www.genderwork.ca/cpd/?page_id=42.

Relevant Websites

Comparative Perspective on Precarious Employment Database (CPD): www.genderwork.ca/cpd
Gender and Work Database (GWD): www.genderwork.ca/gwd

CHAPTER 13

Unpaid Health Care: An Indicator of Equity[1]

Pat Armstrong

Introduction

Unpaid health care is a gender issue, an equity issue, and a human rights issue. It is a gender issue because women and girls throughout the world do the overwhelming majority of unpaid health care. It is an equity issue not only because women do more of this labour than men and more of the labour that is most demanding and daily. It is also an equity issue because women with the fewest economic resources are the most likely to do the heaviest work, and because those who need care experience inequities in the amount and quality of care they receive as a result. If we are to recognize, as the Universal Declaration of Human Rights (1948) does, that everyone has the right to health, then unpaid health care is a human rights issue as well because those who provide unpaid care too often suffer disproportionately from ill health as a consequence of this work and are thus themselves denied the highest attainable physical and mental health. This applies also to the many children, and especially girls, who often do such work. The right to health requires the right to provide or not provide unpaid health care, and thus access to the conditions that support this right.

Unpaid health care is complex in terms of the contexts, the activities, the actors, and the issues. It includes help with the activities of daily living and with personal care, nursing care, health care management, and advocacy for services as well as social and emotional support. It is becoming increasingly complex as demand for such care grows alongside fundamental alterations in the nature of the care required. Although it is difficult to capture unpaid health care in all its complexity—in part because unpaid care has not been a top priority of governments—there is more than enough evidence to identify the main factors that are shaping unpaid health care, the consequences for different populations, and the urgency of developing policies in this field. As the United Nations' *Human Development Report 2010* (UNDP, 2010) makes clear, "people are the real wealth of a nation" (p. iv). Assessing "whether people can lead long and healthy lives, whether they have the opportunity to be educated and whether they are free to use their knowledge and talents to shape their own destinies" is a critical measure of a country's success (p. iv). Unpaid health care serves as both a reflection and a gauge of a nation's human development. It provides an indicator of the growing inequalities between women and men as well as among them. It is a means of addressing inequities for both those who need such care and those who provide it. Unpaid health care also has consequences for the formal economy, as well as for the future of women, of families, and of the next generation. As a result, governments everywhere have a responsibility to take action.

This chapter makes the case for understanding unpaid health care labour as an indicator of equity in health services, and identifies strategies for addressing the inequities that result from the current nature and distribution of unpaid care work. It is intended to provide an integrated picture of the factors shaping changes in unpaid health care work; in the nature, extent, and distribution of this work; and of the consequences not only for individuals doing the work but also for the labour force, for those with care needs, and for societies in general. It seeks to contribute not only to analysis of health policies but also to the development of new approaches to equity in the health field.

Unpaid Health Care Activities

Unpaid health care involves a host of overlapping and increasingly complex activities. The six identified here cover broad categories that are involved to varying degrees depending on the location within the country and the person with care needs (Armstrong & Kits, 2004). Understanding what constitutes unpaid health care provides a basis for understanding the scope of what needs to be done, who does it, and what is required to promote equity.

The most common form of care work required is what in the literature is called Instrumental Activities of Daily Living (IADL). These activities primarily involve those usually provided in and by households. They include cooking, shopping, cleaning, and laundry as well as home maintenance tasks and any other work frequently done in and around the home. In some countries or households it may also include work such as feeding and tending to animals, carrying water, or other forms of household production. Some of these tasks must be done on a daily basis and at specific times, but many of them are more flexible, allowing care providers to undertake them when their schedules allow. Many mean adding to the usual daily tasks, although the workload is often more intense and the tasks frequently take more time. If the person providing care does not live in the household, travelling is added to the work time. Equally important, the tasks may have a significantly different form and even dangerous consequences for both worker and the person needing care when they are provided for someone who is ill or disabled. For example, clothes from those with infectious diseases may have to be washed separately and in particular ways and diets may require special preparation, as is the case with diabetics. As a result, the quality and the risks of care become the responsibility of the person—usually a female—doing the tasks rather than of the health system.

A growing number of people require more than assistance with these instrumental activities however. What are termed activities of daily living (ADL) refer to much more personal and increasingly medical aspects of health care work. These include assistance with dressing, bathing, eating, using the toilet, brushing teeth, and combing hair. Incontinence care is increasingly common, as is the need to lift and move people in and out of bed. In short, this work involves the direct, personal care that individuals who are able usually do for themselves. Those who return from day surgery, have disabilities, or have become frail in old age may also require assistance getting around the house or moving outside it. Most of these tasks must be done on a daily basis and many must be done according to a strict schedule. Some must be done around the clock and may be made more difficult by the need to travel to provide care. All require extra effort and some skill when they are done for others and when those others are frail, disoriented, or disabled.

There is a third set of tasks that are also becoming more visible as health reforms and new technologies are put in place. They include giving medications, inserting needles, changing dressings, monitoring temperature or blood pressure, and using a variety of equipment such as catheters, oxygen masks, and feeding tubes. These tasks could be defined as *nursing care*, even though they are seldom carried out by people with formal nursing credentials. Nurses not only have the education to ensure they know how to do the work, but they also have a professional code of ethics covering their practices and often some form of collective organization to protect their rights, while those doing unpaid health care work seldom have any of these.

A fourth, less visible but increasingly important form is *health care management*. While most care providers do some care management, some are primarily managers and care navigators. They investigate and arrange for more formal care services, as well as ensure that such services are provided. In effect, unpaid providers act as what in the formal system are called case managers, determining hours of service and eligibility, making appointments, and convincing care recipients to participate. They mediate between the formal and informal system, as well as between the system and the person with care needs. Managing money, completing forms, assembling documents, investigating options, and tracking tests results are all part of care management. Some aspects of care management are possible to do from a distance and offer considerable flexibility in terms of when they must be done. However, other aspects can only be done at the convenience of the formal system. The program and office support provided by volunteers in hospitals and other health care facilities could also be classified as management work. Similarly, the fundraising done for various health care services could also fit in this category (Mellow, 2011). It is work that requires both knowledge of the system and equipment such as computers in order to do some of the tasks.

A fifth form of care work has to do with associated activities done in relation to those outside the home. Care providers often have to spend considerable time and energy *advocating*, individually and through organizations, for care and supports. They frequently have to educate others about the particular health issues faced by their disabled children or older relatives (Home, 2002). This advocacy work is time consuming and, like other aspects of unpaid health care work, requires considerable knowledge and time to do effectively.

Finally, there is a form of unpaid health care work that should pervade all other forms but may constitute the primary aspect. Everyone requires *social and emotional support*. But those who have undergone surgery, live with disabilities, or live into frail old age have particular needs for companionship, for touch, for listeners and talkers. This is especially the case if they are not able to leave their beds or their homes. The need is particularly great for those requiring palliative care. Such support may be combined with other tasks; it may be done from a distance and does not necessarily have to be done at specific times. It is work that is often assumed to come naturally to women, but it is a skill taught to formal care providers because it is both an essential and learned capacity for health care work.

These various aspects of care may be provided by the same person, by different people, or by more than one person at a time and for more than one person. The location of the unpaid work also varies. It is not necessarily provided in homes. Not everyone has a home and the homeless may receive some unpaid support on the street or in the shelters where they live. Not everyone in a health care facility receives the full range of support, creating the need within these facilities for various forms of unpaid health care (Mellow, 2011). Emotional and social support has long been expected from families and friends regardless of location, and this is especially the case for women. Contemporary communication technologies increase both the opportunity and expectation that people are available to provide support 24/7. Increasingly, however, paid workers in facilities are unable to carry out the full range of tasks required and must leave them to be done by unpaid providers or work unpaid overtime themselves in order to get the job done (Armstrong & Daly, 2004). Unpaid workers empty bedpans and feed patients, fetch warm blankets and supervise exercises, to name only some of the tasks done by unpaid workers within care facilities. It is also important to note that while it is possible to identify the needs for and aspects of unpaid health care work, there is no guarantee that such work is done or provided well and willingly.

Who Provides

Families, relatives, friends, neighbours, and volunteers individually or through organizations constitute the unpaid health care labour force. Who does what for how long each day and over time is difficult to determine (Budlender, 2007). When unpaid care is counted, time may be underestimated or unrecorded when it is an extension of existing work, as in the case of women doing more cleaning or laundry when people are ill; or it may be overestimated if it is unusual, as might be the case when men take their mothers to the doctor or clean their toilet. Moreover, "unpaid care work is not identical to unpaid work since there are some types of activities that are not care work" (Budlender, 2007, p. 3) and care work encompasses work for children that would not usually be defined as health care. In short, unpaid health care work is difficult to count and often goes uncounted, especially for women.

Nevertheless, there are enough data to demonstrate that women do the bulk of the unpaid health care work and that this is especially the case for activities of daily living, which are the most regular, time consuming, and demanding. As Duxbury et al. (2009, p. 33) put it, the "research is clear about the persistence of a gendered division of labour in the allocation of caregiving work, with women, regardless of employment status, income and family structure, being more likely than men to perform the more intensive personal and physical care tasks." In Canada in 2007, "nearly 40% of women caregivers and fewer than 20% of men caregivers provided personal care" for the elderly, while women were twice as likely as men to perform regular tasks inside the house (Cranswick & Dosman, 2007, p. 54). Men did more work outside the house, work that was more flexible in terms of when and for how long it was done. Women were much more likely than men to do high-intensity, unpaid health care work (Pyper, 2006).

The male/female gap is especially wide when it comes to the care and supervision of disabled people, which is work that is likely to last for years and require support every day, even all day. Canadian research also indicates that women, unlike the men who were primary care providers, said there were no substitutes available to do the work when they took on the responsibility (Lilly, Laporte, & Coyte, 2010). They have no alternatives. This lack of substitutes builds on and reinforces women's sense of responsibility for care at the same time as it reflects their limited economic and power resources as well as assumptions about women's work (Cranswick & Dosman, 2007). It is women with the least education and the lowest incomes who have no alternatives to doing the unpaid health care work. It is the most vulnerable women who carry the heaviest loads, even though they do so with the fewest supports and the least visibility.

Most unpaid health care labour is provided to close family members, but unrelated others also participate in health care work. Although half of elder care is provided to parents or in-laws, nearly 20 percent is provided to a neighbour or friend (Cranswick & Dosman, 2007, chart 1). Women are more likely than men to receive care from a friend—a friend who is female (p. 54). As is the case with all data on unpaid care, however, the failure to recognize care as work must be taken into account. It is both the women who do the work and those who do the counting who fail in this way. That only 7 percent of survey respondents report they care for a spouse may reflect women not considering the work they do for their partner as extra or even unpaid care work. It may also be a result of the way the questions are asked. Nevertheless, almost half of Canadian men report that their main provider is a spouse, while this is the case for only one in five women (Statistics Canada, 2007, Table 13). Care for younger people with disabilities is also disproportionately done by women and for partners or close relatives. Their numbers are growing, as is the time they spend daily and over the years in doing unpaid health care work. But here, too, others are often involved.

Those living outside the household and family who provide care may be acting as individuals. But some at least are connected through community organizations. Religious groups in particular are active in organizing volunteer help in various countries and in providing social support for caregivers. A range of other community organizations are also involved, sometimes providing both paid and unpaid health care services. Many volunteers do unpaid care work within facilities. While similar numbers of women and men are counted as volunteering, women do most of the volunteer direct health care work. Research in three hospitals indicated women made up between two-thirds and more than three-quarters of those providing volunteer care. When men were involved in direct care, they tended to seek work in the emergency department, although more volunteered for fundraising work (Mellow, 2011, pp. 221–222). Not to be forgotten are those paid workers who put in unpaid time in order to make up for the care deficit (Baines, 2004). Their work goes uncounted in all the data and it is women who do most of this form of labour, both because they comprise most of the paid health care labour force and because they are held responsible and feel responsible for the care deficit.

While adults provide most of the unpaid care, it is important to note the role children as young as five years old play. Data on children who do unpaid health care work may be even less reliable and more underestimated than those on adults because they rely mainly on parents' reports. Parents may not recognize their children's care work (Becker, 2007, p. 27). Nevertheless, there is enough information to suggest there are a significant number of children who do this work and the numbers may well be growing. A 2012 study indicated that more than one in four Canadians between the ages of 15 and 29 provided some form of unpaid health care, with 31 percent of young women and 24 percent of young men recorded as doing so (Statistics Canada, 2014).

> In 2012, 1.9 million (27%) of young Canadians between the ages of 15 and 29 provided some form of care to a family member or friend with a long-term health condition, disability or aging need . . . with 31% of women under the age of 30 providing care compared with 24% of young men. (Statistics Canada, 2014)

In sum, the daily work of providing unpaid health care and especially the personal care is disproportionately done by women in every country for which we have data. Men are more likely to do the work that is most flexible in terms of when and where it can be done.

Children, too, provide care and so do neighbours, volunteers, and some workers otherwise paid to do the work. However, there is research to indicate that there are differences within these patterns depending on location, culture, and economic status. But it is also the case that the overwhelming majority of health care work in the home is unpaid and that even when some paid care is provided, unpaid work is still required and is still done. For instance, close to 97 percent of all those receiving paid home care services also have an unpaid care provider. Four in 10 of these providers report they are distressed and more than a quarter say they cannot continue (CIHI, 2011a, Table 9).

The Contexts Shaping Unpaid Health Care

There are demographic, economic, technological, political, health, and value factors shaping the changing demand for and nature of unpaid health care. While the impact of any specific factor varies within Canada and the various factors interact in different ways, there are some common patterns.

Demographic changes are both the most discussed and the most obvious factor influencing demand for unpaid care. Living to be over 70, as more women especially now do, does not necessarily mean health care dependency or even significant care needs, but even if the proportion of the older population requiring care remains the same, the actual numbers will increase significantly in the next two decades with the aging of the postwar generation. Whether the aging population will need care and of what kind is partly shaped by the kinds of lives these older people have experienced as well as by the nature and the range of alternative supports available. More women are likely to need care and for a longer time period at the same time as they are expected to do the care work. Income is a critical factor in the need for unpaid health services, with higher income associated with better health as well as with more opportunities to hire health services. Because women are more likely than men to be poor, they are less likely to be able to either pay for care or hire substitutes for their labour.

Households are also changing in ways that have profound implications for unpaid care provision. Although it is important to avoid assuming that all families, and especially the women and girls within them, have traditionally provided unpaid health care willingly and well, it *can* be assumed that most of the unpaid care provided in households has in the past been provided by the females within them. And although it is also important to avoid assuming that traditionally all households had an earning husband and a wife and/or daughters—along with other extended family members—available to provide care, it can be assumed that new patterns in household formations alter who is available or able to provide care.

Extended families have become less common, with fewer people per household, while same-sex marriages that tend to involve few children have become more common (Statistics Canada, 2012). Fertility decline means there will be fewer children around to do care work for aging parents or other siblings with disabilities, even assuming children did so in the past and would or could do so now (Statistics Canada, 2013a). Moreover, children and even spouses are increasingly likely to seek employment far from their family of origin, making intergenerational unpaid care difficult, if not impossible, to perform, and disturbing family and neighbour connections that are often sources of support. Because women tend to marry men older than themselves and to live longer than men, they tend to be without that male partner in old age even if they stayed married. Meanwhile, more divorces and more never-married women parenting alone often mean female-headed families with low income (Statistics Canada, 2013b). Remarriage after divorce may create larger households, but reconstituted families can also bring more people requiring care. In addition, a growing number of women are migrating within and across national boundaries to do care work, in the process leaving their own families without access to any unpaid care contribution from them. Immigrants, too, often find themselves without familiar family supports. Finally, the growing numbers of homeless are usually without family or estranged from them, and thus are unlikely to have family willing or able to provide care.

Neighbourhoods and other social networks are also changing. If you Google "social engagement," the most common sites talk about social media and the ways people connect over the web. While such technologies expand acquaintance networks and may link families, there is little indication that they could or would provide a source of unpaid health care. Half the respondents to a Canadian study did not know their neighbours and only a minority belong to the kinds of community and religious organizations that provide volunteer health care services, including the kinds of social support networks essential to health (Statistics Canada, 2004).

With the exception of changes in women's growing labour force participation, *economic factors* shaping the growing demand for unpaid work have received less attention than demographic ones. A majority of women are now in the paid workforce and most are there full-time, leaving them little time or energy for unpaid health care work (Statistics Canada, 2013b). Most women enter the labour force because they need the money (Armstrong & Armstrong, 2010a) and even with women's pay, income inequality has been growing among households in the wake of the most recent economic crisis (Statistics Canada, 2013c). Moreover, increasing numbers of women are the sole economic support because either they do not have a partner or their partner is unemployed. And these figures do not consider the women who work in the underground economy, but this work, too, has an impact on the time available for unpaid health care.

But the economic issues shaping unpaid health care are about more than women's growing labour force participation. With the emergence of managerial practices justified in terms of global competition and flexibility, work itself is changing. As a result, women and men are working longer hours in their paid jobs and they move from job to job more frequently. Women especially often work irregular hours that make it difficult for them to take on regular and unpaid health care work involving heavy time commitments (Vosko, 2006). Indeed, with employment becoming more precarious for both women and men, few may be willing to leave work or refuse overtime in order to provide care because they may fear losing their jobs. For many, technology and pressures to compete combine to extend the paid work day into the home as employees are increasingly expected to answer emails after their paid work hours. Moreover, although technology may make it possible to do more jobs from home, suggesting women could combine paid work with unpaid health care, the combination may make it difficult to do either job well. With paid work becoming more demanding, neither women nor men may have energy left to take on unpaid care work at home. This is especially the case for the women who make up the majority of those who provide paid health care as well as for those who have to take on more than one job to make ends meet (Armstrong & Armstrong, 2010b; Vosko, 2006).

Technological advances, including mechanical, medical, and therapeutic ones, also contribute not only to the growing demand for unpaid health care but also to its changing nature. New technologies have made it possible to do more day surgeries, sending people home for their recovery while still in need of considerable and complicated care. Technologies have also been critical in allowing people to live after severe injuries or with chronic illnesses, often at home. Yet such conditions often require extensive and daily support. Equally important, technologies have made it possible to send home the kind of care previously possible only in hospitals. People now go home with catheters, monitoring devices, and oxygen masks; have dialysis and a wide range of injections; and frequently require a variety of therapies and complex equipment. Technologies can also be used as well to link patients at home with professionals outside it or to family members, reducing the need for transport to services while increasing the amount of care left to be done at home. This is not sending care back home but rather using technologies to relocate care, mostly to unpaid providers, who usually receive little training for the increasingly complicated care work required of them.

More babies are surviving with disabilities, thanks in part to new technologies and health services for pregnant women. Others become disabled in later years as a result of injury or illness, malnutrition, lack of health services, abuse, and alcohol or drug addiction, to name only some of the major causes. War is also a significant factor in the growing number of disabled in Canada. All these developments mean there are a growing number of young people who need care on a daily basis (Employment and Development Canada, 2013). Those with disabilities are less likely than others in the population to have higher education or paid jobs that would allow them to purchase care. And women are more likely than men to live with disabilities (see Pinto in this volume), often making it more difficult for them to provide care for others.

Political developments influence the demographic, economic, and technological factors shaping demand for unpaid health care. The decades-old emphasis on market strategies has had a profound impact. Tax cuts intended to promote competition, combined with an emphasis on smaller government and concern over rising government debt, have resulted in smaller and fewer public health and social services. Most of those who provide these public services and most of those who use them are women. Meanwhile, the market strategies applied to the public services that remain have resulted in women especially losing paid work in the public sector at the same time as they have been pressured to take on more unpaid health care work that has been sent home. A report for the United Nations (2008, p. 9) identifies the "ever growing gap in services and safety nets on the part of governments associated with health sector reforms, decentralization, privatization and cuts to social spending" as critical factors in the increase in demands for unpaid care work. To varying degrees, governments have promoted responsibilization, encouraging the voluntary sector, families, and individuals to take responsibility for their own care in ways that increase the amount of unpaid care required (Ilcan & Basok, 2004).

Values also have an impact on the demand for unpaid care. There are a host of often contradictory developments in expressed and assumed values that influence the demand for unpaid health care. What is consistent is the increasing emphasis placed by governments and economic leaders on individual and family responsibility for care. This responsibilization is often characterized as choice, but without options this choice may reflect "compulsory altruism" (Land & Rose, 1985) or "conscription" (National Forum on Health, 1997) into unpaid health care work, especially for the women and girls who are assumed to be natural caregivers. Furthermore, choice is often equated with having services available for hire and thus with the ability to purchase—an ability that many, and especially many women, do not have. At the same time, women are described as choosing to take on paid work, even though economic need is the primary motivation for women's paid employment. Increasingly, governments have been promoting a restriction of public services to governments' "core business" and the transfer of services to the private, often for-profit, sector where costs are higher and access more limited. This emphasis has coincided with a strong critique of institutionalization as oppressive and hospitals as dangerous places in terms of infections, malnutrition, and loss of mobility. The critique is linked in turn to stress on the value of independent living for those with disabilities.

There is, as well, a widespread belief that the best and preferred care is at home, assuming there is a home, and that families—or more particularly the women within them—want to and can provide quality care. And there is also an assumption that most people want to die at home. Yet Canadian research "offers little empirical evidence that the first choice of most frail elderly is to depend on family for hands-on caregiving, nor that most family members would freely and willingly choose to do so" (Guberman et al., 2006, p. 74). Indeed, income and education matter at least as much as culture in terms of the kinds and amounts of unpaid health care women provide. Those who can afford to buy services or can access public services do so (Chubachi, 1999; Guberman, 2004). Caution is needed in assuming not only that some cultures or genders naturally want to provide unpaid care or that providing care means it is a choice, but also in assuming that stated values match practices or that practices result in quality care.

In addition, there has been a growing conviction that markets and for-profit practices provide the most effective and efficient services and supports. This is combined with the assumption that private delivery and the right to buy allows more choice. However, like the belief that all women can and want to provide unpaid, appropriate care, it is a value that tends to be based on belief rather than evidence. Unquestionably, when services must be bought, there are those who cannot afford to buy. Moreover, there is little evidence to demonstrate that the quality is better when access declines as a result or that the for-profit sector provides better care. As markets increasingly dominate in health services, they become luxury, private goods rather than accessible public ones and access to health care is no longer a human right or even understood as such. Women especially suffer as a result.

At the same time, there is growing demand for more and better services or supports of various kinds from governments. According to a European Commission report (Braun et al., 2009), "the number and influence of vocal patient groups and self-help groups is likely to increase and the trend towards internationalizing health interest groups is set to grow" (p. 13). Alongside these value shifts is the continuing belief in the importance of encouraging the education and labour force participation of women and a commitment to equity, both of which depend to some extent on government intervention and which cannot be easily combined with more unpaid health care. This contrasts with the persistent idea that care is women's responsibility and that care is about "love, attachment, duty and reciprocity" and not about work (Becker, 2007, p. 23). Without pay in a world where more and more services are valued in monetary terms, the unpaid labour in health care has less value than other work. Without supports, those who do want to provide care find it difficult to do and to do well.

In sum, a growing number of people require unpaid health care and the care they require is more complex than in the past, even though few have the necessary training to do the work effectively. At the same time, fewer women or other family members are available to provide unpaid care and governments have not only failed to fill the gap, they have cut back on services and introduced reforms in ways that increase demand. Meanwhile, shifting values simultaneously promote individual responsibility for economic survival and health care while emphasizing women's place in the home in providing unpaid health care.

Consequences of Unpaid Health Care

Unpaid health care has consequences for both the individuals who need care and for those who provide it. It has an impact on families and on the next generation as well as on social relationships between families and others. Governments, too, are affected, as are employers and the labour force. Unpaid health care has an impact on health and costs, on social solidarity, and on equity. Given that women and girls bear the primary responsibility for the most intense and long-term unpaid health care, it is their health and future that are most at risk as the pressure to do the work and the work itself increases.

The *health* consequences of unpaid care work for individual providers are well documented. There are rewards to providing care, but these rewards may well be outweighed by burdens that can be especially heavy in the absence of economic and other supports. The health impact varies with the nature of the care demands. Overall, "Employees who provide caregiving for elderly dependents who live with them experience the highest levels of financial strain, physical strain and emotional strain." (Duxbury et al., 2009, p. 63) Age, too, makes a difference, with older providers at greater risk of injury (Jull, 2010). The impact varies as well with how much time is involved on a daily basis and over the lifespan. However, most unpaid providers experience physical changes when considerable time or particular illnesses are involved. More than a third of Canadians doing this work experienced moderate to high levels of physical strain (Duxbury et al., 2009, p. 60). Fatigue is especially common, and is combined with difficulty sleeping. Headache, back pain, weight loss, colds, and worsening of a health condition are also common (Jull, 2010, p. 8). Physical injury is frequent, especially if the person needing care is violent or particularly difficult to move. Mental health consequences may be even more likely and less varied in their impact. In Canada, "across caregiving types, ethnic groups and geographic location, many women reported that caregiving led to feelings of depression and helplessness" (Brannen, 2006, p. 12). The more hours involved, the greater the stress. The more severe the health problems of those with care needs, the more severe the health consequences for those doing the unpaid care work (CIHI, 2010).

Women's health is more likely to suffer because they do most of the heavy, primary health care labour that is most commonly associated with negative health outcomes (Lee, 1999). And women are more likely than men to be poor. "The strong association between increased financial and emotional caregiver strain and poorer physical and mental health does not, however, vary with caregiver group" (Duxbury et al., 2009, p. 74). Women in older age groups who cannot afford to either buy support or quit their paid jobs are most at physical risk while emotional strain is highest for women with little money who do unpaid care work for elderly dependants (p. 85). Lack of choice contributes to these feelings of depression and helplessness. "Three out of six factors that appear to be determinants of a woman's decision to provide care represent external or structural constraints: the inadequacy of institutional and community resources, the imposition of the decision by the dependent person and woman's economic dependency" (Guberman, 2004, p. 81). Although Canada has, at least in theory, universal access to doctor and hospital care, other supports such as mental health services, residential care, respite care, and home care are much more limited, more privatized, and inaccessible, and so are income and employment supports. In other words, unpaid health care workers often have little choice and it is women who have the fewest choices and supports.

Lack of financial resources exacerbates the health consequences and those providing care worry about money. Those particularly subject to physical strain were older women who lived with those for whom they provided care and who were unable to pay for support or quit their paid work. Emotional strain was highest for women with little money, without children, and providing care for elderly dependants. With the work characterized as high demand and low job control, it is not surprising that the health of these women suffers when they provide unpaid care (Duxbury et al., 2009). Many are themselves frail or in ill health, and the extra work may not only exacerbate their conditions but also mean they are unable to provide adequate care. The lack of financial resources, combined with new managerial practices, put into public health services contributes to the growth of unpaid work in the formal sector as women employees in particular seek to make up for the care deficit by putting in uncompensated overtime. While it is difficult to determine with any precision how much this overload accounts for the high and growing rates of absences due to illness and injury in health services, it seems more than likely it is a factor (Armstrong, Armstrong, & Scott-Dixon, 2008). For other women with paid work, there is added stress of doing unpaid care work for which they are not trained.

The impact on the *next generation* may be most obvious for the children who themselves are directly involved in the unpaid health care work. On the one hand, children who provide care may develop skills and capacities that are useful to them as adults and their labour can also make it easier for employed adults to juggle demands (Duxbury et al., 2009, p. 64). On the other hand, children who provide considerable care "can experience significant restrictions in their development, participation and opportunities, and educational attainment, even when there may be some 'positives' associated with caring—such as enhanced coping mechanisms, the development of life, social and other skills, maturity, as sense of purpose and closer attachments" (Becker, 2007, p. 25). Less obvious are the ways the devotion of time and resources to health care for one or two family members may mean others have little support. The presence of people with heavy care needs can also result in social exclusion, both as a result of stigmatizing attitudes and because there is no time for developing or maintaining social networks (Home, 2002).

Care provided in the *family and community* can bring people closer together as they share and learn from each other. However, the emotional stress that is a frequent consequence of unpaid health care may play out in family dynamics and in community relations. When many unpaid health care providers give up their leisure time to provide care, families have less time to have fun together (Cranswick, 2003). Emotional strain in particular appears to have a negative impact on families (Duxbury et al., 2009, p. 71). Heavy unpaid care workloads also mean care providers have less time to be involved in building communities. It also often means many women end up parenting alone.

Care may be unpaid, but it is not without direct economic costs. Equipment, pharmaceuticals, and supplies must be purchased. Renovation to housing is often required.

Transportation to and from services adds to expenses, as does responding to special dietary needs. Often there are direct payments for health services involved. These costs, combined with restrictions on employment resulting from the workload, can move women especially into poverty. Technologies have also increased some of the costs of care, both for the individual and for health systems. The extra expenses are the most common problem for those providing unpaid care (Keefe, 2011, Figure 2) and the problems increase if those doing unpaid care work live at a distance. "Even after other socioeconomic factors and the number of caregiving hours were taken into account, the odds of having extra expenses were three times higher for caregivers living more than half a day's journey away than for those in the same neighbourhood," and this was especially the case for women (Statistics Canada, 2010).

One clear impact on the *economy* is the reduction in labour force participation by those who take primary responsibility for the unpaid care work. While a survey of the literature shows that working-age unpaid care providers are as likely as non-providers to take paid work, it also shows that they often reduce their hours when they take on unpaid health care work and that the heavy work of a primary caregiver frequently results in withdrawal from the labour force entirely (Lilly, Laporte, & Coyte, 2010). Given that women usually take on the heavy personal care loads that are difficult to combine with regular paid work, and given that women on average earn less than men, it is mainly women who withdraw or reduce hours. It is mainly women who feel the emotional and physical consequences of the stress, stress that can also be felt in their families when women take the stress home. Unpaid health care work not only influences whether and how much women participate in the labour force, it also has an impact on the way they participate and on their future, not only in the labour force but also in terms of support in old age. Involvement in unpaid health care often restricts women's employment options, encouraging them to take paid work close to home and with hours that can fit in with their unpaid work demands. It can make it too difficult to accept promotion or increased responsibility, to accept overtime or uneven work demands. It can also mean they become ineligible for pensions and new jobs after their unpaid care work is over, jeopardizing their future and reducing the flexibility of the labour force overall (Duxbury et al., 2009). Those who reduce their hours have pensions based on lower earnings. Indeed, with many rights of citizenship and benefits linked to full-time employment, women with few options other than withdrawing from the labour force or reducing their time there in order to do their unpaid care work end up with fewer social rights and benefits now and in the future. At the same time, the double workload of women continues to be used as a justification for the segregation of women into the lowest-paid jobs (Armstrong, 2011).

Employers feel the impact as heavy unpaid workloads are associated with high absenteeism and turnover (Duxbury et al., 2009, p. 68). Unpaid care work shows up in stress at work. Stressed workers are "more likely to be unhealthy, poorly motivated, less productive, and less safe at work. And their organizations are less likely to succeed in a competitive market" (Park, 2007, p. 5). In addition, those with heavy unpaid care work responsibilities may come in late or leave early, or take calls from home while at work and lose their concentration. Among those providing four or more hours of care a week, approximately two-thirds of the women and nearly half of the men experienced significant job-related consequences (Pyper, 2006). In addition, conferences and training are less possible, making these workers and their organization less adaptable to change. Lack of investment in supporting paid and unpaid health care now could mean higher costs for employers in the future in terms of the labour force supply as well as in terms of medical costs.

Government costs may be directly influenced by rising demands on those providing unpaid care. Some health care costs rise. Those unpaid care providers who are under financial strain visit emergency rooms more often than others, and those experiencing physical or emotional strain see their family physician more often (Duxbury et al., 2009, p. 71). The risk of poverty increases with heavy unpaid workloads, as does withdrawal from the labour force, leading to increasing demands on governments for economic support in the future. Governments that fail to provide supports for those doing unpaid care work may find that those in need are abandoned entirely, leaving them to the formal system. Moreover, there is no clear evidence that post-acute care or home care for the severely disabled is cheaper at home even without factoring in the economic value of unpaid care (Keefe et al., 2007, p. S66). And there may be political consequences resulting from the failure to provide supports for those doing the unpaid work. For example, exposure of neglect for those needing care and of the health consequences for unpaid health care workers can contribute to election defeats.

The changing nature of unpaid health care work means that providers need more *skills*. New managerial skills are required to coordinate, record, and arrange care, giving those with more formal education and language skills, as well as cultural ones, an advantage. Nursing work, which in hospitals is done only by those with formal training, is being transferred to the home, often with little formal training. But it is not only nursing work that requires new skills. The work involved in providing IADL also requires training in lifting, for example. Even those aspects most closely associated with women's domestic tasks, such as laundry and cooking, require new skills when the person needing health care has an infectious disease, such as HIV/AIDS, or is old and especially vulnerable to infections. And the skills involved in providing social and emotional support cannot be considered natural or usual for women either. Alzheimer's provides just one example of conditions that demand particular relational skills. At the same time, the transfer of so much work more often defined as skilled when done for pay can denigrate the skills of both paid and unpaid providers. If it is assumed that anyone, and especially any woman, can take up the tasks or at least can be quickly taught them, then the skills of paid workers is undermined. Indeed, the result may be less paid care work. Given that women make up the overwhelming majority of those providing both the paid and unpaid care work, the impact is felt primarily by women.

The undermining of skills and the transfer of care work to the household goes hand in hand with the increasing demand for *migrant female labour*. The lack of supports for care work sent home encourages the employment of the cheapest available labour, labour made cheap by the denigration of the skills required and by those government policies that simultaneously allow their employment and fail to protect them from poor conditions of work (Spencer et al., 2010). It is made cheap as well by the assumption that any woman can do the work by virtue of being a woman (Armstrong, 2013). Discrimination against these migrant workers can increase the risk to them while reinforcing the notion that any woman can do the work.

Linked to skills are the consequences for *those needing unpaid health care*. Unskilled assistance can put both the provider and patient at risk, resulting in poor-quality care. Pressures on providers contribute to making direct abuse, or indirect abuse as a result of neglect, not uncommon. The person who needs care may have little choice about having the most intimate personal care provided by a daughter, even when they would prefer a professional provider and even when the work is done badly. They may also have little say about when and how care is provided if the daughter is employed in a job with fixed time demands that also leave her with little energy. The dependency involved may create depression, especially if the person feels like a burden, a risk to the care provider, or that the nature of care puts the person at risk. Given that women make up the majority of the elderly who need care, and are more likely to live in poverty in old age, women are particularly vulnerable to being financially dependent in ways that give them little choice about who provides what kinds of care (CIHI, 2011b).

In sum, unpaid health care work may be done willingly and well. And it may be rewarding for both those who need the services and those who provide them. However, this is most likely to be the case when alternatives and supports are in place. Otherwise, the consequences are more likely to be negative. Given that women bear the primary responsibility for the most intense and long-term unpaid health care, it is women's health and future that are most at risk as the pressure to do the work and the work itself increases. In addition, the unpaid work limits women's labour force participation in ways that can make them more economically dependent on men, limiting their power in the household and beyond. It is not only the women doing the unpaid work who are at risk, however. Men who take the primary responsibility for providing intensive care also experience negative consequences. Employers and governments can also face rising costs as a result, and so can the next generation. What suffers as well is equity, with women who are poor in particular losing out and differences among women increasing.

Unquestionably the demands for unpaid health care are increasing, and the work itself is becoming more demanding in both time and skills. While more men are providing such care, it is women who have the major responsibility for the heaviest and most time-consuming labour even as the majority of women also have paid employment. While this may be a labour of love, it is still labour. These trends have profound consequences for women as a group and for particular groups of women as well as for those for whom they provide care.

Even if we are willing to countenance the impact on equity, we cannot ignore the significant negative consequences of this growing workload for individuals, families, communities, employers, and governments.

Governments and employers have a responsibility to develop strategies to provide services to reduce the demand for unpaid health care and to provide both accommodations and supports for those who willingly provide such care. Any approach must recognize that unpaid care workers are often disadvantaged to start with and the intensification of unpaid work too often leads to further disadvantage for them as well as for those for whom they do the care work. The market mechanisms must be carefully scrutinized for their impact on the nature and distribution of both care services and care work. Research to date indicates they tend to increase inequality while sending more care to communities and households where the time, the skills, and the stress involved in the care work become invisible. In planning government strategies, critical questions need to be asked about who pays for care and at what cost to which women, even when our focus is unpaid care. How payment is made or not made, and under what criteria for what care are issues that have significant consequences not only for access to formal care but also for costs to caregivers, both paid and unpaid. Payment for women providing care for relatives in the home, for example, may reinforce women's responsibility for such work without providing them with adequate supports.

It is also important to understand women's paid and unpaid care work as integrally linked. Public services simultaneously create paid jobs for women and reduce their unpaid health care work. As cutbacks in public care, combined with new technologies and new ideas about where care should be provided, move care into households, the skills and the labour time become much harder to see. Women's paid work also suffers and some women even withdraw from care at significant costs to their income now and in the future. Employers have an interest in ensuring a supply of effective women workers, and this requires supports and accommodations from employers. Inequality affects us all and unpaid health care work is a critical indicator of equity.

The complexity of unpaid health care, combined with the significant variation in demands and supports, mean other patterns are less clear and vary more by location. This unpaid care work may be provided in homes, on the street, or in facilities of multiple kinds, and it may be provided by relatives, friends, or volunteers who are strangers. Different conditions exist in urban and rural areas, for those with families and for those without. Governments shape what unpaid care is required, how it is provided, by whom, for how long, and in what ways. For-profit and not-for profit service organizations also play a role, as do people paid to offer care. Employers, governments, families, and communities all feel the consequences of the growth and change in unpaid care work demands, and the consequences are often negative.

There are no simple answers to the question of how to support unpaid health care work and how to reduce the load. There are multiple tensions that shape alternatives in every country and for every group. There are, however, many strategies currently in place that can be evaluated in terms of their efficacy in any specific place and in terms of their consequences for equity. It is clear that, regardless of location, the right to care for both providers and recipients requires structural supports especially from governments, but also from employers and communities. The right to care also requires real alternatives to unpaid health care work for those who now provide or are pushed to provide the labour and for those who need the care. And these alternatives must take culture, location, age, and resources into account. Without them, inequalities will increase not only between women and men but also among women and men.

Note

1. This chapter is based on a paper originally commissioned by the Pan American Health Organization, which has given permission for publications out of that work. For the full paper, see http://new.paho.org/hq/index.php?option=com_content&view=article&id=2680&Itemid=4017. The responsibility for content is mine.

References

Armstrong, P. (2011). Pay Equity: Yesterday's Issue? In L. Tepperman & A. Kalyta (Eds.), *Reading Sociology: Canadian Perspectives* (2nd ed., pp. 211–214). Oxford: Oxford University Press.

Armstrong, P. (2013). Puzzling Skills. Special Issue, 50th Anniversary of the *Canadian Review of Sociology* 53(3): 256–283.

Armstrong, P., & H. Armstrong. (2010a). *The Double Ghetto: Canadian Women and Their Segregated Work.* Toronto: Oxford University Press.

Armstrong, P., & H. Armstrong. (2010b). *Wasting Away: The Undermining of Canadian Health Care.* Toronto: Oxford University Press.

Armstrong, P., H. Armstrong, & K. Scott-Dixon. (2008). *Critical to Care: The Invisible Women in Health Services.* Toronto: University of Toronto Press.

Armstrong, P., & T. Daly. (2004). *"There Are Not Enough Hands": Conditions in Ontario's Long-Term Care Facilities.* Report prepared for the Canadian Union of Public Employees. Toronto: CUPE.

Armstrong, P., & O. Kits. (2004). One Hundred Years of Caregiving. In K. R. Grant et al. (Eds.), *Caring for/Caring About: Women, Home Care, and Unpaid Caregiving* (pp. 45–74). Aurora, ON: Garamond Press.

Baines, D. (2004). Caring for Nothing: Work Organization and Unwaged Labour in Social Services. *Work, Employment and Society* 18(1): 29–49.

Becker, S. (2007). Global Perspectives on Children's Unpaid Caregiving in the Family. *Global Social Policy* 7(1): 23–50.

Brannen, C. (2006). Women's Unpaid Caregiving and Stress. *Centres of Excellence for Women's Health Research Bulletin* 5(1): 12–13. Retrieved from http://www.cewh-cesf.ca/PDF/RB/bulletin-vol5no1EN.pdf.

Braun, A., et al. (2009). *Special Issue on Healthcare. Healthy Aging and the Future of Public Healthcare Systems.* Luxembourg: European Commission.

Budlender, D. (2007, June). *A Critical Review of Selected Time Use Surveys.* Gender and Development Programme Paper No. 2. Geneva: United Nations Research Institute for Social Development.

Canadian Institute for Health Information (CIHI). (2010). *Supporting Informal Caregivers—The Heart of Home Care.* Ottawa: Author. Retrieved from www.cihi.ca/cihi-ext-portal/internet/en/document/types+of+care/hospital+care/continuing+care/release_cont_26aug10.

Canadian Institute for Health Information (CIHI). (2011a). NCRS QuickStats Table 9. *Informal Care of Assessed Home Care Clients 2010–2011.* Retrieved from www.cihi.ca/CIHI-ext-portal/xls/internet/HCRS_Quickstats_2010-2011_en.

Canadian Institute for Health Information (CIHI). (2011b). *Health Care in Canada, 2011: A Focus on Seniors and Aging.* Ottawa: Author.

Chubachi, N. (1999). *Geographies of Nisei Japanese Canadians and Their Attitudes towards Elderly Long-Term Care* (MA thesis). Queen's University, Kingston, Ontario.

Cranswick, K. (2003). *General Social Survey, Cycle 16: Caring for an Aging Society.* 89-582-XIE. Ottawa: Statistics Canada, Housing, Family, and Social Statistics Division.

Cranswick, K., & D. Dosman. (2007). Eldercare: What We Know Today. *Canadian Social Trends* 86(1): 49–57.

Duxbury, L., C. Higgins, & B. Shroeder. (2009). *Balancing Paid Work and Caregiving Responsibilities: A Closer Look at Family Caregivers in Canada.* Ottawa: Human Resources and Skills Development Canada.

Employment and Development Canada. (2013). *Disability in Canada: A 2006 Profile.* Retrieved from www.esdc.gc.ca/eng/disability/arc/disability_2006.shtml.

Guberman, N. (2004). Designing Home and Community Care for the Future: Who Needs to Care? In K. R. Grant et al. (Eds.), *Caring for/Caring About: Women and Unpaid Caregiving* (pp. 75–90). Aurora, ON: Garamond Press.

Guberman, N., et al. (2006). Families' Values and Attitudes Regarding Responsibility for Frail Elderly: Implications for Aging Policy. *Journal of Aging and Social Policy* 18(3/4): 59–78.

Home, A. (2002). Challenging Hidden Oppression: Mothers Caring for Children with Disabilities. *Critical Social Work* 3(1): 1–6. Retrieved from www.uwindsor.ca/criticalsocialwork/.

Ilcan, S., & T. Basok. (2004). Community Government: Voluntary Agencies, Social Justice, and the Responsibilization of Citizens. *Citizenship Studies* 8(2): 129–144.

Jull, J. (2010). *Seniors Caring for Seniors.* Ottawa: Canadian Association of Occupational Therapists. National Alliance for Caregiving.

Keefe, J. (2011). *Supporting Caregivers and Caregiving in an Aging Canada.* Montreal: Institute for Research on Public Policy.

Keefe, J., J. Légaré, & Y. Carriére. (2007). Developing New Strategies to Support Future Caregivers of Older Canadians with Disabilities: Projections of Need and Their Policy Implications. *Canadian Public Policy* 23(Suppl.): S65–S80.

Land, H., & H. Rose. (1985). Compulsory Altruism for Some or an Altruistic Society for All? In P. Bean, J. Ferris, & D. Whynes (Eds.), *In Defense of Welfare* (pp. 74–96). London: Tavistock.

Lee, C. (1999). Health, Stress, and Coping among Women Caregivers: A Review. *Journal of Health Psychology* 4(1): 27–40.

Lilly, M. B., A. Laporte, & P. C. Coyte. (2010). Do They Care Too Much to Work? The Influence of Caregiving Intensity on the Labour Force Participation of Unpaid Caregivers. *Canadian Journal of Health Economics* 29(6): 895–903.

Mellow, M. (2011). Voluntary Caregiving? Constraints and Opportunities for Hospital Volunteers. In C. Benoit & H. Hallgrimsdóttir (Eds.), *Valuing Care Work: Comparative Perspectives* (pp. 215–235). Toronto: University of Toronto Press.

National Forum on Health. (1997). *Value Working Group Synthesis Report in Canada Health Action: Building on the Legacy.* Synthesis Report and Issues Papers. Ottawa: Public Works and Government Services.

Park, J. (2007, December). Work Stress and Job Performance. *Perspectives on Labour and Income* 8(12): 5–17. Retrieved from www.statcan.gc.ca/pub/75-001-x/2007112/article/10466-eng.htm.

Pyper, W. (2006, Winter). Balancing Career and Care. *Perspectives on Labour and Income* 18(4): 5–15. Retrieved from www.statcan.gc.ca/pub/75-001-x/11106/9520-eng.pdf.

Spencer, S., et al. (2010). *The Role of Migrant Care Workers in Aging Societies: Report on Research Findings in the United Kingdom, Ireland, Canada, and the United States.* Geneva: International Organization for Migration.

Statistics Canada. (2004). *2003 General Social Survey on Social Engagement, Cycle 17: An Overview of Findings.* Retrieved from www.statscan.gc.ca/pub/89-598x2003001-eng.pdf.

Statistics Canada. (2007). *Women and Men Aged 65 Years and over Who Received Assistance Because of a Chronic Health Problem, by Relationship to Main Caregiver, Canada, 2007.* Table 13. Retrieved from www.statcan.gc.ca/pub/89503x/2010001/article/11441/tbl/tbl013-eng.htm.

Statistics Canada. (2010). Study: Consequences of Long Distance Caregiving. *The Daily.* Retrieved from www.statcan.gc.ca/daily-quotidien/100126/dq100126a-eng.htm.

Statistics Canada. (2012). *2011 Census of Population: Families, Households, Marital Status, Structural Type of Dwelling, Collectives.* Retrieved from www.statcan.gc.ca/daily-quotidien/120919/dq120919a-eng.htm.

Statistics Canada. (2013a). *Births and Total Fertility Rate, by Province and Territory (Births).* Summary table. Retrieved from http://www.statcan.gc.ca/tables-tableaux/sum-som/l01/cst01/hlth85a-eng.htm.

Statistics Canada. (2013b). *Women in Canada: A Gender-Based Statistical Report.* Ottawa: Statistics Canada. Retrieved from www.statcan.gc.ca/pub/89-503-x/89-503-x2010001-eng.htm.

Statistics Canada. (2013c). Average Income after Tax by Economic Family Types (2007 to 2011). Retrieved from www.statcan.gc.ca/tables-tableaux/sum-som/l01/cst01/famil21a-eng.htm.

Statistics Canada. (2014, September 24). Study: Young Canadians Providing Care, 2012. *The Daily.* Retrieved from www.statcan.gc.ca/daily-quotidien/140924/dq140924a-eng.htm.

United Nations Development Programme (UNDP). (2010). *Human Development Report 2010. 20th Anniversary Edition. The Real Wealth of Nations: Pathways to Human Development.* New York: Palgrave Macmillan.

United Nations Joint Programme on HIV/AIDS and the United Development Fund for Women. (2008). *Caregiving in the Context of HIV/AIDS.* Paper prepared for the CSW Expert Group Meeting, United Nations Economic Commission for Europe, Geneva, 6–9 October.

Vosko, L. (Ed.). (2006). *Precarious Employment: Understanding Labour Market Insecurity in Canada.* Montreal & Kingston: McGill-Queen's University Press.

Further Reading

Keefe, J. (2011). *Supporting Caregivers and Caregiving in an Aging Canada*. Montreal: Institute for Research on Public Policy.

Lilly, M. B., A. Laporte, & P. C. Coyte. (2010). Do They Care Too Much to Work? The Influence of Caregiving Intensity on the Labour Force Participation of Unpaid Caregivers. *Canadian Journal of Health Economics* 29(6): 895–903.

Benoit, C., & H. Hallgrimsdóttir. (Eds.). (2011). *Valuing Care Work: Comparative Perspectives*. Toronto: University of Toronto Press.

Spencer, S., et al. (2010). *The Role of Migrant Care Workers in Aging Societies: Report on Research Findings in the United Kingdom, Ireland, Canada, and the United States*. Geneva: International Organization for Migration.

Relevant Websites

Maritime Data Centre for Aging Research and Policy Analysis: www.msvu.ca/en/home/programsdepartments

Pan American Health Organization: women as caregivers: www.paho.org/

World Health Organization: www.who.int/en/

CHAPTER 14

Where Policy Meets the Nursing Front Line

Linda Silas and Carol Reichert

Introduction

The Canadian Federation of Nurses Unions (CFNU) represents close to 200,000 Canadian nurses (registered nurses [RNs], licensed practical nurses [LPNs], and registered psychiatric nurses [RPNs]) and student nurses working in hospitals and long-term care facilities within communities or in patients' homes in eight provinces (the exceptions are Quebec and British Columbia). Our members are first-hand witnesses to the impacts of short staffing: stress in the workplace, absenteeism, injury, burnout, and staff turnover.

This chapter will examine the human resource needs of a health care system from the perspective of front-line nurses who provide direct care in Canadian health care settings on a 24/7 basis. It will consider the issues nurses face on a daily basis and how these challenges impact the health of patients and nurses. It will then detail the role nurses' unions are playing in protecting both health care providers and their patients.

Introduction

In January 2014, the CFNU attended the Canadian Nursing Students' Association annual conference, where we listened to young student nurses talk about their concerns about the future. What we heard repeatedly was that students were afraid they would not get jobs in nursing within their struggling provincial economies; they were concerned about the shift of resources away from the delivery of care and they were worried about the workplace itself. Their fears are justified. Many of their friends who had graduated found few permanent full-time jobs, and took temporary or part-time work. The stress of excessive overtime and heavy workloads were already taking their toll. Some had also experienced the effects of workplace bullying, a symptom of the current state of the nursing workplace. In Canada, 40 percent of workers have experienced bullying on a weekly basis (CIHR, 2012). The evidence suggests that bullying is more prevalent in nursing than in other areas of the health care sector (Sandercock & Butt, 2012).

Although over 11,000 registered nurses (RNs) graduated in 2012 (CASN, 2013), it still takes a full four years from graduation for RN graduates to reach the average RN full-time employment rate (CIHI, 2014a, p. 5). Meanwhile, many of the RNs, who make up the majority of the nursing workforce, are on the cusp of retirement. The number of RNs age 60 and older more than doubled between 2003 and 2013. In 2003, 17,871 RNs in Canada were age 60 and older; by 2013, that number had reached 40,625 (CIHI, 2014a, p. 9).

Gaining a full and accurate picture of the nursing workforce, which would account for both new graduates and retirement trends, is difficult. A 2014 review of human resource

Box 14.1

Canada's Nurses

- In 2013, 375,768 Canadians were employed as regulated nurses (CIHI, 2014b, Table 4); over 90 percent were women (CIHI, 2014b, tables 9, 22, 31, 45). Compared to physicians, who have seen a dramatic shift from a predominantly male workforce—women now comprise almost 40 percent of physicians, and the majority in some specialities—nursing remains a field largely dominated by women. The seismic shift in physician gender is most apparent when age groups are considered: women comprise the majority of physicians in the youngest age group (Canadian Medical Association, 2014).
- In 2013, there were 276,914 registered nurses (RNs) in the regulated nursing workforce in Canada, accounting for almost three-quarters of Canada's regulated nurses (CIHI, 2014b, Table 6). Another quarter (93,585) were licensed practical nurses (LPNs) (CIHI, 2014b, Table 28). The small remainder was comprised of registered psychiatric nurses (RPNs).
- In 2013, there were 3,477 nurse practitioners (NPs) in the nursing workforce (CIHI, 2014b, Table 20); the supply of NPs grew by 15.7 percent between 2009 and 2013 (CIHI, 2014a, p. 4).
- Most of Canada's regulated nurses provide direct patient care. About 60 percent of Canada's nurses work in hospitals (CIHI, 2014b, tables 13, 26, 35, and 49) and RNs represent the majority of this workforce (CIHI, 2014b, Table 13). Just below 50 percent of LPNs are employed in hospitals (CIHI, 2014b, Table 35); between 2012 and 2013 this percentage increased by 5 percent.
- The average age of RNs was 45.1, of LPNs it was 42.3, and of RPNs it was 47.2 years (CIHI, 2014b, tables 10, 32, and 46). More than 25 percent of RNs, who make up the majority of the workforce, are 55 or older (CIHI, 2014b, Table 11).

planning commissioned by the CFNU found an absence of pertinent, quantified data on the nursing workforce (Janowitz, 2014).

Drawing on the recommendations of the Canadian Nursing Advisory Committee, the CFNU advocates for a 70 percent full-time employment rate (Canadian Nursing Advisory Committee, 2002, p. 16), with additional hires to make up for the shortfall of nurses on units, which leads to staffing inefficiencies (excessive overtime, absenteeism) on wards across the country. In addition to ensuring greater continuity in terms of patient care, a higher proportion of full-time nurses is associated with lower nurse turnover rates (CNA, 2009), allowing for a stable cohesive workforce, improved collaborative teamwork, and better work-life balance. As workforce restructuring increasingly shifts care from front-line nurses to other providers (such as health care aides, who have significantly less formal training), and graduate nurses find themselves marginalized with few new jobs or casual/part-time positions, the CFNU has called for a moratorium on workforce restructuring, as well as the introduction of new graduate initiatives designed to secure the retention of new graduate classes.

The Nursing Workforce

As of 2013, there were over 375,000 regulated nurses employed in Canada. Nurses make up a third of the health care workforce. They are overwhelmingly female and are in every health care setting—from hospitals to community care settings, to caring for patients in their homes or in long-term care facilities—although approximately six in 10 nurses still work in the hospital sector. Most public sector nurses are members of unions (87 percent) (Informetrica Ltd., 2013), and this rate is almost three times that of the general population (Galarneau & Sohn, 2013).

Over 90 percent of the nursing supply are employed in nursing; the majority have permanent employment. Of those employed in nursing, over 87 percent reported regular full-time or part-time employment (CIHI, 2014b, Table 4). The RN full-time employment rate (58.4 percent; CIHI, 2014b, Table 12) is significantly higher than that of the LPN full-time employment rate (48.8 percent; CIHI, 2014b, Table 34). However, the overall Canadian figures mask significant provincial variability. While Newfoundland and Labrador has had an RN full-time employment rate above 70 percent for a number of years, the western provinces (with the exception of Saskatchewan) have full-time employment rates below 50 percent (CIHI, 2014b, Table 12). British Columbia also shows a trend toward the hiring of casual employees, both among RNs and LPNs (CIHI, 2014b, Table 12, p. 34).

Overall, the nursing workforce is aging. Over 25 percent of all RNs are 55 or older, on the cusp of retirement. Again, this figure hides provincial variability. Among RNs in some provinces, the figure is closer to 30 percent (CIHI, 2014b, Table 11). Of course, for LPNs the picture is very different. LPNs are generally younger. In 2013, the number of LPNs younger than 40 outnumbered those age 60 and older by more than 5.5 to 1 (CIHI, 2014b, Table 33).

	% Full-Time	% Part-Time	% 55 or Older	Hospital	Community Health	LTC
Canada	58.4	29.8	25.9	62.0	15.2	9.2
Newfoundland and Labrador	72.4	13.5	16.0	67.3	13.6	8.1
PEI	53.0	33.7	30.2	58.6	4.1	14.1
Nova Scotia	64.4	23.9	29.8	65.3	12.4	12.2
New Brunswick	64.8	25.1	24.2	66.6	13.5	10.4
Quebec	59.0	32.1	20.1	56.7	11.6	11.3
Ontario	66.8	25.9	29.5	63.5	17.1	8.2
Manitoba	46.9	44.8	27.7	60.8	16.2	11.6
Saskatchewan	59.4	26.9	27.0	59.1	18.4	10.9
Alberta	40.5	45.5	25.1	63.5	16.5	6.6
BC	48.0	22.7	28.8	67.3	16.2	7.3

TABLE 14.1: National and Provincial Data by Selected Characteristics, RNs, 2013

Source: CIHI, 2014b, *Regulated Nurses, 2013: Data Tables*, tables 11, 12, 13. Retrieved from https://secure.cihi.ca/estore/productFamily.htm?locale=en&pf=PFC2646&lang=en.

	% Full-Time	% Part-Time	% 55 or Older	Hospital	Community Health	LTC
Canada	48.8	37.3	18.4	49.8	11.5	31.0
Newfoundland and Labrador	65.0	4.2	14.0	41.3	4.2	52.9
PEI	49.1	38.9	28.3	49.8	15.3	32.7
Nova Scotia	52.2	26.6	22.7	49.9	13.9	34.3
New Brunswick	54.4	32.7	19.2	53.4	5.5	39.6
Quebec	39.7	49.8	12.8	68.1	1.5	14.4
Ontario	56.8	34.6	21.8	42.3	14.7	37.5
Manitoba	34.1	51.5	28.2	38.7	14.1	42.5
Saskatchewan	53.3	27.8	18.8	59.0	21.8	18.2
Alberta	43.2	42.8	18.6	44.4	26.3	25.7
BC	43.6	24.0	15.7	39.9	8.9	43.6

TABLE 14.2: National and Provincial Data by Selected Characteristics, LPNs, 2013

Source: CIHI, 2014b, *Regulated Nurses, 2013: Data Tables*, tables 33, 34, 35. Retrieved from https://secure.cihi.ca/estore/productFamily.htm?locale=en&pf=PFC2646&lang=en.

This finding is borne out by the inflow/outflow statistics for the nursing workforce. While the supply of RNs entering and leaving the profession was relatively flat with the outflow rate slowly increasing since 2009, the percentage of LPNs entering the profession in 2013 was almost double the outflow rate indicated in 2012, resulting from a sharp rise in the number of new LPN graduates (CIHI, 2014b, Table 5). Between 2009 and 2013, average annual growth rates in the supply of LPNs were 5.7 percent for LPNs, compared to 1 percent for RNs/NPs combined (CIHI, 2014c, p. 9). Although the number of NPs in the workforce remains relatively small, the NP supply has increased dramatically over the past five years.

As noted, despite the emphasis by several provincial governments on a shift away from the hospital sector to home, community, and long-term care, the majority of RNs continue to work in a hospital setting. LPNs are more likely to be found in the community or long-term care sector; in British Columbia, Alberta, Manitoba, Ontario, and Newfoundland and Labrador, the majority of LPNs work in community or long-term care rather than in a hospital setting (CIHI, 2014b, Table 35). Nevertheless, nationally the percentage of LPNs working in hospitals grew between 2012 and 2013 by 5 percent.

Work Environment and the Health of Nurses

Nurses are the backbone of the Canadian health care system, but nurses are more stressed, injured, or sick, and work more overtime on a regular basis than most other Canadian workers. As nurses find themselves isolated, especially within community or long-term care settings, workplace violence and workplace mental health issues are emerging as priority occupational health and safety issues. Ironically, health care workers experience one of the least healthy workplaces.

Nurses have seen a significant increase in workloads as a result of health care restructuring due to fiscal constraints and budget cuts. This trend has occurred as the Canadian population continues to age, resulting in a growing demographic living with chronic illness. Hospitals and facilities faced with a budget crunch prioritize the most acute patients for admission. In-patient hospital stays are also shortened with care transferred to out-patient and community settings, ultimately leading to a rise in the level of acuity of residents in long-term care facilities. Concurrently, nurse staffing has been reduced as have nursing management, support staff, and ancillary services. Staff mix has been diluted with the hiring of health care aides, with less formal training, to replace RNs/LPNs as workforce restructuring has occurred. In short, fewer nurses are looking after sicker patients while nursing responsibilities and accountabilities have increased. To keep budgets in check, the strategy is often to overuse the available nurses, requiring overtime and extra shifts.

As CFNU's publication *Valuing Patient Safety: Responsible Workforce Design* describes in case studies of workforce restructuring in Australia, New Zealand, the United Kingdom, the United States, and Canada, if this trend continues, patient safety will suffer (MacPhee,

2014). Numerous studies have shown that there is a link between excessive workloads and increased patient mortality (Needleman, Buerhaus, Mattke, Stewart, & Zelevinsky, 2001; Aiken, Clarke, Sloane, Sochalski, & Silber, 2002; Aiken et al., 2014).

Overtime, as CFNU's 2013 report on overtime and absenteeism details, is costly both in human and financial terms. Excessive workloads and overtime contribute to burnout and to a potential decline in nurses' health. In 2012, an average of almost 19,000 public sector nurses were absent on a weekly basis due to their own illness or disability at an estimated cost of $734.3 million. Absenteeism rates for the provinces varied between 5 percent and 10 percent with overtime rates of 20 percent to 35 percent. Overtime is also financially costly. In 2012, nurses worked over 21.5 million hours of overtime, the equivalent of almost 12,000 full-time jobs, at an estimated cost of $952.5 million annually. New graduates are deprived of potential full-time jobs, and overtime costs the health care system almost $1 billion per year (Informetrica Ltd., 2013). Such staffing inefficiencies need to be mitigated through proper health human resources planning.

Between 2000 and 2006, there were 10 major national reports published in Canada that addressed health human resource planning and the major challenges facing front-line nursing. Among the issues identified: frequent interruptions, role confusion, limited technical and human support, lack of integration and coordination, and ever-increasing patient acuity, as well as overwork. Two decades of research show that nursing workload and quality practice environments have a direct, measurable impact on patient health outcomes with implications for patient and provider safety (Berry & Curry, 2012).

Most recently, a comprehensive study published in *The Lancet*, conducted in 300 hospitals in nine European countries, reiterated the message that an increase in nurses' workloads increased the likelihood of in-patient deaths. The same study found that a rise in the number of nurses with a bachelor's degree was associated with a decrease in hospital deaths (Aiken et al., 2014).

The effects on patient safety are evident in the National Health Service (NHS), England, where workforce redesign began over a decade ago with the elimination of LPNs and the replacement of RNs with care aides. These cuts, focused solely on budgetary constraints, led to substandard care, patient neglect, and high patient mortality rates, which were revealed in a high-profile public inquiry into the Mid Staffordshire NHS Foundation Trust. The public inquiry's final report, dubbed the *Francis Report*, serves as a wake-up call for Canadians (Francis, 2013). The report—along with two related studies in response to its findings (Keogh, 2013; Berwick, 2013)—identifies the need for clear staffing requirements and professional standards, and proposes tools to assess the needs of patients to match them to staffing decisions. Taken together, the reports highlight the need for better data on outcomes, adverse events, care delivery, and staff mix to inform future decisions about patient care.

Increases in workload and inadequate staffing also have implications for provider safety. Violence is endemic in the health care workplace. Nurses are more likely than prison guards or police to be assaulted on the job. WorkSafeBC reports that approximately 40 percent of all violence-related claims come from health care workers even though they make up less than

5 percent of the total BC workforce (WorkSafeBC, 2005, p. 8), and violence-related lost-time claims among health care workers are 11 times those for public administration (which includes law enforcement) (WorkSafeBC, 2009). In Manitoba, where the government has recently introduced a workplace violence-prevention program, 56 percent of Manitoba's nurses report being physically assaulted, and more than 9,000 have been verbally abused (MNU, n.d.). The situation with respect to nurses' health is similar across Canada: according to the Association of Workers' Compensation Boards of Canada, the health and social services sector has the highest rate of lost-time injuries in Canada (AWCBC, 2013). Depending on the definition of violence—if it is inclusive of physical, verbal, and emotional abuse—as well as the time frame and sectors studied, "studies have reported a wide range of incidence rates of workplace violence, between 20%-90%," despite the fact that underreporting is common since many nurses are hesitant to report incidents (Wang, Hayes, & O'Brien-Pallas, 2008, p. 3).

Working conditions in home care are also difficult and exacerbated by increased outsourcing and the pressures of competitive bidding. Most organizations keep a small staff and bring in nurses, as needed, limiting the continuity of care for patients. Nurses who work outside of hospitals tend to earn less than their colleagues employed in a hospital setting. In general, their benefits packages are also lower. Nurses in long-term care institutions face high patient workloads, and increasingly the residents have complex health care needs with multiple co-morbidities. A study comparing the situations for Canadian long-term care workers with

	Absenteeism Rate (%)	Overtime Rate (%)	Union Members (%)
Canada	7.5	28.8	87
Newfoundland and Labrador	8.4	21.7	92
PEI	—	26.4	90
Nova Scotia	8.0	25.6	88
New Brunswick	10.1	23.5	92
Quebec	6.7	35.3	91
Ontario	6.8	26.2	79
Manitoba	10.0	27.9	93
Saskatchewan	5.5	30.7	93
Alberta	7.5	30.9	86
BC	9.1	25.7	93

TABLE 14.3: Provincial Public Sector Health Care Nurses, Rates of Overtime, Absenteeism, Unionization, 2012

Source: Data from Informetrica Ltd., 2013, *Trends in Own Illness or Disability-Related Absenteeism and Overtime among Publicly-Employed Registered Nurses—Quick Facts*. Report prepared for CFNU. Retrieved from https://nursesunions.ca/report-study/absenteeism-and-overtime.

that of selected Nordic countries found that Canadian long-term care workers, 43 percent of whom report actual violence "more or less everyday," "are nearly seven times more likely to experience daily violence than workers in Nordic countries" (Banerjee et al., 2008, p. 8).

Retention and Recruitment

Deteriorating working conditions ultimately affect job satisfaction and the quality of patient care. Many nurses leave the profession because they are unable to reconcile accepting larger patient caseloads while still maintaining their own health and providing quality care to ensure patient safety. The ability of an organization to retain staff is strongly linked to job satisfaction and better health outcomes for patients.

Unfortunately, in many workplaces, the emphasis has been on short-term planning, with an eye on the bottom line. Financial administrators view nurses as an expense rather than a critical component in patient care. They also fail to take into account the overall costs of turnover, nurse training, and preventable patient safety incidents, adverse events, or readmissions. Institutions that experience high rates of turnover as a result of job dissatisfaction have higher costs per discharge, increased lengths of patient stays, and higher rates of undesirable outcomes (Curtin, 2003). One study commissioned by the Canadian Patient Safety Institute (CPSI) found that globally adverse events account for "at least one dollar in every seven dollars spent on hospital care" (Jackson, 2009, p. 2). In Canada, the CPSI reports that preventable patient safety incidents account for an estimated \$397 million on an annual basis (CPSI, 2012). The economic argument is clear: the cost of appropriate nurse staffing based on a formal real-time needs assessment of patients on a ward-by-ward basis could be largely recouped through a reduction in the number of adverse events.

Given the current demographics, many RNs will be eligible for retirement over the next five years, raising concern about Canada's lack of a health human resources planning. The data suggest that nurses may be delaying retirement, and a recent U.S. study confirms this may be the reality across North America (Rand Health, 2014). However, without sufficient Canadian data, it is unknown whether this is a long-term trend or merely a response to the current economic uncertainty. Retaining new graduates also presents a challenge. Despite the fact that more than 10,000 new RNs are graduating each year, many are not finding permanent, full-time employment (CASN, 2013; CIHI, 2014a), and even among those who do, many may leave the nursing workforce due to the stressful workplace environment. Overall nursing turnover rates are 20 percent, at an average cost of \$25,000 per nurse (with much higher costs for critical care areas) (CNA, 2009), but for new graduates these numbers are much higher. Cho, Laschinger, and Wong (2006) found that 66 percent of new graduates were experiencing severe burnout, and that burnout was associated with negative workplace conditions. Another report identified an actual turnover rate for new graduates of 30 percent in the first year and 57 percent after two years. These results are alarming since the future of professional nursing depends on finding ways to create high-quality work environments that retain newcomers to the profession (as cited in Laschinger, Finegan, & Wilk, 2009).

A 2009 study on intergenerational diversity found that younger nurses have different expectations and attitudes toward the workplace than the generation that preceded them. They place a greater emphasis on work-life balance, expect greater control over their hours of work and overtime, want greater levels of autonomy, and respond well to mentoring initiatives. The report concludes that retaining younger nurses may mean adopting workplace strategies to take into account the needs of all four generations currently in the nursing workforce (Wortsman & Crupi, 2009).

The report *Valuing Patient Safety: Responsible Workforce Design*, which focuses on recommendations to ensure patient safety by providing appropriate staffing based on patient needs, also considers the role of workplace environments in recruitment and retention. It recommends that health care organizations and their leadership strive for Magnet-like work environments for best possible quality, safe care delivery. Magnet-like environments are known for effective nursing leadership at all levels of the organization, collaborative teamwork, staffing adequacy, effective communications, and nurse control over practice. Magnet hospitals go through a rigorous accreditation process to attain their status and are known to attract and retain nurses, have greater nurse job satisfaction, lower nurse burnout, and better patient outcomes (MacPhee, 2014, p. 17).

The challenge of retention and recruitment may be even greater in community and long-term care, where pay rates and benefits are less generous, and the workplace may be subject to the whims of the marketplace, making the workplace less attractive to health care workers. Underwood and Mowat (2010) note that the "move to community health requires careful human resources planning to ensure adequate skilled staff are available to deliver services and are used to their full potential" (p. 1). Their report focuses on how to retain community health nurses: "Community health nursing needs to be seen as a desirable and fulfilling career to continue to attract and keep nurses and to meet the growing demand for community-based care" (Underwood & Mowat, 2010, p. 1). Long-term care faces a similar question: How can it be promoted as a rewarding career specialty (Long-Term Care Task Force on Resident Care and Safety [Ontario], 2012)? The evidence suggests that in Canada, "Despite shrinkage in the hospital sub-sectors, hospitals remained highly sticky. The expanding sub-sectors, in general, appear relatively unattractive to nurses" (Alameddine et al., 2006, p. 2310). "It is likely to remain difficult to recruit and retain competent direct care workers . . . because of the negative industry image, non-competitive wages and benefits, a challenging work environment, and inadequate education and training" (Stone & Bryant, 2012, p. 188).

Given these ongoing challenges, a long-term national health human resources plan needs to be developed that includes a more equitable and efficient distribution of nurses, support for the current workforce through safe staffing and safer workplace measures to protect patient safety, and initiatives that ensure permanent stable employment for new graduates.

Box 14.2

Nurse Staffing and Retention

- Average turnover rate = 20 percent
- Turnover rates in intensive-care units = 26.7 percent
- Cost of turnover per nurse = $25,000
- Turnover rate for new graduates in their first year = 30 percent
- Turnover rate for new graduates in their second year = 57 percent
- Each 10 percent increase in turnover = 38 percent more medical errors

Sources: Data as cited in Laschinger, Finegan, Wilk (2009); O'Brien-Pallas, Murphy, Shamian (2009); CNA (2009).

Box 14.3

Workplace Challenges Facing Nurses

Research confirms that nursing today presents many challenges including:

- heavy workloads;
- excessive overtime;
- unpredictable and inflexible scheduling;
- health and safety issues, including violence and bullying;
- security concerns;
- inadequate support from management;
- role blurring due to scope of practice issues;
- lack of opportunities for leadership and professional development; and
- lack of meaningful engagement of direct-care nurses in decision-making processes that directly impact their work and patient safety.

Role of Nurses' Unions

Nurses' unions have a central and vital role to play. While there has been a decline in unionization rates in the overall workforce, more than 80 percent of nurses are members of a union. Unions provide a vehicle for women to address issues affecting both their home and work lives, including access to child care, pay equity, and the elimination of sexual harassment. Nurses' unions continue to advocate for these issues, but with an increasing focus on improving working conditions, improving nurse-patient ratios, ensuring that the staff mix meets the identified needs of patients, and ensuring the workplace is safe and secure.

Nurses' unions are concerned that governments and employers continue to be reluctant to implement the program and policy recommendations resulting from evidence-based research. Despite the extensive research that shows there is a correlation between work environments and good health care, there continues to be a gap between the recognition of good ideas and their implementation in practice. Reducing workloads, improved nurse-patient ratios, appropriate staff mix, and providing a safe and secure workplace are critical to attracting and retaining nurses and safeguarding patient safety.

The Canadian Federation of Nurses Unions and its provincial member organizations have been actively working on ways to address the staff shortfall and staff dilution on wards across the country, as well as stressful working conditions, through a number of initiatives.

Nursing Awareness Campaigns

The CFNU and its provincial affiliates have several active campaigns to raise public awareness about the health care system and the role of nurses. Among these campaigns' goals are:

- to raise the profile of nurses' role in health care by educating the public about research that shows the essential role and knowledge of nurses and their critical decision-making skills;
- to ensure that nurses guide health care practices to help raise the standard of patient care across Canada;
- to articulate nurses' common identity through educating the public, other health care providers, health care administrators, and decision-makers about what nurses contribute to the health care system on a daily basis; and
- to articulate nurses' common identity through visual identifiers and/or by encouraging nurses to proactively identify themselves as nurses.

A number of nurses' unions have launched campaigns to renew and reinforce the common sense of identity of nurses through creating a common professional visual image—for example, through standardized uniforms or pins, so that nurses are distinguished from other health care staff.

Improvements through Collective Bargaining and Legislation

Unions have traditionally used collective bargaining as a means to improve the working lives of their members. The collective-bargaining process now addresses issues that range far beyond wages and benefits, such as workplace health and safety, workload measures, staff mix, and alternative work arrangements. Collective agreements include articles on flexible staffing and scheduling, parental and education leave, measures to reduce violence in the workplace, mentoring, full-time and part-time ratios, and ways to increase professional development and training.

Nurses' unions are routinely bringing workload issues into contract negotiations. Many provinces' collective agreements provide legal mechanisms for nurses to address staffing issues, workload, and professional practice through filing workload situation reports and through independent assessment committees (IAC) to review RN concerns. In Ontario, the latest contract creates a workload/professional responsibility review tool, which mandates the employer to disclose all relevant information and base any subsequent recommendations on this information in areas where improper workload assignment forms are completed (ONA, 2014).

In Nova Scotia, insufficient staffing can be addressed directly through a clinical capacity report filled out by an RN or LPN who believes that patient safety is affected by staffing levels, including the failure to replace scheduled staff with similarly qualified staff. This new approach goes beyond the traditional work situation report because it includes patient acuity measures, clearer timelines, and a mandate to go higher up the institutional ladder (MacPhee, 2014).

As in Ontario and Nova Scotia, nurses can fill in workload situation reports, but RNs in Saskatchewan can also document situations that prevent them from carrying out the highest-quality, expert care for patients. Workload issues in Saskatchewan can then end up before an independent assessment committee, but uniquely, in Saskatchewan the IAC's decisions are binding insofar as they relate to nurse workload concerns (MacPhee, 2014).

Similar language and processes to report unsafe staffing and unsafe working conditions can be found in provincial collective agreements in other Canadian provinces.

Nurses' unions have also been instrumental in shaping provincial legislation. All provinces have occupational health and safety laws that provide varying levels of protection to workers from unsafe work. The Manitoba Nurses Union recently convinced their government to introduce a Violence Prevention Program, with strict new regulations to protect nurses and other health care workers (MNU, n.d.). In Ontario, The Excellent Care for All Act was the first of its kind in Canada to statutorily require research and evidence to inform health care planning (MacPhee, 2014).

Improvements through Research and Policy

In December 2013, the CFNU partnered with the Canadian Nurses Association, Accreditation Canada, and the Canadian Patient Safety Institute to hold a pan-Canadian roundtable with four principle objectives:

1. Identify enablers of quality and safety in patient care.
2. Discuss and better understand the reported realities of health care workplaces and the contributing factors identified through the Accreditation Canada (AC) work life standards.

3. Achieve consensus on key priorities for improving quality and safety in patient care.
4. Develop a framework and action strategies for a pan-Canadian action plan to achieve improved quality and safety in patient care, and define the roles of nurses in this plan.

The roundtable resulted in four key priorities:

1. Empower patients and the public through education and supports that are the key enablers of quality and safety.
2. Support nursing students and nurses.
3. Promote evidence-based staffing practices.
4. Promote strong nursing leadership.

The result was the CNA/CFNU Joint Initiative *Quality and Safety in Patient Care: Summary of Pan Canadian Roundtable* (CNA & CFNU, 2014). In response to this, CNA and the CFNU developed a concept proposal for an evidence-based Safe Staffing Toolkit comprised of several online modules. Both boards have endorsed this proposal, and a full project plan is being developed. The first module will present information about evidence-based staffing.

Innovative Workplace Practices

The CFNU, the federation that represents provincial nursing unions, and the CFNU affiliates, have expressed concern that there are inadequate and unsafe staffing levels in Canada's hospitals and that employers are trying to save money by diluting the staff mix of our workforce.

Despite extensive research showing the correlation between healthy work environments and good health care, a gap exists between the recognition of good ideas in research and policy and their implementation. How do we move from promise to practice to improve health workplaces for both health care workers and their patients?

In an effort to make the link, in 2008–2009, CFNU's Research to Action (RTA, 2011) Project funded by Health Canada ran 10 provincial pilots in which nurses implemented specific activities (e.g., mentoring, leadership, and orientation). The resulting evaluation revealed a 10 percent reduction in overtime, absenteeism, and turnover costs, and a 147 percent increase in the number of nurses reporting a high level of leadership and support (CFNU, 2011).

One RTA initiative in Winnipeg, Manitoba, was so successful that it has since been widely replicated. Recognizing that pressure on the long-term care (LTC) sector is growing with the aging demographic, and that it is often difficult to retain and recruit nurses in this sector, the Winnipeg Regional Health Authority (WRHA), Manitoba Health, and Manitoba Nurses Union piloted a project entitled Enhanced Orientation for Nurses New to Long-Term Care. The project involved the introduction of a mentorship program and a series of six clinical workshops designed to provide nurses in long-term care with the supports needed to excel in their work, to develop greater leadership capacity, to better serve residents' needs, and to become more satisfied with their work. The response to both initiatives was extremely positive (Research to Action, 2011).

The CFNU believes that nurses need to stand united and be recognized for our leadership in health care. In 2014, we still lag behind in terms of our impacts on budgets, safe staffing, or positioning ourselves as important players within the health care system. Why this failure to recognize nurses' leadership? The lack of a united voice and a united sense of identity within the many organizations representing nurses remains an ongoing obstacle. Canada's nurses' unions are asking: How can we create a better understanding of the nurses' role and value to our health care system? Renewing and reinforcing our common sense of identity as nurses is a priority for our nurses' unions.

One aspect of identity is creating a common professional visual image so that nurses are distinguished from other health care staff. Recently, a number of nurses' unions have negotiated the use of distinctive uniforms to stand out from other workers. For example, in Nova Scotia and Newfoundland and Labrador their contracts now contain language identifying the standardized uniform for nurses to distinguish them from other workers. In Saskatchewan and in Alberta (on Wear White Wednesdays) nurses are encouraged to wear the traditional white top to assert their professional presence.

Returning to the traditional "branded" image of nurses is a way of raising awareness among the public, other health care workers, and health care administrators about both the role and the numbers of nurses in hospitals and other health care institutions. Nurses report that they feel proud wearing their uniforms, which identify them as registered nurses, licensed practical nurses, registered psychiatric nurses, or nurse practitioners. The campaign has also met with a favourable reaction from patients, families, and other health care professionals, with many patients now proactively requesting nurses. This effort to make nurses more visible has also highlighted how few nurses are actually present on hospital wards, raising the question of patient safety.

Unions from coast to coast are designing campaigns to educate the public, other health care professionals, and health care administrators about the unique contributions nurses make to our health care system. In eastern Canada, the Newfoundland and Labrador Nurses' Union designed The Clarity Project, which aims to help RNs in the province clarify their common identity by proactively identifying themselves and articulating what they contribute to our health care system. Other Atlantic Canada nurses' unions, such as the Nova Scotia Nurses' Union's Nursing Led by Nurses campaign and the PEI Nurses' Union's RNs Invaluable/Irreplaceable Leaders in Health Care campaign, aim to assert the role of practising nurses to guide health care practices and raise the standard of patient care across Canada through their essential knowledge and critical decision-making skills.

New Brunswick Nurses Union RN Campaign's message, "There is no substitute for an RN," addresses directly the issue of RNs replacement on hospital wards. In central Canada, the Ontario Nurses' Association led a successful More Nurses campaign in 2014, calling for more RNs, highlighting the fact that Ontario has the second-lowest provincial ratio of RNs-to-population and that despite this, it continues with RN cuts to administrators and front-line workers. The wealth of research that shows how essential nurses are to patient safety and health outcomes is showcased by the Saskatchewan Union of Nurses' Making the Difference campaign. In Alberta, an education campaign about the need for more nurses formed part of the union's collective bargaining efforts.

To exert influence, nurses must be one voice, conveying confidence and pride in their identity, and educating others about their essential contributions to our health care system so that the public, employers, other health care professionals, and decision-makers will develop a greater understanding and appreciation for nurses and what they bring to our health care system on a daily basis as direct care providers on the front line.

More information about Canadian nurses' unions' campaigns can be found at the union websites listed at the end of the chapter.

Conclusion

Increased workloads, excessive overtime hours, illness- and injury-related absenteeism have negative consequences for the health care system, patients, nurses, and their families. The welfare of patients and that of providers are closely linked. Safe and appropriate nurse staffing is critical to patient health, safety, and well-being since nurses deliver more individual health care than any other health care provider. There are many examples of innovative projects underway that have produced positive changes for front-line nurses in workplaces across Canada. Yet, we are a nation of pilot projects. Once the pilot project ends, often it dies, no matter how successful it may have been, and too often the final report is relegated to the bookshelf. The challenge is to ensure that successful pilots become practices permanently embedded into the health care system.

The provincial unions that make up the CFNU have considerable expertise in health care and workplace issues and, as such, understand the reality and challenges of health human resources planning. With more manageable workloads, better staffing ratios, and increased support from employers, managers, and decision-makers, there will be decreased overtime, absenteeism, injury, and burnout, and this will translate into better retention and facilitate recruitment. A healthier workplace will pay dividends for government and employers in improved quality of patient care and a more sustainable workforce. As a representative of the front line of health care, the Canadian Federation of Nurses Unions' message to the premiers, who make up the Council of the Federation's Health Care Innovation Working Group, calls for a united front to do the following:

1. Oppose the federal government's continued erosion of health care funding to the provinces which has—and will continue—to result in negative health outcomes for all Canadians, ultimately leading to a dramatic loss of nurses for our treasured national health care system.
2. Develop a long-term national health human resources (HHR) plan that includes a more equitable and efficient distribution of nurses, support for the current workforce through safe staffing, safer workplace measures to safeguard patient safety, and initiatives that ensure permanent stable employment for new graduates.
3. Support and improve front-line patient care in all sectors of our health system by basing direct staffing decisions on patient needs, best practices, and evidence-based research rather than focusing solely on short-term measures such as ill-conceived budget cuts.
4. Encourage nurse-led innovations within the public system, and include front-line nurses as partners in discussions on system design and innovation, in order to facilitate the successful implementation of long-term, effective solutions.
5. Call for the development and implementation of innovative federal programs, such as a national pharmacare program in this country; this measure alone could save over $11 billion annually (Gagnon, 2014), savings that could then be reinvested in our health care system.

References

Aiken, L. H., S. Clarke, D. Sloane, J. Sochalski, & J. Silber. (2002). Hospital Nurse Staffing and Patient Mortality, Nurse Burnout, and Job Dissatisfaction. *JAMA* 288(16): 1987–1993.

Aiken, L. H., et al. (2014). Nurse Staffing and Education and Hospital Mortality in Nine European Countries: A Retrospective Observational Study. *The Lancet.* doi: org/10.1016/S0140-6736(13)62631-8.

Alameddine, M., et al. (2006). "Stickiness" and "Inflow" as Proxy Measures of the Relative Attractiveness of Various Sub-Sectors of Nursing Employment. *Social Science and Medicine* 63(9): 2310–2319.

Association of Workers' Compensation Boards of Canada (AWCBC). (2013). *2012 Injury Statistics.* Retrieved from http://awcbc.org/?page_id=14.

Banerjee, A., et al. (2008). *"Out of Control": Violence against Personal Support Workers in Long-Term Care.* Toronto & Ottawa: York University and Carleton University.

Berry, L., & P. Curry. (2012). *Nursing Workload and Patient Care.* Ottawa: CFNU.

Berwick, D. (2013). *A Promise to Learn—A Commitment to Act: Improving the Safety of Patients in England.* National Advisory Group on the Safety of Patients in England. Retrieved from https://www.gov.uk/government/uploads/system/uploads/attachment_data/file/226703/Berwick_Report.pdf.

Canadian Association of Schools of Nursing (CASN). (2013). *2011–2012 Nursing Education Statistics Report.* Retrieved from https://www.casn.ca/en/Surveys_112/items/15.html.

Canadian Federation of Nurses Unions (CFNU). (2011). *Research to Action. CFNU Backgrounder.* Retrieved from http://nursesunions.ca/sites/default/files/2011.backgrounder.rta_.e.pdf.

Canadian Institute for Health Information (CIHI). (2014a). *Regulated Nurses, 2013: Chartbook.* Retrieved from https://secure.cihi.ca/estore/productFamily.htm?locale=en&pf=PFC2646&lang=en.

Canadian Institute for Health Information (CIHI). (2014b). *Regulated Nurses, 2013: Data Tables.* Retrieved from https://secure.cihi.ca/estore/productFamily.htm?locale=en&pf=PFC2646&lang=en.

Canadian Institute for Health Information (CIHI). (2014c). *Regulated Nurses, 2013: Report.* Retrieved from https://secure.cihi.ca/estore/productFamily.htm?locale=en&pf=PFC2646&lang=en.

Canadian Institutes of Health Research (CIHR). (2012, September 24). *Experts Discuss the Health Consequences of Bullying.* Press release. Retrieved from http://www.cihr-irsc.gc.ca/e/45820.html.

Canadian Medical Association. (2014). Percent Distribution of Physicians by Age, Sex, Province/Territory, Canada. Retrieved from http://www.cma.ca/Assets/assets:library/document/en/advocacy/85AgeSexPrv.pdf.

Canadian Nurses Association (CNA). (2009). *Costs and Implications of Nurse Turnover in Canadian Hospitals.* Retrieved from http://cna-aiic.ca/~/media/cna/page-content/pdf-en/roi_nurse_turnover_2009_e.pdf.

Canadian Nurses Association (CNA) & Canadian Federation of Nurses Unions (CFNU). (2014). *Quality and Safety in Patient Care: Summary of Pan-Canadian Roundtable.* Retrieved from http://cna-aiic.ca/~/media/cna/page-content/pdf-en/quality_and_safety_in_patient_care_roundtable_report_summary_e.pdf.

Canadian Nursing Advisory Committee. (2002). *Our Health, Our Future: Creating Quality Workplaces for Canadian Nurses.* Final Report of the Canadian Nursing Advisory Committee. Retrieved from http://www.hc-sc.gc.ca/hcs-sss/pubs/nurs-infirm/2002-cnac-cccsi-final/index-eng.php.

Canadian Patient Safety Institute (CPSI). (2012). *Economics of Patient Safety.* Retrieved from http://www.patientsafetyinstitute.ca/english/research/commissionedresearch/economicsofpatientsafety/pages/default.aspx.

Cho, J., H. K. Laschinger, & C. Wong (2006). Workplace Empowerment, Work Engagement, and Organizational Commitment of New Graduate Nurses. *Nursing Research* 19(3): 43–60.

Curtin, L. (2003, September 30). An Integrated Analysis of Nurse Staffing and Related Variables: Effects on Patient Outcomes. *Nursing World* 8 (3).

Francis, R. (2013). *Mid Staffordshire NHS Foundation Trust Public Inquiry Final Report.* Retrieved from http://www.midstaffspublicinquiry.com/.

Gagnon, M.-A. (2014). *A Roadmap to a Rational Pharmacare Plan.* Ottawa: CFNU.

Galarneau, D., & T. Sohn. (2013). *Long-Term Trends in Unionization.* Ottawa: Statistics Canada.

Informetrica Ltd. (2013). *Trends in Own Illness or Disability-Related Absenteeism and Overtime among Publicly-Employed Registered Nurses—Quick Facts.* Report prepared for CFNU. Retrieved from https://nursesunions.ca/report-study/absenteeism-and-overtime-quick-facts-2013.

Jackson, T. (2009). *One Dollar in Seven: Scoping the Economics of Patient Safety.* Ottawa: CPSI.

Janowitz, S. (2014). *Nursing Workforce: Retirement and New Graduate Employment Trends.* Unpublished research, CFNU, Ottawa.

Keogh, B. (2013). *Review into the Quality of Care and Treatment Provided by 14 Hospital Trusts in England: Overview Report.* Retrieved from National Health Service England http://www.nhs.uk/nhsengland/bruce-keogh-review/documents/outcomes/keogh-review-final-report.pdf.

Laschinger, H., J. Finegan, & P. Wilk. (2009). *New Graduate Burnout: The Impact of Professional Practice Environment, Workplace Civility, and Empowerment.* Retrieved from http://www.medscape.com/viewarticle/719035.

Long-Term Care Task Force on Resident Care and Safety (Ontario). (2012). *An Action Plan to Address Abuse and Neglect in Long-Term Care Homes: Executive Summary.* Retrieved from http://www.longtermcaretaskforce.ca/.

MacPhee, M. (2014). *Valuing Patient Safety: Responsible Workforce Design.* CFNU. Retrieved from http://nursesunions.ca/news/valuing-patient-safety-responsible-workforce-design.

Manitoba Nurses Union (MNU). (n.d.). *Reducing Workplace Violence.* Retrieved from http://manitobanurses.ca/workplace-priorities/reducing-workplace-violence.html.

Needleman, J., P. I. Buerhaus, S. Mattke, M. Stewart, & K. Zelevinsky. (2001). *Nurse Staffing and Patient Outcomes in Hospitals.* Final Report for Health Resources and Services Administration. Boston: U.S. Department of Health and Human Services.

O'Brien-Pallas, L., G. T. Murphy, & J. Shamian. (2009). *Nurses' Turnover in Canadian Hospitals.* Retrieved from http://www.stti.iupui.edu/pp07/vancouver09/11536.O'Brien-Pallas,%20Linda-I%2002.pdf.

Ontario Nurses' Association (ONA). (2014). *Highlights of the Kaplan Award between ONA and Participating Hospitals.* Retrieved from http://www.ona.org/documents/File/bargaining/ONA_HospitalCentralCollectiveAgreement_HighlightsOfArbitratorAward20140502.pdf.

Rand Health. (2014, July 16). *Registered Nurses' Delayed Retirement Helps to Boost Nursing Supply in the U.S.* Press release. Retrieved from http://www.rand.org/news/press/2014/07/16.html.

Research to Action (RTA). (2011). *Applied Workplace Solutions for Nurses.* Retrieved from http://www.thinknursing.ca/rta.

Sandercock, K., & N. Butt. (2012, February 7). *Presentation on Bullying in the Workplace.* Ontario Nurses Association Teleconnect. Retrieved from http://www.ona.org/documents/File/humanrightsequity/ONA_HRETeleconnect_BullyingWorkplace_20120207.pdf.

Stone, R., & N. Bryant. (2012). The Impact of Health Care Reform on the Workforce Caring for Older Adults. *Journal of Aging & Policy* 24 (2): 188–205.

Underwood, J., & D. Mowat. (2010). *Building Community and Public Health Nursing Capacity.* Ottawa: Canadian Health Services Research Foundation.

Wang, S., L. Hayes, & L. O'Brien-Pallas. (2008). *A Review and Evaluation of Workplace Violence Prevention: Final Report.* Toronto: Nursing Health Services Research Unit.

WorkSafeBC. (2005). *Preventing Violence in Health Care: Five Steps to an Effective Program.* Retrieved from http://www.worksafebc.com/publications/health_and_safety/by_topic/assets/pdf/violhealthcare.pdf.

WorksafeBC. (2009). *Violence in Health Care and Social Assistance in BC: Fact Sheet.* Retrieved from http://www2.worksafebc.com/PDFs/healthcare/fact_sheet_violence.pdf.

Wortsman, A., & A. Crupi. (2009). *From Textbooks to Texting: Addressing Issues of Intergenerational Diversity in the Nursing Workforce.* CFNU. Retrieved from https://nursesunions.ca/report-study/textbooks-texting-addressing-issues-intergenerational-diversity-in-the-nursing-workplac.

Further Reading

Baumann, A., et al. (2001). *Commitment and Care: The Benefits of a Healthy Workplace for Nurses, Their Patients, and the System—a Policy Synthesis*. Ottawa: Canadian Health Services Research Foundation.

Canadian Nurses Association. (2008). *Code of Ethics for Registered Nurses*. Ottawa: Author.

Canadian Nurses Association and Canadian Federation of Nurses Unions. (2006). *Joint Position Statement on Practice Environments: Maximizing Client, Nurse, and System Outcomes*. Retrieved from https://nursesunions.ca/position-statement/practice-environments-maximizing-client-nurse-and-system-outcomes-joint-position-.

Canadian Nurses Association and Canadian Federation of Nurses Unions. (2007). *Joint Position Statement on Workplace Violence*. Retrieved from https://nursesunions.ca/position-statement/workplace-violence-joint-position-statement-cfnucna.

Cho, J., H. K. Laschinger, & C. Wong (2006). Workplace Empowerment, Work Engagement, and Organizational Commitment of New Graduate Nurses. *Nursing Research* 19(3): 43–60.

International Council of Nurses (ICN). (2006). *Abuse and Violence against Nursing Personnel*. Geneva: Author.

Quality Worklife Quality Healthcare Collaborative. (2007). *Within Our Grasp: A Healthy Workplace Action Strategy for Success and Sustainability in Canada's Healthcare System*. Ottawa: Canadian Council on Health Services Accreditation.

Registered Nurses Association of Ontario. (2011). *Healthy Work Environments Best Practice Guidelines: Preventing and Mitigating Nurse Fatigue in Health Care*. Toronto: Author.

Relevant Websites

Canadian Federation of Nurses Unions and Member Affiliates Websites

Canadian Federation of Nurses Unions: www.nursesunions.ca
Manitoba Nurses Union: http://manitobanurses.ca/
New Brunswick Nurses Union: https://www.nbnu.ca
Newfoundland and Labrador Nurses' Union: http://www.nlnu.ca
Nova Scotia Nurses' Union: https://www.nsnu.ca
Ontario Nurses' Association: http://www.ona.org
Prince Edward Island Nurses' Union: http://peinu.com
Saskatchewan Union of Nurses: http://sun-nurses.sk.ca
United Nurses of Alberta: www.una.ab.ca

Other Websites

British Columbia Nurses Union: https://www.bcnu.org/
Canadian Foundation for Healthcare Improvement: http://www.cfhi-fcass.ca
Canadian Nurses Association: http://www.cna-aiic.ca
Fédération Interprofessionnelle de la santé du Québec : http://www.fiqsante.qc.ca
International Council of Nurses: http://www.icn.ch

CHAPTER 15

Midwifery in Ontario: Opportunities for Women's Health Policy Research

Wendy Katherine

Introduction

In the 20 years since Ontario became the first province in Canada to introduce regulated midwives into the health system, we have seen great strides in integration and a tenfold expansion of the profession. It is an opportune time to look at evidence generated about midwifery and to examine opportunities for further research.

Background

Following a ministry review of the Regulated Health Professions Act and an organized consumer lobby for better access to midwifery care, the Government of Ontario proclaimed the Midwifery Act on December 31, 1993, providing the first 70 registered midwives the opportunity to offer funded services to women and families. Many other pieces of coinciding legislation—acts respecting hospitals, care during transport, prescription authority, birth registration, and lab testing—were amended to enable midwives to implement their scope of practice. Ontario established an autonomous College of Midwives to govern the new profession in the public interest and designed a scope of practice that enables midwives to be comprehensive primary care providers for healthy women and newborns.

The Ontario midwifery scope is aligned with the Definition of the Midwife, adopted by the International Confederation of Midwives:

> A midwife is a person who, having been regularly admitted to a midwifery educational programme, duly recognised in the country in which it is located, has successfully completed the prescribed course of studies in midwifery and has acquired the

> requisite qualifications to be registered and/or legally licensed to practice midwifery.
>
> The midwife is recognised as a responsible and accountable professional who works in partnership with women to give the necessary support, care, and advice, during pregnancy, labour, and the postpartum period, to conduct births on the midwife's own responsibility and to provide care for the newborn and the infant. This care includes preventative measures, the promotion of normal birth, the detection of complications in mother and child, the accessing of medical care or other appropriate assistance and the carrying out of emergency measures.
>
> The midwife has an important task in health counselling and education, not only for the woman, but also within the family and the community. This work should involve antenatal education and preparation for parenthood and may extend to women's health, sexual or reproductive health and child care.
>
> A midwife may practice in any setting including the home, community, hospitals clinics, or health units. (International Confederation of Midwives, 2014)

Ontario established a four-year baccalaureate Midwifery Education Program (MEP) by a consortium of three Ontario universities as well as an additional route of entry to practice for midwives prepared in other jurisdictions. Candidates entering midwifery practice through these two routes have combined to increase the number of registered midwives from 70 in 1994 to over 680 in 2013 (Canadian Association of Midwives, 2014). The province also amended the Midwifery Act, effective September 1, 2011, to expand the scope of practice of midwives working in Ontario. Funding for the Ontario Midwifery Program increased from $23.7 million in 2002–2003 to approximately $117.6 million in 2012–2013 (Ontario Midwifery Program, Ministry of Health and Long-Term Care, 2014).

Midwives function as primary maternity care providers within a provincial system in which most births are attended by physician-nurse teams. Midwifery clients typically receive care from uni-professional groups of their chosen care providers, who adapt care to each woman's/infant's needs. Prenatal care is most often delivered in a neighbourhood clinic with each practice group of two to 12 midwives sharing 24-hour, on-call care for between 80 and 400 women (and their infants) per year. While midwives offer clients the choice of either a home or hospital birth setting, approximately 82 percent give birth in hospitals or birth centres (Better Outcomes Registry and Network, 2013–2014), where midwives maintain admitting privileges. Approximately two-thirds of Ontario birthing hospitals have granted admitting privileges to registered midwives, enabling them to function as full partners with other hospital staff. However, the Association of Ontario Midwives reports that in some hospitals, limitations on the number of midwives or on their scope restrict expansion of the profession. Services for women and newborns whose care becomes complicated are obtained as per College of Midwives' protocols by local obstetricians, family physicians, pediatricians, anesthetists, nurse practitioners, nurses, and other health care professionals.

Midwives continue with follow-up care in both the home and hospital settings, providing well-woman and well-newborn care until six weeks postpartum.

In addition to home and hospital births, Ontario established a third setting in the form of three midwifery-led birth centres in Toronto, Ottawa, and Ohsweken, delivering similar care in scope to home births.

Building a Foundation for Midwifery Research

Ontario is fortunate to stand on the foundation of a worldwide movement, led by the World Health Organization (WHO), to support the proliferation of quality, effective, and efficient midwifery services. However, an additional body of provincial evidence on health outcomes naturally follows the introduction of a new health profession. A small but growing number of midwife academics and other scholars looking at the introduction of midwifery in Ontario are contributing scholarship to the current literature pool. As midwifery has expanded, the profession has been understandably focused on education, expansion, and integration in new communities and hospitals. An increasing focus will be on the development of independent research opportunities stimulated by the growing number of midwives with graduate and post-graduate research experience and linkages with academic/tertiary institutions, research sponsors, perinatal partners, and others.

Until 2009, when the Better Outcomes Registry and Network (BORN) was established as Ontario's registry of maternal and child information, lack of a reliable, comprehensive, provincial, clinical outcomes data set contributed to the difficulty in studying provincial maternity care in general. This dramatically changed with the inception of BORN, improving the forecast for analysis, reporting, and research. Researchers into maternity care had primarily studied unlinked databases, including Vital Statistics, the Discharge Abstract Database, or the Ontario Health Insurance Plan database, and conducted original research projects such as the women's health report card. BORN, a partnership between the Niday Perinatal Database, the Ontario Midwifery Program, the Newborn Screening and Prenatal Screening Ontario, and the Fetal Alert Network yielded, in 2005–2006, the first provincial report on maternity care outcomes.

BORN's ongoing commitment to achieving 100 percent collection of Ontario birth data (over 140,000/year), along with its status as a prescribed registry under the Office of the Information and Privacy Commissioner of Ontario authorizing it to collect, protect, and disclose personal health information, makes BORN a powerful tool through which scientists, clinicians, policy-makers, and others can study perinatal outcomes. As the existence of the BORN data holding has become more well known, there has been a marked increase in research queries and an interest in studying the demographic characteristics of women in care, hospital designations, prevalence of particular risk factors among the maternity care population, access measures, prenatal and newborn screening data, and midwifery.

Increasing reliability of information and effective models for dissemination have created opportune conditions for linking of data sets, hypothesis-generating research, administrative analysis, and discrete data collection into areas such as non-quantitative measures of midwifery care, including historical accounts, women's personal accounts, and the experiences of midwives. As the number of years of complete data collection grows, BORN will become an increasingly important foundation of longitudinal health research by which to compare birth outcomes, key measures of the ongoing health of Ontario children and youth.

Research Infrastructure

At present, midwifery education programs in Ontario extend only to the undergraduate level, limiting midwives' capacity to access research infrastructure within their own faculties. A growing number of midwives are seeking graduate and post-graduate education in other disciplines, enabling them to study research methods within faculties such as sociology, nursing, education, ethics, health care policy, and management and epidemiology. Exploration of the feasibility of establishing a midwifery graduate and post-graduate program through existing midwifery education program faculties, or in partnership with interdisciplinary programs, continues.

Emerging Clinical Issues for Research

Healthy diversification of research interests has followed growth in the number of midwives. With more women in midwifery care each year, research questions are increasingly being focused not only on the uniform cohort of midwifery clients, but smaller groups within the cohort, e.g., Aboriginal families, socio-economic status quintiles, and disease groups.

Longitudinal Health Status

Links between both child and adult onset chronic disease and birth outcomes are clearer as we learn more about the origins of disease in the human reproductive cycle. This places increased pressure on women and families to adopt healthy behaviours prior to pregnancy. Maternity care providers are also building education on complex topics into early stages of care to enable women to consider maternal–fetal screening tests for an increasing number of risk factors in pregnancy that can contribute to poor long-term maternal–child health. As we look for upstream responses to higher rates of obesity and chronic disease in the population, access to quality public health programs, early primary prenatal care, birth care, and postnatal care (including breastfeeding support) plays an increasingly significant role. Linking of indicators between women's health, maternity care, and child health over a long time period will generate a rich resource for the study of population health across the maternity care continuum and even across generations. It will enable the coordination of maternal–newborn care with existing health care strategies on diabetes and other chronic diseases, healthy weight, asthma, smoking cessation, HIV, and public health.

Models of Midwifery and Maternity Care

During the drive toward implementation of midwifery in Ontario, the Task Force on the Implementation of Midwifery in Ontario (TFIMO) was appointed to provide advice on a proposed provincial model. The TFIMO conducted comparative research on midwifery models from countries with well-established professions: Denmark, Holland, New Zealand, and Britain (TFIMO, 1987), and surveyed College of Nurses of Ontario registrants on their level of desire to practise midwifery in Ontario. In addition to its alignment with the international Definition of the Midwife, the report emphasized three key points that were incorporated into the Ontario model. One was continuity of care, defined as services to each woman delivered by a small group of midwives in order to ensure a birth caregiver who is known to the woman. The second was informed choice. Midwives discuss evidence, community standards, and options with each woman and include her as a primary decision-maker in her care. The third was choice of birthplace. Midwives attend normal births in the woman's planned choice of home, hospital, or birth centre setting.

The practice of midwifery in Ontario has remained loyal to the above tenets as evidence has grown documenting the model's success. Based on a program evaluation of midwifery in Ontario in 2003, midwifery care was associated with low Caesarean section and instrumental birth rates (forceps and vacuum extractions), low rates of episiotomy (a surgical cut to enlarge a woman's vaginal opening at birth), short hospital stay rates, and high rates of breastfeeding and consumer satisfaction (Ontario Midwifery Program, Ministry of Health and Long-Term Care, 2014). Performance measurement of midwifery care in subsequent years has continued to show favourable results. However, with the growth of midwifery has come pressure to diversify the model to meet population health needs from proponents with a variety of compelling rationales. The College of Midwives and stakeholder groups are exploring recommendations by provincial and national reports to adapt the model to enable more integration between midwives and other maternity care professionals, and for special situations where the scope could be expanded to better enable midwives to serve specific populations.

Following consultation with Aboriginal communities, the TFIMO also recommended an exemption for Aboriginal midwives from Ontario regulations. Evidence of the exemption can be seen in the successful implementation of a model of Aboriginal midwifery in the First Nations community of Six Nations. Ongoing development of Aboriginal midwifery in Ontario may lead to a range of culturally specific models in First Nations communities. A variety of service-delivery models and emerging action-based research methodologies present opportunities for scholars interested in midwifery in Aboriginal contexts to develop culturally competent models of maternity care, and measure the performance of services for Aboriginal women in comparison with other populations.

Integration of Midwifery: Impact on Women and Families, Health Care Providers, and the Health Care System

Integration of midwifery in Ontario began with the first 70 midwives organizing themselves into mainly group practices, with new midwife graduates being absorbed into those groups. New midwives gradually established secondary groups in communities that had never received midwifery services before; these have become platforms for further expansion into smaller urban and remote centres. Currently there are approximately 90 midwifery practice groups in Ontario, with service areas spread across urban, rural, and remote locations.

Community-generated proposals, in addition to proposals by midwives, are invited by the ministry annually for consideration of further expansion. Human resources criteria—such as access to obstetrical care, unmet demand for midwifery services, demographics of the population to be served, and availability of financial resources—are factored into the allocation-approval process for new midwifery practice groups. As a managed program with the capacity to target resources to particular communities in need of improved access to maternity care, midwifery differs from physician programs that rely on the professionals themselves to determine where to set up practice.

Although integration has taken place rapidly and smoothly in most communities, midwifery services are curtailed where hospitals have imposed caps on the number of midwives or the number of births permitted to be attended by them, or where hospitals limit the midwife's scope by implementing protocols requiring women's care to be transferred to physicians in some situations (such as when an epidural or induction is done). With Ontario being joined in recent years by other provinces with regulated midwifery, it is an opportune time to examine the root causes of disrupted midwifery integration in order to improve the forecast for access to midwifery care in Ontario and Canada.

Emerging Sociological Research Issues Access to Midwifery Care

Since midwifery care has been funded in Ontario, demand for services has exceeded the supply of midwives, even though the number of practice groups has more than tripled. Expansion of the profession now permits midwives to deliver services to over 19,000 women per year, which represents over 10 percent of the Ontario women giving birth each year. However, 70–80 percent of women in Ontario could be considered within the midwifery scope (WHO, 1997). Approximately 8,000 additional women requested midwifery care, but were unable to be accommodated due to full practice groups (Better Outcomes Registry and Network, 2013–2014).

Further research into targets for access to midwifery care at the provincial level, as well as the right mix and distribution of midwives among other maternity care providers, would be advantageous in addressing regional access issues and in stabilizing access for communities with declining physician, nurse, and/or hospital capacity.

Care to Diverse and Vulnerable Populations

Although data are beginning to be available to study provincial-level midwifery performance measures and some regional access measures, contemplation of service delivery to specific populations in Ontario has gone largely unpublished to date. Research that creates linkages between Ontario's population needs and existing frameworks for the study of culturally competent care, care in rural and remote settings, and the qualitative aspects of women's experience will enrich the current pool of research, which emphasizes clinical outcomes and economic measures.

Emerging Issues for Policy and Planning

Health Human Resources Planning

The growth of midwifery and our emerging ability to study midwifery practice patterns and career enablers/constraints will improve planning capacity in the future. Scholars interested in health human resources planning will be interested in midwifery as a homogeneously female profession with a dynamic tension between the needs of the client and the carer. Work in the subject area of midwifery would augment emerging areas of research looking at uptake of evidence-based health policy and knowledge transfer between academic and public policy sectors. Research into labour issues related to the differential pay rates between largely female and other maternity care professions would be particularly timely, given a recent human rights complaint by the Association of Ontario Midwives charging systemic gender-based pay rate discrimination by the province.

Health Economics

Financial cost efficiency is an increasingly influential factor in policy decisions about health care services generally, and access to maternity care specifically. Costs in maternity care are not easy to track, with large elements spread between provider compensation, direct and indirect hospital costs at birth, community programs, lab and ancillary costs, public health, emergency room, transport, pediatric, and private health care. Cost drivers include hospital-stay rates for women and infants, liability insurance costs, childbirth intervention rates (including how often inductions, Caesarean sections, and epidurals are done), and whether complex medical or social services are required during maternity care or afterwards for complications associated with birth outcomes. Comparative cost analysis between maternity care models can be difficult due to nuanced differences in models and challenges in capturing all related costs in traditional case-costing projects.

Value-based maternity care must also factor in human as well as financial costs, which are difficult to quantify in traditional forms of research. For example, the vast geography of Ontario combines a small number of high-volume hospitals with a large group of dispersed smaller-volume hospitals. As in most non-urban settings in Canada, hospital birth volumes in less densely populated communities in Ontario are substantially lower than in urban hospitals. Some have characterized this as "less cost-efficient." However, cost-effectiveness and human impact must be balanced in determining how far families must travel to obtain basic primary care maternity services. New models of analysis that incorporate the relative human costs—such as the impact of a poor birth outcome, family separation during the weeks of evacuation when women are flown from their communities to give birth in distant communities (in a second language, without relatives or support), and/or the process of transport for women and newborns travelling longer distances to give birth in larger urban hospitals—should be developed that provide for these issues to be factored into funding decisions about maternity care in local communities.

Conclusion

Midwifery advocates and Ontario midwives can be proud of the strides made by the profession in establishing itself and demonstrating high-quality services while managing an ambitious expansion effort. Researchers into women's health, and specifically maternal–newborn health, will find a wealth of opportunities to interpret these excellent clinical outcomes and document the knowledge gained by midwifery's integration into the Ontario health system. The development and publication of locally generated midwifery knowledge will be the task of midwives and women's health scholars, standing on the shoulders of the profession's first advocates and leaders.

References

Better Outcomes Registry and Network (BORN). (2013–2014). *LinkedIn*. Retrieved from https://www.linkedin.com/company/better-outcomes-registry-&-network-born-ontario.

Canadian Association of Midwives. (2014). *Ontario Midwives—Midwifery in Ontario, Canada*. Retrieved from http://www.canadianmidwives.org/province/Ontario.html?prov=10.

International Confederation of Midwives. (2014). *Definition of the Midwife*. Retrieved from http://www.internationalmidwives.org/who-we-are/policy-and-practice/icm-international-definition-of-the-midwife/.

Ontario Midwifery Program, Ministry of Health and Long-Term Care. (2014). *Results-Based Plan Briefing Book 2013-2014*. Retrieved from http://health.gov.on.ca/en/common/ministry/publications/plans/rbplan13/#2.1.

Task Force on the Implementation of Midwifery in Ontario (TFIMO). (1987). *Report of the Task Force on the Implementation of Midwifery in Ontario*. Toronto: Government of Ontario.

World Health Organization (WHO). (1997). *Safe Motherhood: Care in Normal Labour: A Practical Guide*. Geneva: WHO Division of Reproductive Health.

Further Reading

Bourgeault, I. L., C. Benoit, & R. Davis-Floyd (Eds.). (2004). *Reconceiving Midwifery*. Montreal & Kingston: McGill-Queen's University Press.

Canadian Women's Health Network. (1999). Special Delivery: The Midwifery and Childbirth Issue. *The Canadian Women's Health Network Publication* 2(3). Retrieved from www.cwhn.ca/network-reseau/2-3/default.html.

Carroll, D., & C. Benoit. (2001). Aboriginal Midwifery in Canada: Blending Traditional and Modern Forms. *The Canadian Women's Health Network Publication* 4(3). Winnipeg: Network/Le Réseau. Retrieved from www.cwhn.ca.

Hackett, L. L. (1998). *Midwifery in Canada, 1980-1997: A Brief History and Selective Annotated Bibliography of Publications in English*. Halifax: School of Library and Information Studies, Dalhousie University.

Relevant Websites

Association of Ontario Midwives: www.aom.on.ca
Canadian Women's Health Network: www.cwhn.ca
College of Midwives of Ontario: www.cmo.on.ca
National Aboriginal Council of Midwives: www.aboriginalmidwives.ca/

SECTION FOUR

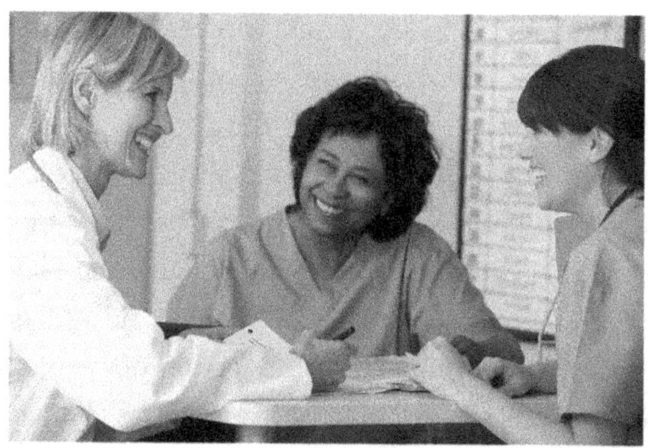

Linking Research, Policy, and Practice

The fourth, and final, section considers ways of using research to influence policy and practices. While earlier sections also propose means of moving research into action, this section makes such a move the central theme. The first chapter in this section, Chapter 16, is co-written by an Ontario researcher and activist, most recently serving as head of both the Canadian Women's Health Network and the National Network for Environments in Women's Health and by a health policy and research analyst from Nova Scotia. Using the example of environmental and occupational influences on the development of breast cancer, Anne Rochon Ford and Ellen Sweeney challenge the dominant discourse on breast cancer. The example is particularly important given the popularity of the run-for-a-cure approaches to policy and practices. They go on to explore the critical role that government regulation and health policy can play in protecting women's health and preventing detrimental health outcomes rather than in focusing almost exclusively on cures and individual prevention efforts.

Chapter 17 is written by an Ontario Health Council Chair in Women's Health, a medical doctor who is in the Dalla Lana School of Public Health, Institute of Health Policy, Management, and Evaluation, and Lawrence S. Bloomberg Faculty of Nursing at the University of Toronto. Using the specific example of chronic care, Arlene Bierman suggests how research can influence change, and explores the impact of policy on health outcomes. In doing so, she proposes using a chronic care model and tools for monitoring and improving women's health.

Julie Maher and Sara Mohammed are researchers and activists with the Ontario Women's Health Network, an organization explicitly devoted to communicating research and other information to a broad range of women and especially to the most marginalized in order to promote change. In Chapter 18, they use the project Our Words, Our Health to discuss the health concerns and priorities identified by diverse women in Ontario. But they do more than describe the methods used to ensure these voices are heard; they reflect upon the constraints of meeting their health care preferences in the current context of cutbacks, financial cutbacks, and a general loss of support for "women's health" initiatives, structures, and programs in the province.

The final chapter in this section, Chapter 19, is a particularly moving piece about using film to make change. Laura Sky is an award-winning filmmaker who has been creating films about women for over 30 years. She has an honorary doctorate in recognition of her work. In the last decade or so, she has focused more specifically on women's health. All of her films are based on thorough research, much of it original for the purposes of the film, and all of it intended to provide a venue for women's voices and to use these voices to make change. In this chapter, she uses her personal journey to explore a participatory model of research and documentary production based on research and the development of long-term relationships with individuals and groups committed to equity and social justice. She explains how Skyworks developed a method of film dissemination built on the principles of contributing to community engagement for purposes of social change.

The last section, then, returns us to the first, where Lorraine Greaves writes about the origins of gender-based analysis in the women's health movement and about the efforts to use research to make change. The chapters in this section specifically focus on turning research into action, but, in a sense, this is a consistent message throughout the book. Indeed, all the authors in this book are making changes in policy, in research, and in practices through their own work on gender. The intent of this book is not only to share their expertise in specific areas but to demonstrate how gender-based analysis can be done, and done in ways that make a difference. There is still a long way to go and many gaps in our analysis. After all, women's work is never done.

These chapters raise multiple issues about the role research plays in policy and about how to make change. Some questions that come to our minds are:

1. What means are effective in putting research into practice?
2. How should we ensure marginalized women have their voices heard in both research and policy?
3. Who and what are missing when we focus on cures?
4. Is the personal political? Do we have shared policy concerns as women?

CHAPTER 16

Missing in Actions: The Critical Role of Environmental and Occupational Exposures in the Development of Breast Cancer in Women[1]

Anne Rochon Ford and Ellen Sweeney

> From the right to know and the duty to inquire
> flows the obligation to act.
>
> —STEINGRABER, 2010, p. 122

Introduction

The role played by environmental and occupational exposures to toxic compounds in the development of breast cancer is frequently absent from discussions of this now very public disease. Forces around the world are mobilized every October to raise millions of dollars for *the cure*, with remarkably little attention to *the cause*. Research dollars spent on better understanding the causes and prevention of breast cancer pale in comparison with amounts spent on finding a cure. Medical school and other health profession curricula routinely leave out or provide comparatively little detail on environmental and occupational influences on disease. Popular education and media implore women to eat more healthily, exercise, not smoke, drink less alcohol, and get regular mammograms, but rarely is there discussion about where they work, where they grew up, the neighbourhoods they live in, and the everyday exposures to toxic substances, including mammary carcinogens and endocrine-disrupting chemicals. This chapter will examine the critical emergence of understanding about environmental and occupational influences on the development of breast cancer, why this challenges the dominant discourse on breast cancer, and the critical role that government regulation and health policy can play in protecting women's health and preventing detrimental health outcomes.

Environmentalism and Occupational Health: Women Making Their Mark

> All over this world—as wonderful as it is polluted, as peace loving as it is violent, and as beautiful as it is scarred—there is a groundswell of indomitable, persistent, committed untiring women who struggle to make this a healthier place . . . women are naming the problems in their communities, asking about others' experiences, and fighting for answers. (Wyman, 1999, p. 18)

The call for prevention and recognizing the environmental and occupational links to breast cancer can be situated in the history of women's involvement in environmental and occupational health movements. From the early twentieth century pioneering occupational health work of Alice Hamilton (her examination of toxins in the workplace helped to put industrial hygiene on the map) to Rachel Carson's seminal work on harms caused by pesticides in the 1950s and 1960s, to the Indigenous Water Walk Grandmothers who circled the Great Lakes to raise awareness about the importance of protecting sacred water for future generations, women in North America—and internationally—have been at the forefront of movements linking our environment and our workplaces to our health (Wyman, 1999; Messing, 2014; Rahder & Peterson, 2000).

Occupational and environmental research and activism have often coalesced around the issue of breast cancer and its genesis, with both these areas of study having a focus on primary prevention.

Box 16.1

Key Milestones in Canada

1975: At the First World Conference on Women, Mexico City, Indian-born, Canadian-trained environmental activist and scholar Vandana Shiva introduces the issue of women and the environment in an international context.

1976: *Women and Environments International* magazine, housed at York University, is created.

1980s: Women and Environments Education and Development (WEED) Foundation Canada is created.

1985-1990: L'Institut de recherche en santé et en sécurité du travail du Québec (IRSST) at l'Université du Québec à Montréal is created; in 1987 it becomes Centre de recherche sur les interactions biologiques entre la santé et l'environnement (CINBIOSE).

1990: Women and the Environment: Changing Course is Canada's first conference to bring together women involved in environmental activity.

1991: Women's Network on Health and the Environment in Toronto (which later became Women's Healthy Environment Network) is created with an initial focus on cancer prevention.

1991: Labour Canada and Health Canada jointly commission a research report on women's occupational health, encouraging a gender-based analysis.

1992: The former Women's Health Bureau of Health Canada sponsors a research round table on gender and occupational health for researchers and policy-makers.

1992: The Sub-Committee on the Status of Women of the House of Commons Standing Committee on Health and Welfare, Social Affairs, Seniors, and the Status of Women released its report, *Breast Cancer: Unanswered Questions*.

1993: A National Forum on Breast Cancer is held in Montreal, a collaborative effort of Health Canada, the National Cancer Institute of Canada, the Medical Research Council, the Canadian Cancer Society, and cancer-survivor organizations; the issue of environmental contaminants is given time on the conference agenda.

1993: A group of Montreal-based breast cancer survivors create Breast Cancer Action Montreal, promoting a focus on prevention (currently Breast Cancer Action Quebec).

1994: Sharon Batt's *Patient No More: The Politics of Breast Cancer* is published, offering a message that political interests are keeping us from "conquering the disease."

1995: Messing et al. publish *Invisible: Issues in Women's Occupational Health/La santé des travailleuses*.

1996: The former Women's Health Bureau of Health Canada sponsors a Canada–USA Women's Health Forum at which there are workshops on occupational health.

1996: The National Network on Environments and Women's Health (at York University), one of five federally funded Centres of Excellence in Women's Health, is created and mandated to carry out policy-based research examining the social, economic, and physical environments that affect women's health.

1997: The First World Conference on Breast Cancer, held in Kingston, Ontario, linked breast cancer to environmental issues affecting health; it is co-sponsored by Women's Network on Health and the Environment and the Women's Environment and Development Organization (WEDO).

1997: The Canadian documentary film *Exposure: Environmental Links to Breast Cancer* is released.

1998: The Elizabeth May Chair in Women's Health and the Environment is endowed at Dalhousie University, recognizing the work of environmental activist Elizabeth May.

2006: Elizabeth May is named first leader of the Green Party of Canada.

2009: The CIHR Team on Gender, Environment, and Health, created to contribute to the development of new approaches and methods for the integration of sex and gender in environmental and occupational health research, is announced.

2013: Federal government withdraws all funding from the National Network on Environments and Women's Health, and all programs affiliated with Health Canada's Women's Health Contribution Program.

2013: The creation of nine CIHR Chairs in Gender Work and Health is announced.

Environmentalism and Occupational Health: Necessary Partners in the Same Discussion

There does not appear to be any definitive history on how and when activist and scholarly work in the fields of women's occupational health and environmental health converged in Canada. In a 1997 review of the literature related to research on women's health, health and environment, and women and environments, Rebecca Peterson found "very little overlap or knowledge of the other fields" (Peterson, 1997, cited in Rahder & Peterson, 2000, p. 4).

In 2003, organizers of a series of women's health events in Canada decided to include environmental health in discussions of occupational health problems reflecting the growing interest in the research community. A special issue of *Environmental Research* included equal amounts of research on occupational exposures as well as harms from environmental and household chemicals. The editors agreed that with respect to these overlapping fields, "the pathways that explain gender differences are rarely examined, even though it is through the understanding of these pathways and the underlying mechanisms that adequate prevention and therapy can be put in place" (Messing & Mergler, 2006, p. 147).

Researchers in these two areas of study brought to their work some commonalities in approach: (1) a commitment to applying a gender lens to their work, including accumulating information on gender-differentiated exposure to environmental and occupational hazards; (2) an understanding of the importance of community-academic partnerships and a commitment to participatory research; (3) the involvement of women in the formulation and implementation of policy related to these two areas of study; (4) an acknowledgement that the impact of different environments on women's health and well-being varies by age, class, race, ethnicity, and other cultural factors; and (5) a commitment to the precautionary principle as a baseline for prevention and treatment.

Breast Cancer and Plastics: An Illustrative Vignette

A Canadian case-control study by Brophy et al. (2012) found an increased risk of breast cancer among women working in certain occupations, including farming, automotive, food canning, metal working, and bars, casinos, and racetracks. Women who worked for 10 years in occupations where they were exposed to high levels of cancer-causing substances and endocrine-disrupting chemicals were found to have a higher risk of developing breast cancer. Women working in the automotive industry are routinely exposed to plastics, which release estrogenic and carcinogenic chemicals, and were found to be more than twice as likely to develop breast cancer; pre-menopausal women were five times more likely to develop the disease.[2]

Why have these findings and related research not become part of the current discourse about breast cancer or a dominant theme in "awareness-raising pink ribbon" activities? What factors play a role in preventing environmental and occupational links to breast cancer from being part of the discussion about women's health?

Background to the 2012 Study

Breast cancer is the most commonly diagnosed cancer in women worldwide (WHO, 2014). Breast cancer rates in Canada are among the highest in the world with incidence rates similar to those in the United States, northern Europe, and Australia (CCS and NCIC, 2007). One in nine women will develop breast cancer in her lifetime and approximately 67 Canadian women are diagnosed with breast cancer every day. An estimated 24,400 women in Canada will be diagnosed this year and 5,000 will die as a result (BCSC, 2014).

While breast cancer is most often attributed to a family history or lifestyle factors such as diet, these factors account for less than half of diagnosed cases. Rather, breast cancer is caused by a combination of genetic, hormonal, lifestyle, and environmental factors (Gray, 2010; Parkin et al., 2011). The traditional risk factors are unable to account for the increased incidence of breast cancer in industrialized countries since World War II as thousands of new chemicals with unknown health effects were being introduced and women were entering the workforce in record numbers.

The 2012 Study of Workers in Essex and Kent Counties, Ontario

> I worked at the plastic plant for five years and then developed breast cancer when I was 32. There are six or seven breast cancers that we know of. They are all younger than 50. (Focus group participant, in DeMatteo et al., 2012, p. 438)

Women's occupational health has not traditionally been a priority for researchers and regulators despite the fact that many workers are regularly exposed to cancer-causing agents and endocrine-disrupting chemicals at work (Sweeney, 2012). Advances in recent research are shedding important light on the relationship between chemical exposures and disease by highlighting the complex interaction in the human body between cancer-causing and hormone-disrupting agents in which the endocrine system plays an important role (Darbre & Fernandez, 2013; Grossman, 2012; Rudel et al., 2014; Vandenberg et al., 2012). This case study was conducted in Essex and Kent counties in southern Ontario, where there are extensive manufacturing and agriculture industries. This study involved 1,006 women with breast cancer and 1,146 women without the disease who provided detailed occupational histories in order for the researchers to identify potential exposures to carcinogens and endocrine-disrupting chemicals. Participants also provided information on reproductive risk factors, including the number of pregnancies, the history of breastfeeding, the age at start of menstruation and menopause, as well as risk factors such as level of physical activity, alcohol use, and smoking history. In addition to the exposure to chemicals in the everyday environment, consumer products, and dietary sources, some workers face the additional toxic burden of multiple chemicals in their paid employment. Airborne exposures are of particular concern as women in some of the industries examined in this study described their workplace as a "toxic soup" of chemicals (Sweeney, 2012).

Through the personal stories and observations of workers who participated in focus groups and through a collection of hygiene reports, it was learned that

> women in the study area . . . held a wide range of jobs in the plastics industry dating back to the 1960s; the majority of automotive plastics manufacturing workers in the study area were women; the work environment is heavily contaminated with dust, vapours and fumes; there has been historic failure by government regulators to control exposures; workers receive a steady dose of mixtures of chemicals through inhalation, absorption and ingestion; workers are getting sick; and society is largely unaware of their plight. The apparent invisibility of blue-collar women raises issues of gender and class bias and discrimination. (Brophy et al., forthcoming)

The significance of this case study lies in both the findings, which conclude that women are at an increased risk for developing breast cancer in the automotive plastics industry, and in highlighting the lack of attention paid to environmental and occupational exposures to chemicals and the gaps in the regulatory system that place women at risk.

Context: Breast Cancer Research

The dominant approach to studying breast cancer is based on the biomedical model of disease, which attributes causation to individual-level factors, including diet, exercise, age at first menstruation, and genetics (Brown, 2007). This approach places an emphasis on personal approaches to prevention, detection, and treatment, including lifestyle changes such as diet; use of mammograms to detect tumours; and treatment options, which include surgery, radiation, and chemotherapy. The biomedical community, various levels of government, and the mainstream breast cancer movement frame breast cancer as a preventable disease by placing the onus of responsibility on the individual in terms of managing individual risk factors and behaviours, and downplaying social, structural, political, economic, and environmental factors that influence the disease (Zavetoski et al., 2004; Orsini, 2007).

There are multiple symbolic meanings associated with women's breasts in Western society, including representations of sexual pleasure and desire, nurturing and motherhood. However, women's breasts are also now associated with notions of danger and risk: the "risk of disease, risk of defeminisation, risk of deformity, [and] risk of death" (Klawiter, 2008, p. xx). The predominant view of cancer prevention focuses "almost exclusively on individual lifestyle changes" (Chernomas & Donner, 2004, p. 4). This view is promoted by Health Canada, the Public Health Agency of Canada, and mainstream cancer and breast cancer organizations, including the Canadian Cancer Society, the Canadian Breast Cancer Foundation, the Breast Cancer Society of Canada, and the Canadian Breast Cancer Network (BCSC, 2013a, 2013b; Canadian Cancer Society, 2008, 2013; CBCF, 2012a, 2012b; CBCN,

2013; Health Canada, 2012; PHAC, 2009, 2012). The "risky behaviours" include using tobacco; consuming alcohol; not engaging in physical activity; excessive exposure to the sun; and a diet high in fat, red meat, sugar, and processed foods.

What is remarkable about the long history of focus on modifiable risk factors such as lifestyle and diet is that the official narrative rarely concedes that these factors account for only a fraction of breast cancer incidence. Even a *Canadian Cancer Statistics* report, which *does* acknowledge this, places the onus of responsibility on the individual with its emphasis on personal behaviours (CCS and NCIC, 2007). This individualization of health, also referred to as the "responsibilization paradigm," places the onus of responsibility on the individual and suggests that the risk factors for health are controllable if one makes the appropriate lifestyle choices (Orsini, 2007, p. 349). It is no surprise, then, that when one "behaves accordingly" and still becomes ill, blame is often targeted at the individual and a sense of shame and guilt can easily ensue (Batt, 1994; Deacon, 2014).

The mainstay of breast cancer prevention remains early detection and treatment (Shah, 2003, p. 221). However, measures of detection and prevention are often conflated in the discourse surrounding breast cancer. In the United Kingdom, the United States, and Canada, public health policy has a very clear directive promoting detection over primary prevention (Potts, 2004). McCormick et al. (2003, p. 550) note that the American Cancer Society and the National Cancer Institute have a long history arguing that "mammography is the best form of prevention." Breast cancer organizations promote mammography as part of "preventive health care" (CBCF, 2012c). The Breast Cancer Society of Canada (2013a) promotes early detection as a means of prevention, including breast self-exams, clinical breast exams, and mammography. However, once a tumour has been detected, prevention has ultimately failed.[3]

A truly primary prevention-focused approach involves attempting to prevent the disease before it develops. Primary prevention may be broadly defined as "the protection of health by personal and community-wide efforts . . . [which] consist of measures aimed at preventing the . . . occurrence of disease" (Tomatis & Huff, 2001, p. 458). A primary prevention approach to breast cancer would "aim to reduce and eliminate as far as possible, human exposures to all substances or agents that are known to be, or suspected of being, implicated in the disease process" (UK Working Group on the Primary Prevention of Breast Cancer, 2005, p. 10).

In the United States, the President's Cancer Panel produced a report in 2009 that calls for reducing the risk of developing cancer associated with the widespread and ubiquitous exposure to toxic substances. The panel was "particularly concerned to find that the true burden of environmentally induced cancer has been grossly underestimated" (Reuben, 2010, p. 5). Director of the Science and Environmental Health Network, Dr. Ted Schettler, suggested that the panel "underscored that regulatory agencies should reduce exposures even when absolute proof of harm was unavailable," drawing on the precautionary principle (Cone, 2010). Similarly, the Interagency Breast Cancer and Environmental Research Coordinating Committee published a report in 2013 that recognizes environmental contaminants and calls for making prevention as the key to reducing the burden of breast cancer (IBCERCC, 2013). Jeanne Rizzo, co-chair of the committee and president and CEO of the Breast Cancer Fund, states that the report demonstrates that research and programs "focused on preventing breast cancer need as much attention as treatment and a cure" (Goldman, 2013). Rizzo notes that

> [w]e're extending life with breast cancer, making it a chronic disease, but we're not preventing it. We have to take a look at early life exposures, *in utero*, childhood, puberty, pregnancy and lactation. Those are the periods when you get set up for breast cancer. How does a pregnant woman protect her child? How do we create policy so that she doesn't have to be a toxicologist when she goes shopping? (Grady, 2013)

The committee found that identifying and mitigating the environmental causes of breast cancer is the key to reducing the number of new cases (IBCERCC, 2013). "Prevention requires we close the knowledge-to-action gap and translate science into preventive public health actions that can impact breast cancer incidence in the future" (Rizzo, 2013).

By recognizing the carcinogenic, bio-accumulative, and persistent nature of environmental contaminants, there is a clear need for prevention and action related to protecting women's health in Canada. Thus, it becomes necessary to consider environmental links to breast cancer—and how we might prevent them—including mammary carcinogens and endocrine-disrupting chemicals through occupational and everyday exposures to industrial chemicals and toxic substances in consumer products. But that preventive action must not be confined to "buying one's way to prevention." Sociologist Norah MacKendrick introduced the notion of "precautionary consumption" to describe "the practices of individuals trying to reduce their body burdens by purchasing environmentally friendly products. The premise is that individual consumer action is the primary mode of responding to these risks as opposed to changing government regulation" (MacKendrick, 2010; see also Lee & Scott, 2014). The promotion of precautionary consumption practices acknowledges the potential role of toxic substances in health outcomes. However, risk is still framed as something that can be controlled by individual citizens through acts of green consumption in order to avoid everyday exposures to toxic substances. This practice is also highly problematic in placing the onus of responsibility at the level of the individual and in dismissing other social determinants of health, including socio-economic status, education, and literacy level, as well as creating a gendered and disproportionate burden on women.

The Pinking of Breast Cancer

> What a change. We used to march in the streets and now we're supposed to run for a cure. . . . The effect of the whole pink ribbon culture was to drain and deflect

> the kind of militancy we had as women who were appalled to have a disease that is epidemic and yet that we don't even know the cause of. (Barbara Ehrenreich, author and breast cancer survivor, in *Pink Ribbons Inc.*, 2011)

The now widely recognizable and corporate-influenced pink ribbon has its origins within a grassroots movement. Inspired by the red ribbon associated with the HIV/AIDS movement, in 1992, Charlotte Haley began distributing peach ribbons to raise awareness about breast cancer and funds for the prevention of the disease (Harvey & Strahilevitz, 2009; Moffett, 2003). She distributed postcards with the peach ribbons that stated: "The National Cancer Institute's annual budget is $1.8 billion, only 5 percent goes for cancer prevention. Help us wake up our legislators and America by wearing this ribbon" (BCA, 2011, p. 2). However, Haley was not interested in commercializing her efforts and refused to partner with cosmetics company Estée Lauder. Based on focus group research, Estée Lauder created, produced, and marketed the *pink* ribbon, with the colour choice representing conventional notions of femininity and hope (Estée Lauder, 2010; Jain, 2007).

There is very little transparency in terms of the revenues that corporations donate from purchases of pink-ribbon products during Breast Cancer Awareness Month to breast cancer research, treatment, screening, prevention, or education (Harvey & Strahilevitz, 2009; Moffett, 2003). Questions that may be asked when purchasing pink-ribbon products include: Is there a cap on the amount of money the company will donate and has the maximum amount already been met? Is the company contributing to the increasing incidence rates of breast cancer through everyday exposures to their products? What organization will receive the funds and how will they be used? (BCA, 2011). Indeed, King (2010, p. 108) argues that there is "nothing inherently uncontroversial about breast cancer. . . . [T]he disease has been manufactured as such over two decades of organizing that has gradually been incorporated into conservative political agendas, the programs of large nonprofits in partnerships with the cancer industries, and corporate marketing strategies."

Pharmaceutical company AstraZeneca is the primary sponsor of National Breast Cancer Awareness Month and fundraising events such as Run/Race for the Cure involve thousands of participants across Canada and the United States each year. Feminist environmental activists have brought a critical perspective to National Breast Cancer Awareness Month. They maintain that it legitimizes and promotes early-detection programs as the only public health approach to breast cancer and does not recognize a causal link between environmental contaminants and breast cancer (Klawiter, 2008). For instance, AstraZeneca has the authority to approve or disapprove all printed materials for the month-long campaign and, not surprisingly, this literature does not include mention of the potential role of environmental contaminants in causing breast cancer (Sherwin, 2006; Wilkinson, 2007). They further maintain that the very multinational corporations that participate are also contributing to the development of cancer through the production of toxic products, including pesticides, plastics, and their industrial by-products, such as dioxin. In particular, AstraZeneca is critiqued because it produces pesticides, including the carcinogen acetochlor, and one of its manufacturing plants is reportedly the third largest source of airborne carcinogenic pollution in the United States (Klawiter, 2008; Wilkinson, 2007, p. 424). Finally, certain corporations, such as pharmaceutical companies, profit from both the diagnosis *and* the treatment of breast cancer, and this information is concealed from the public (Klawiter, 2008, p. 201).

Jain (2007, p. 519) contends that the use of pink-ribbon campaigns to increase profits and build name recognition among consumers, while "cover[ing] up their production of carcinogens bears the name 'pinkwashing'. . . which obscures the links among the production, suffering and obfuscation of disease." The term "pinkwashing" is used to describe a company or organization that claims to care about breast cancer by promoting a pink-ribbon product, but at the same time produces, manufactures, and/or sells products that are linked to disease (BCA, 2011). Pink-ribbon culture has become more than a successful cause-related marketing campaign:

> [I]t has become a distinct cultural system that is integrated into the fabric of [North] American life. Grounded in advocacy, deeply held beliefs about gender and femininity, mass-mediated consumption, and the cancer industry, pink ribbon culture has transformed breast cancer from an important social problem that requires complicated social and medical solutions to a popular item for public consumption. (Sulik, 2011, p. 9)

King further adds that:

> Many women actually feel alienated by the overly-optimistic approach. They feel like they can't have their feelings of anger or despair or helplessness and feel like a legitimate person with breast cancer. In order to be a survivor you must maintain this optimistic outlook and participate in what I call the tyranny of cheerfulness. (*Pink Ribbons, Inc.*, 2011)

Women would benefit from a re-politicization of breast cancer in order to shift away from the fundamental emphasis on lifestyle and behavioural risk factors, as well as from the widespread and consumption-based pink-ribbon campaigns, which are designed to raise a very specific type of "awareness." Pink-ribbon campaigns have resulted in the commercialization of breast cancer, which presents the disease through a very restricted and narrow lens. The efforts to raise awareness about breast cancer present a particular framing of the disease and do not encourage a more critical examination around the messaging of the campaigns, a lack of transparency in donated funds, and instances of pinkwashing. These pink-ribbon campaigns divert attention from the realities of the disease, environmental and occupational links to breast cancer, and calls for primary prevention.

Placing Women at Risk: Gaps in Health Policy and Legislation

The primary prevention of environmental and occupational health outcomes has not been a strong feature of public health policy and legislation in Canada, despite the efforts of environmental, occupational, and breast cancer activists who advocate for a precautionary approach. Greaves (2009) notes that gender was first introduced into health research by social philosophers and social scientists. Since then it has become an important consideration in health research, policy, programming, and service development, particularly as the health determinants model gains more widespread acceptance and support, and gender has been identified as a key determinant of health. The analysis of sex and gender in health research has emerged as an increasingly important methodology that necessitates the consideration of impacts on both men and women, as well as identifying the shortcomings that emerge as a result.

In the case of environmental and occupational exposures to toxic substances, both sex and gender play a key role in the development of breast cancer. It is important to account for levels of susceptibility, body size, or sex-linked differences, which contribute to sex-specific variations in disease. For instance, women may be at higher risk for health issues related to exposure to environmental contaminants, which tend to concentrate in body fat and are often related to estrogen receptors such as the case of endocrine-disrupting chemicals (Clow et al., 2009; Women's College Hospital, 2013). Cumulative exposures to toxic substances during key windows of susceptibility experienced by women throughout their lives also place them at increased risk for developing breast cancer. The role of gender becomes evident when considering that gender stratification takes place within the trades in Canadian industry. The plastics automotive industry is predominantly staffed by women, who experience a multitude of chemical exposures both in their workplace and through everyday exposures. Many of these women also experience higher amounts of everyday exposures as a result of their roles as caregivers in their personal lives and gendered divisions of labour.

Advocates of sex- and gender-based analysis contend that it is essential for improving the health of Canadians and the development and implementation of health programs and policies. The "integration of a sex- and gender-based analysis makes for better science and more inclusive policies" (Lewis, 2011, p. 5). Based upon a recommendation from the House of Commons Standing Committee on the Status of Women in April 2008, the auditor general of Canada conducted an audit of the implementation of sex- and gender-based analysis policy by the federal government (Minister of Public Works and Government Services Canada, 2009). The audit found that "despite the government commitment to GBA [(gender based-analysis)] since 1995, there is no government-wide policy requiring that departments and agencies perform it" (Minister of Public Works and Government Services Canada, 2009, p. 2). Importantly, sex- and gender-based analysis was found to be inadequately integrated into policy development. Despite a formal commitment to sex- and gender-based analysis in the health portfolio of the federal government, the audit revealed that there were zero cases in Health Canada where sex- and gender-based analysis was performed and integrated into policy options development.

The audit clearly demonstrates that sex- and gender-based analysis is not being adequately incorporated in health policy or legislation in Canada. Sex and gender must be accounted for in public health policy and legislation as the lack of implementation can have real implications for health outcomes among Canadian citizens (Butler-Jones, 2012). This discussion raises important questions about where the burden of risk and responsibility is presumed to lie in the prevention of disease. The Government of Canada (2011) promotes risk as being within the control of Canadian citizens in suggesting that "we are all risk managers." However, the predominant focus on lifestyle and behavioural factors in cancer research and public health policy has resulted in gaps, including the prevention of exposure to toxic substances and the resulting detrimental health outcomes such as the development of breast cancer in environmental and occupational settings.

Policy and the Issue of Exposures

The majority of exposure standards for occupational, environmental, and consumer health and safety are still based on the toxicology model, which is insufficient in accounting for endocrine-disrupting chemicals and low-dose cumulative exposures. Recent research demonstrates that low-dose exposures to endocrine-disrupting chemicals (EDCs)can have effects that are not predicted at higher doses (Vandenberg et al., 2012). These chemicals can have effects at low doses. Brophy et al. (2013) suggest that "[i]f there are no 'thresholds' for certain substances at which no effects are observed, no 'safe' limit can be established." There is a significant critique from the field of epidemiology of reliance on the dose-response relationship, which is based on principles from toxicology and is utilized in risk assessment processes. Vandenberg et al. (2012, p. 378) argue that whether low doses of endocrine-disrupting chemicals "influence certain human disorders is no longer conjecture, because epidemiological studies show that environmental exposures to EDCs are associated with human diseases. Thus, fundamental changes in chemical testing and safety determination are needed to protect human health." The role of scientists in influencing law, policy, and practice of the federal government has been diminishing in recent years in Canada,[4] raising greater concerns than ever about the regulation of hazardous chemicals in the environment and in the workplace. This is reflected in the 700 jobs cuts at Environment Canada in 2011 and repeated accusations of "muzzling" federal scientists from speaking publicly about peer-reviewed research results (Chung, 2014; Gatehouse, 2013; Magnuson-Ford & Gibbs, 2014). However, the current regulatory regime remains highly dependent on very specific types of expertise, including the exclusive reliance on toxicology for the risk assessment processes associated with toxic substances.

Workers' Compensation

The Canadian case study which determined that women workers have an increased risk of developing breast cancer also presents clear challenges to the workers' compensation system (Brophy et al., 2013). It is understood that assessing and managing occupational diseases is a complex process that is influenced by social, cultural, and political issues, as well as medical knowledge and theories (Watterson, 1999). The difficulties in establishing a direct and causal link between a particular substance and a specific health outcome are complicated by a variety of factors. For example, lengthy latency periods are often required in order to establish a statistically significant correlation between an exposure to a toxic substance and an increased incidence of disease in a particular population. The contested nature of environmental health outcomes may mean that it is not possible to establish a connection conclusively and to the satisfaction of the entire scientific community (Markowitz & Rosner, 2002, p. 6).

Health outcomes as a result of environmental and occupational exposures have traditionally been framed as contested and are surrounded by questions of uncertainty and accountability. In cases concerning occupational exposures and breast cancer, the existence of the disease itself is not contested, but its causation and issues of accountability are continually surrounded by scrutiny and debate. Many of the endocrine-disrupting chemicals and mammary carcinogens of concern in the development of breast cancer have come into widespread use over the past 30 years and women in Canada are exposed to these toxic substances on a regular basis.

> Based on the mounting evidence, this widespread introduction of toxic chemicals into various work environments, and particularly new pesticides into agriculture and plastics into automotive manufacturing, will likely result in escalating numbers of claims for workplace compensation for women who have developed breast cancer from these new technologies. (Brophy et al., 2013)

To date there have been no workers' compensation claims upheld in Canada in cases of toxic exposures linked to breast cancer (Keith, 2013). Manitoba became the first jurisdiction in Canada to "enact a firefighter's disease presumption" when it added breast cancer to its list of compensable diseases for firefighters in 2011 (Government of Manitoba, 2010). Ten primary-site cancers were listed in the original legislation in 2002, including brain, bladder, kidney, lung, ureter, colorectal, esophageal, and testicular cancers, non-Hodgkin's lymphoma, and leukemia. The amendments proposed in 2010 apply to volunteer, part-time, and full-time firefighters and included four additional cancers, including multiple myeloma, primary-site prostate, skin, and breast cancer (Government of Manitoba, 2010). The risk of a female firefighter developing breast cancer is three to five times higher than the general population as a result of exposure to more than 200 known carcinogens connected to breast cancer at every fire (CBC, 2010). Thus far, other provinces and territories have not included the breast cancer category for firefighters or any other specific occupational group. A workers' compensation claim was initially granted to health care workers who experienced a breast cancer cluster in a hospital laboratory in British Columbia and claimed they were exposed to carcinogens. However, this claim was appealed by the employer, who argued that there was insufficient evidence to demonstrate that the claimants' cases of breast cancer were caused by occupational factors. The claim was overturned by the provincial Supreme Court, though the case has been left open if new evidence becomes available in the future (BC Justice, 2013).

Meek and Armstrong (2007, p. 593) note that the definition of environment in the Canadian Environmental Protection Act, 1999 (CEPA 1999) is broad enough to encompass the occupational environment. However, the federal regulatory regime that is designed to protect human health, including CEPA 1999 and the Chemicals Management Plan, does not encompass occupational health, which instead falls under provincial and territorial legislation in the form of Occupational Health and Safety Acts. The research conducted by Brophy et al. (2012) linking increased incidence rates of breast cancer to occupational exposures of toxic substances raises important questions about the adequacy of existing chemical-testing protocols in workplaces under provincial occupational health and safety standards. The Association of Workers' Compensation Boards of Canada recently listed breast cancer as an emerging issue, citing the Brophy et al. (2012) study and its findings that the risk of breast cancer is higher in workers in automotive plastic manufacturing (Association of Workers' Compensation Boards of Canada, 2013). The growing body of epidemiological and laboratory research has the potential to impact the workers' compensation system and frame breast cancer as a compensable occupational disease (Brophy et al., 2013).

Conclusion

Neither the federal regulatory nor provincial occupational health and safety regimes adequately protect women and prevent detrimental health outcomes, including the development of breast cancer as a result of exposure to toxic substances. The Government of Canada contends that "[n]ational consistency secures the same level of environmental and human health protection for all Canadians" (Environment Canada and Health Canada, 2006, p. 18). However, the federal regulatory regime does not account for women as a susceptible population who are at risk as a result of everyday exposures to toxic substances, and the influence of sex- and gender-related determinants of health are not adequately considered. At the same time, there is a gendered burden that places the onus of responsibility for preventing disease on individual women. The risk assessment and management frameworks do not adequately account for the effects of low-dose, cumulative, and synergistic effects of exposure to complex mixtures of toxic substances. These frameworks do not currently account for the emerging understandings of the long-term health effects of endocrine-disrupting chemicals, despite the "abundant scientific evidence of the harmful effects by EDCs [which] has accumulated to support a swift change in public health and environmental policies aimed at protecting the public in general, and, in particular, the developing fetus and women of reproductive age" (Soto & Sonnenschein, 2010, p. 7).

Only a truly precautionary approach can be effective in protecting women's health. This approach would require shifting debates around causation upstream to focus on everyday exposures to toxic substances, while concurrently shifting the focus away from individual-level factors.

Notes

1. Much of the content of this chapter was produced as part of Ellen Sweeney's doctoral dissertation research in the Faculty of Environmental Studies, York University. More information on the breast cancer pink-ribbon campaigns is found in a forthcoming article in *Women's Studies* by Sonja Killoran-McKibbin and Ellen Sweeney, entitled "Selling Pink: Feminizing the Non-Profit Industrial Complex from Ribbons to LemonAid."
2. A few key concepts are critical background to the Brophy et al. (2012) research, including:

   Carcinogens: There are several stages involved in the development of cancer, including initiation, promotion, and progression. The complex mixture of chemical exposures in the industrial workplace may have an impact on each of these stages.

   Endocrine-disrupting chemicals: Synthetic chemicals can disrupt a variety of essential endocrine functions in the body. Disruption of the delicate hormone balance can result in reproductive disorders, immune system dysfunction, some cancers, birth defects, and neurological effects. In traditional toxicology, a higher dose of a substance is expected to produce a greater effect. This is not necessarily the case with endocrine-disrupting chemicals, which can have health effects even at very low levels.

   Windows of susceptibility: The timing of chemical exposure and the stage of biological development can have an impact on a woman's risk of developing breast cancer. Women are more susceptible to the effects of endocrine-disrupting chemicals before breast tissue is fully matured. This study considered cumulative exposures during four critical windows: (1) before menstruation; (2) menstruation to the first full-term pregnancy; (3) first full-term pregnancy to menopause; and (4) after menopause (Sweeney, 2012).
3. Degrees of prevention include primary, secondary, and tertiary prevention and are well utilized in the field of health promotion. Primary prevention promotes the prevention of disease among specific populations and is most relevant for this research in its potential to truly prevent disease from a public health perspective. In an environmental health framework, these strategies would include the objective of reducing human exposure to environmental contaminants. Secondary prevention efforts promote access to screening measures, early detection of disease, and timely intervention. For breast cancer, measures of secondary prevention include breast self-examination, biopsy, and mammography. Finally, tertiary prevention efforts attempt to minimize the health effects of disease. Efforts of tertiary prevention in breast cancer involve the traditional interventions, including surgery, radiation, chemotherapy, and medication (Brown et al., 2006, pp. 511–512).
4. Note the complete de-funding in 2013 of the Women's Health Contribution Program, which supported policy-based research in Centres of Excellence in Women's Health across Canada for 17 years.

References

Association of Workers' Compensation Boards of Canada. (2013). *A National Resource on Workers' Compensation: Emerging Issues.* Retrieved from http://www.awcbc.org/en/print_page.asp?pagename=emergingissues.asp&.

Batt, S. (1994). *Patient No More: The Politics of Breast Cancer.* Charlottetown: Gynergy Books.

BC Justice. (2013). *Fraser Health Authority v. Workers' Compensation Appeal Tribunal: FHA is Seeking to Set Aside the Original Decisions and Reconsideration Decisions on the WCAT, Which Found that the Respondents' Breast Cancers are Occupational Diseases Corrected Judgment.* Retrieved from http://www.bcjustice.com/index.php?option=com_content&view=article&id=10304:fraser-health-authority-v-workers-compensation-appeal-tribunal-fha-is-seeking-to-set-aside-the-original-decisions-and-reconsideration-decisions-of-the-wcat-which-found-that-the-respondents-breast-cancers-are-occupational-diseases-&catid=413:employment-08&Itemid=1165.

Breast Cancer Action (BCA). (2011). *Think Before You Pink Toolkit.* 2011. San Francisco: Author.

Breast Cancer Society of Canada (BCSC). (2013a). *Prevention Methods.* Retrieved from http://www.bcsc.ca/p/43/l/101/t/Breast-Cancer-Society-of-Canada---Prevention.

Breast Cancer Society of Canada (BCSC). (2013b). *Healthy Living.* Retrieved from http://www.bcsc.ca/p/208/l/239/t/Breast-Cancer-Society-of-Canada---Healthy-Living.

Breast Cancer Society of Canada (BCSC). (2014). *Breast Cancer Statistics.* Retrieved from http://www.bcsc.ca/p/46/l/105/t/Breast-Cancer-Society-of-Canada---Statistics.

Brophy, J., R. DeMatteo, M. Keith, & M. Gilbertson. (2013, April 3). New Occupational Breast Cancer Study Challenges the Cancer Establishment. *Socialist Project, E-Bulletin* 796. Retrieved from http://www.socialist project.ca/bullet /796.php#fn3.

Brophy, J., M. Keith, R. DeMatteo, M. Gilbertson, A. Watterson, & M. Beck. (Forthcoming). Plastics Industry Workers and Breast Cancer Risks: Are We Heeding the Warnings? In D. Scott (Ed.), *Consuming Chemicals: Law, Science, and Policy for Women's Health.* Vancouver: UBC Press.

Brophy, J., M. Keith, A. Watterson, R. Park, M. Gilbertson, E. Maticka-Tyndale, M. Beck, H. Abu-Zahra, K. Schneider, A. Reinhartz, R. DeMatteo, & I. Luginaah. (2012). Breast Cancer Risk in Relation to Occupations with Exposure to Carcinogens and Endocrine Disruptors: A Canadian Case Control Study. *Environmental Health* 11(87). Retrieved from http://www.ehjournal.net/content/11/1/87.

Brown, P. (2007). *Toxic Exposures: Contested Illnesses and the Environmental Health Movement.* New York: Columbia University Press.

Brown, P., S. McCormick, B. Mayer, S. Zavestoski, R. Morello-Frosch, R. G. Altman, & L. Senier. (2006). "A Lab of Our Own": Environmental Causation of Breast Cancer and Challenges to the Dominant Epidemiological Paradigm. *Science, Technology and Human Values* 31(5): 499–536.

Butler-Jones, D. (2012). *The Chief Public Health Officer's Report on the State of Public Health in Canada, 2012: Influencing Health—The Importance of Sex and Gender.* Ottawa: Public Health Agency of Canada.

Canadian Breast Cancer Foundation (CBCF). (2012a). *Breast Cancer Risk Factors.* Retrieved from http://www.cbcf.org/central/AboutBreastHealth/Prevention RiskReduction/risk_factors/Pages/default.aspx.

Canadian Breast Cancer Foundation (CBCF). (2012b). *Reduce Your Breast Cancer Risk.* Retrieved from http://www.cbcf.org/central/AboutBreastHealth/ PreventionRiskReduction/ReduceYourRisk/Pages/default.aspx.

Canadian Breast Cancer Foundation (CBCF). (2012c). *Where to Go for a Mammogram.* Retrieved from http://www.cbcf.org/central/AboutBreastHealth/Early Detection/Mammography/Pages/Where-to-Get-a-Mammogram.aspx.

Canadian Breast Cancer Network (CBCN). (2013). *Canadian Breast Cancer Network.* Retrieved from http://www.cbcn.ca.

Canadian Cancer Society. (2008). *The Environment, Cancer, and You.* Toronto: Author.

Canadian Cancer Society. (2013). *How to Reduce Cancer Risk.* Retrieved from http://www.cancer.ca/en/cancer-information/cancer-101/how-to-reduce-cancer-risk/?region=ns.

Canadian Cancer Society and National Cancer Institute of Canada (CCS and NCIC). (2007). *Canadian Cancer Statistics, 2007.* Toronto: Author.

CBC. (2010, December 7). Man.[itoba] Firefighters to Get Breast Cancer Coverage. *CBC News.* Retrieved from http://www.cbc.ca/news/canada /manitoba/story/2010/12/07/mb-breast-cancer-firefighters-manitoba.html.

Chernomas, R., & L. Donner. (2004). *The Cancer Epidemic as a Social Event.* Winnipeg: Canadian Centre for Policy Alternatives.

Chung, E. (2014, October 8). Federal Government Scientists Muzzled by Media Policies, Report Suggests. *CBC News.* Retrieved from http://www.cbc.ca/news/technology/federal-government-scientists-muzzled-by-media-policies-report-suggests-1.2791650.

Clow, B., A. Pederson, M. Haworth-Brockman, & J. Bernier. (2009). *Rising to the Challenge: Sex- and Gender-Based Analysis for Health Planning, Policy and Research in Canada.* Halifax: Atlantic Centre of Excellence for Women's Health.

Cone, M. (2010, May 6). President's Cancer Panel: Environmentally Caused Cancers Are "Grossly Underestimated" and "Needlessly Devastate American Lives." *Environmental Health News.* Retrieved from http://www.environmentalhealthnews.org/ehs/news/presidents-cancer-panel.

Darbre, P., & M. Fernandez. (2013). Environmental Oestrogens and Breast Cancer: Long-Term Low-Dose Effects of Mixtures of Various Chemical Combinations. *Journal of Epidemiology and Community Health* 67(3): 203–205.

Deacon, G. (2014). *Naked Imperfection: A Memoir.* Toronto: Penguin Books.

DeMatteo, R., M. Keith, J. Brophy, A. Woodsworth, A. Watterson, M. Beck, A. Rochon Ford, M. Gilbertson, J. Phartiyal, M. Rootham, & D. Scott. (2012). Chemical Exposures of Women Workers in the Plastics Industry with Particular Reference to Breast Cancer and Reproductive Hazards. *New Solutions: A Journal of Environmental and Occupational Health Policy* 22(4): 427–448. doi: 10.2190/NS.22.4.d.

Environment Canada and Health Canada. (2006). *The Canadian Environmental Protection Act, 1999: Issues Paper.* Prepared for the Parliamentary Five Year Review of CEPA 1999. Ottawa, Ontario.

Estée Lauder. (2010). *Pink Ribbons.* Retrieved from http://www.estee lauder.com/pinkribbon/index.tmpl.

Gatehouse, J. (2013, May 3). When Science Goes Silent. *Maclean's.* Retrieved from http://www2.macleans.ca/2013/05/03/when-science-goes-silent/.

Goldman, L. (2013, February 22). Prevention of Breast Cancer: An Urgent Priority. *The Huffington Post Canada.* Retrieved from http://www.huffingtonpost.com/ lynn-r-goldman/breast-cancer-prevention_b_2733838.html.

Government of Canada. (2011). *What Is Risk Management?* Retrieved from http://www.chemicalsubstanceschimiques.gc.ca/about-apropos/manage-gestion/what-quoi-eng.php.

Government of Manitoba. (2010, December 7). *Amendments Proposed to Workers Compensation Act: Expanded Coverage Would Be for Work-Related Illnesses Affecting Firefighters.* News release. Retrieved from, http://news.gov.mb.ca/ news/?item=10328.

Grady, D. (2013, February 12). Report Faults Priorities in Studying Breast Cancer. *New York Times.* Retrieved from http://www.nytimes.com/ 2013/02/12/health/report-faults-priorities-in-breast-cancer-research.html?_r=0.

Gray, J. (2010). *State of the Evidence: The Connection between Breast Cancer and the Environment* (6th ed.). San Francisco: Breast Cancer Fund.

Greaves, L. (2009). Women, Gender, and Health Research. In P. Armstrong & J. Deadman (Eds.), *Women's Health: Intersections of Policy, Research, and Practice* (pp. 3–20). Toronto: Women's Press.

Grossman, E. (2012, March 19). Scientists Warn of Low-Dose Risks of Chemical Exposure. *Environment* 360. Retrieved from http://e360.yale.edu/feature/scientists_warn_of_low_dose_risk_of_endocrine_blocking_chemical_exposure/2507/.

Harvey, J., & M. Strahilevitz. (2009). The Power of Pink: Cause-Related Marketing and the Impact on Breast Cancer. *Journal of the American College of Radiology* 6(1): 26–32.

Health Canada. (2012). *Cancer.* Retrieved from http://www.hc-sc.gc.ca/hc-ps/dc-ma/cancer-eng.php.

Interagency Breast Cancer and Environmental Research Coordinating Committee (IBCERCC). (2013, February). *Breast Cancer and the Environment: Prioritizing Prevention.* Washington, DC: Author.

Jain, L. (2007). Cancer Butch. *Cultural Anthropology* 22(4): 501–538.

Keith, M. (2013). *Women's Occupational Risk Factors for Breast Cancer: The Need for Research, Regulatory Protection, and Compensation Coverage.* Working document for the National Network on Environments and Women's Health. Toronto, Ontario.

King, S. (2010). Pink Ribbons, Inc: The Emergence of Cause-Related Marketing and the Corporatization of the Breast Cancer Management. In P. Saukko (Ed.), *Governing the Female Body: Science, Media, and the Production of Femininity* (pp. 85–111). New York: SUNY Press.

Klawiter, M. (2008). *The Biopolitics of Breast Cancer: Changing Cultures of Disease and Activism.* Minneapolis: University of Minnesota Press.

Lee, R., & D. N. Scott. (2014, April 30). *Not Shopping Our Way to Safety.* Guest column. Canadian Women's Health Network. Retrieved from http://www.cwhn.ca/en/node/46308.

Lewis, S. (2011). *Sex, Gender, and Chemicals: Factoring Women into Canada's Chemicals Management Plan.* Toronto: National Network on Environments and Women's Health.

MacKendrick, N. (2010). Media Framing of Body Burdens: Precautionary Consumption and the Individualization of Risk. *Sociological Inquiry* 80(1): 126–149.

Magnuson-Ford, K., & K. Gibbs. (2014). *Can Scientists Speak? An Assessment of Media Policies in Canadian Federal Science Departments for Openness of Communication, Protection against Political Interference, Rights to Free Speech, and Protection.* Vancouver: Evidence for Democracy and Simon Fraser University. Retrieved from https://evidencefordemocracy.ca/sites/default/files/Can%20Scientists%20Speak_.pdf.

Markowitz, G., & D. Rosner. (2002). *Deceit and Denial: The Deadly Politics of Industrial Pollution.* Berkeley: University of California Press.

McCormick, S., P. Brown, & S. Zavestoski. (2003). The Personal Is Scientific, the Scientific Is Political: The Public Paradigm of the Environmental Breast Cancer Movement. *Sociological Forum* 18(4): 545–576.

Meek, M. E., & V. C. Armstrong. (2007). The Assessment and Management of Industrial Chemicals in Canada. In C. J. van Leeuwen & T. G. Vermeire (Eds.), *Risk Assessment of Chemicals* (2nd ed.; pp. 591–621). The Netherlands: Springer.

Messing, K. (2014). *Pain and Prejudice: What Science Can Learn about Work from the People Who Do It.* Toronto: Between the Lines Press.

Messing, K., & D. Mergler. (2006). Introduction: Women's Occupational and Environmental Health. *Environmental Research* 101(2): 147–148.

Minister of Public Works and Government Services Canada. (2009). Chapter 1: Gender-Based Analysis. *Report of the Auditor General of Canada to the House of Commons.* Ottawa: Office of the Auditor General of Canada.

Moffett, J. (2003). Moving beyond the Ribbon: An Examination of Breast Cancer Advocacy and Activism in the U.S. and Canada. *Cultural Dynamics* 15(3): 287–306.

Orsini, M. (2007). Discourses in Distress: From "Health Promotion" to "Population Health" to "You Are Responsible for Your Own Health." In M. Smith & M. Orsini (Eds.), *Critical Policy Studies: Contemporary Canadian Approaches* (pp. 347–363). Vancouver: University of British Columbia Press.

Parkin, D. M., L. Boyd, & L. C. Walker. (2011). The Fraction of Cancer Attributable to Lifestyle and Environmental Factors in the U.K. in 2010: Summary and Conclusions. *British Journal of Cancer* 105(52–55): S77–S81.

Peterson, R. (1997). Women, Environments, and Health: Overview and Strategic Directions for Research and Action. In G. S. Shahi, B. S. Levy, A. Binger, T. Kjellstrom, & R. Lawrence (Eds.), *International Perspectives on Environment, Development, and Health: Toward a Sustainable World* (pp. 660–675). New York: Springer Publishing Company.

Pink Ribbons, Inc. (2011). Feature documentary film. Lea Pool (Director). Ottawa: National Film Board of Canada.

Potts, L. (2004). An Epidemiology of Women's Lives: The Environmental Risk of Breast Cancer. *Critical Public Health* 14(2): 133–147.

Public Health Agency of Canada (PHAC). (2009). *Breast Cancer and Your Risk.* Ottawa: Author.

Public Health Agency of Canada (PHAC). (2012). *Breast Cancer.* Retrieved from http://www.phac-aspc.gc.ca/cd-mc/cancer/breast_cancer-cancer_du_sein-eng.php.

Rahder, B., & R. Peterson. (2000). *An Environmental Framework for Women's Health.* Toronto: National Network on Environments and Women's Health.

Reuben, S. (2010, April). *Reducing Environmental Cancer Risk: What We Can Do Now.* President's Cancer Panel 2008–2009 Annual Report. Bethesda, MD: U.S. Department of Health and Human Services, National Institutes of Health, and National Cancer Institute.

Rizzo, J. (2013, April 3). *Analysis of Federal Research Investments in Breast Cancer and the Environment Research. Collaborative on Health and the Environment Partnership Call. Breast Cancer and the Environment: Prioritizing Prevention.* Notes on file with author. Retrieved from http://www.healthandenvironment.org /uploads/docs/ IBCERCCreportslides.pdf.

Rudel, R., J. Ackerman, K. Attfield, & J. Green Brody. (2014). New Exposure Biomarkers as Tools for Breast Cancer Epidemiology, Biomonitoring, and Prevention: A Systematic Approach Based on Animal Evidence. *Environmental Health Perspectives* 122(9). doi: 10.1289/ehp.1307455.

Shah, C. K. (2003). *Public Health and Preventive Medicine in Canada* (5th ed.). Toronto: Elsevier Canada.

Sherwin, S. (2006). Personalizing the Political: Negotiating the Feminist, Medical, Scientific, and Commercial Discourses Surrounding Breast Cancer. In M. C. Rawlinson & S. Lundeen (Eds.), *The Voice of Breast Cancer in Medicine and Bioethics* (pp. 3–20). The Netherlands: Springer.

Soto, A., & C. Sonnenschein. (2010). Environmental Causes of Cancer: Endocrine Disruptors as Carcinogens. *Nature Reviews Endocrinology* 6(7): 363–370.

Steingraber, S. (2010). *Living Downstream: An Ecologist's Personal Investigation of Cancer and the Environment* (2nd ed.). Boston: Da Capo Press.

Sulik, G. (2011). *Pink Ribbon Blues: How Breast Cancer Culture Undermines Women's Health.* New York: Oxford University Press.

Sweeney, E. (2012). *Summary of the Research Findings: Breast Cancer Risk in Relation to Occupations with Exposure to Carcinogens and Endocrine Disruptors: A Canadian Case-Control Study.* Toronto: National Network on Environments and Women's Health in collaboration with the Canadian Women's Health Network.

Tomatis, L., & J. Huff. (2001). Evolution of Cancer Etiology and Primary Prevention. *Environmental Health Perspectives* 109(10): 458–460.

U.K. Working Group on the Primary Prevention of Breast Cancer. (2005). *Breast Cancer: An Environmental Disease. The Case for Primary Prevention.* Annemasse, France: Women in Europe for a Common Future.

Vandenberg, L. N., T. Colborn, T. B. Hayes, J. J. Heindel, D. R. Jacobs Jr., D.-H. Lee, T. Shioda, A. M. Soto, F. S. vom Saal, W. V. Welshons, R. T. Zoeller, & J. P. Myers. (2012). Hormones and Endocrine-Disrupting Chemicals: Low-Dose Effects and Nonmonotonic Dose Responses. *Endocrine Reviews* 33(3). doi:10.1210/er.2011-1050.

Watterson, A. (1999). Why We Still Have "Old" Epidemics and "Endemics" in Occupational Health: Policy and Practice Failures and Some Possible Solutions. In N. Daykin & L. Doyal (Eds.), *Health and Work: Critical Perspectives* (pp. 107–126). London: MacMillan Press.

Wilkinson, S. (2007). Breast Cancer Lived Experience and Feminist Action. In M. Morrow, O. Hankivsky, & C. Varcoe (Eds.), *Women's Health in Canada: Critical Perspectives on Theory and Practice* (pp. 408–433). Toronto: University of Toronto.

Women's College Hospital. (2013). *Why Do Environmental Illnesses Affect Women More than Men?* Retrieved from http://www.womenshealthmatters.ca/ health-resources/environmental-health/why-do-environmental-illnesses-affect-women-more-than-men.

World Health Organization (WHO). (2014). *Breast Cancer: Prevention and Control.* Retrieved from http://www.who.int/cancer/detection/breastcancer/en /index1.html.

Wyman, M. (Ed.). (1999). *Sweeping the Earth: Women Taking Action for a Healthy Planet.* Charlottetown: Gynergy Books.

Zavestoski, S., S. McCormick, & P. Brown. (2004). Gender, Embodiment, and Disease: Environmental Breast Cancer Activists' Challenges to Science, the Biomedical Model, and Policy. *Science as Culture* 13(4): 563–586.

Further Reading

Carson, R. (1962). *Silent Spring.* Greenwich, CT: Fawcett Publications.

Gray, J. (2010). *State of the Evidence: The Connection between Breast Cancer and the Environment* (6th ed.). San Francisco: Breast Cancer Fund.

King, S. (2008) *Pink Ribbons, Inc.: Breast Cancer and the Politics of Philanthropy*. Minneapolis: University of Minnesota Press.

Messing, K. (1998). *One-Eyed Science: Occupational Health and Women Workers*. Philadelphia: Temple University Press.

Steingraber, S. (2010). *Living Downstream: An Ecologist's Personal Investigation of Cancer and the Environment* (2nd ed.). Boston: Da Capo Press.

Relevant Websites

Breast Cancer Action (Montreal): www.bcam.qc.ca
Breast Cancer Action (San Francisco): www.bcaction.org
Breast Cancer Fund: www.breastcancerfund.org
Collaborative on Health and the Environment: www.healthandenvironment.org
National Network on Environments and Women's Health: www.nnewh.org
Women's Voices for the Earth: www.womensvoices.org

CHAPTER 17

Crossing the Chasms: Research, Policy, and Advocacy

Arlene S. Bierman

> All great truths begin as blasphemies.
>
> —GEORGE BERNARD SHAW

Introduction

We can do much better. Inequities in health associated with gender, race/ethnicity, and socio-economic position are ubiquitous. There is enormous untapped potential to improve the overall health and well-being of individuals, communities, and populations while at the same time reducing health inequities. This improvement can be accomplished by translating knowledge into practice, conducting research to expand the evidence base as to what works, and increasing the uptake of evidence by policy-makers and providers. Health inequities are present in societies with very different political systems, public policies, and health care systems. However, the size of the gap in health status between the most advantaged and disadvantaged members of society not only varies greatly between and within countries but also changes over time in response to changing political policies and social conditions (Marmot, 2006). Political, social, and health policies may lead to more or less equitable distribution of health among men and women (Kawachi et al., 1999; Navarro et al., 2006). Thus, health inequities are not inevitable and are amenable to change. Population health and health services research are contributing to a growing body of evidence that can inform the development of policy and are aimed at reducing and ultimately eliminating existing inequities in health.

Achieving equity in health requires both social policy that addresses the social determinants of health and health policy that supports improvements in public health and health care delivery (Bierman & Dunn, 2006). To be successful, these policies must promote gender equity and specifically address health inequities among women, recognizing the contribution of gender roles and relations as central determinants of women's health. Gender-sensitive policy is needed because women and men have very different patterns of illness, morbidity, and mortality, social contexts, and experiences with health care (Bierman & Clancy, 2001). In this chapter the role of research in building the necessary evidence base to inform and evaluate policy interventions aimed at improving health outcomes among all women is examined. Research can be a form of advocacy as well as a tool for advocates. Researchers, policy-makers, providers, and advocates who seek to improve population health and foster health equity work from different vantage points. Partnerships among them have the potential to accelerate the adoption and evaluation of effective strategies to achieve these objectives.

What Is Inequity in Health?

In order to advance the study of health inequities and prioritize policy interventions, it is important to have a clear definition of what constitutes a health inequity. The International Society for Equity in Health (ISEqH) has developed a useful set of definitions that can serve these purposes (International Society for Equity in Health, 2007). They define *inequity in health* as "the systematic and potentially remediable differences in one or more aspects of health across populations or population groups defined socially, economically, demographically, or geographically." *Equity in health* is "the absence of systematic and potentially remediable differences in one or more aspects of health across populations or population groups defined socially, economically, demographically, or geographically." By including "potentially remediable" as a key element of the definition, it focuses attention on identifying and addressing factors amenable to change.

A distinction is made between "equitable" and "equal." Implicit in the definition of equity is the notion of fairness. Achieving gender equity in health will require specifically addressing the causes of these gender inequities and recognizing the different needs of women and men arising from historical, social, and biological factors. Thus, treating men and women equally (the same) will not suffice and is not the objective. Rather, gender equity will require resource allocation and interventions to specifically address the unique needs of women and men.

ISEqH also defines policy and research in relation to equity. *Equity (policy and actions)* are "active policy decisions and programmatic actions directed at improving equity in health or in reducing or eliminating inequalities in health." *Equity (research)* "is research to elucidate the genesis and characteristics of inequity in health for the purpose of identifying factors amenable to policy decisions and programmatic actions to reduce or eliminate inequities" (International Society for Equity in Health, 2007).These definitions suggest that researchers and policy-makers can work synergistically. Both research and policy are integral components that, if aligned, have the potential to accelerate progress. However, there are many barriers to achieving this synergy. Researchers and policy-makers work in very different milieus with different cultures, demands, incentives, and priorities. To have an impact, researchers need not only ask policy-relevant questions, but also develop effective strategies for knowledge translation to policy-makers. Active efforts are needed to bridge the chasm that often separates the two groups.

Gender, Equity, and Health

> All diseases have two causes: one pathological and the other political.
>
> —RUDOLPH VIRCHOW

The social, economic, cultural, and physical environments in which individuals live create the milieus and contexts through which health is determined and mediate the effect of individual level factors on health (Evans & Stoddart, 2003). These social determinants of health are complex, multi-factorial, and act through varied pathways and at different levels to produce health inequities. Living and working conditions are primarily responsible for the production of socio-economic gradients in health. Although gender is routinely acknowledged as a determinant of health, generally insufficient attention is paid to the pathways through which gender determines socio-economic position and intersects with other determinants to influence health. The POWER Study Gender and Equity Health Indicator Framework illustrates the interaction between gender and other health determinants (Clark & Bierman, 2009). Gender serves as a form of social stratification, determining access to resources such as education, employment, and income (Östlin, Sen, & George, 2004). Use of a gender lens in analysis and gender-sensitive policies are therefore needed to foster health equity among women.

Health inequities associated with socio-economic position and ethnicity among women are often greater than overall disparities in health between men and women. In Ontario, women are more likely to have low incomes and less likely to be in the highest income group than men. However, minority men are more likely to be poor and less likely to be affluent than white women, while minority women are the most disadvantaged of the four groups (see Figure 17.1). Gender, race, ethnicity, and class represent a set of social relationships reproduced within local contexts and shaped within historical and contemporary social, cultural, and institutional contexts (Mullings & Schulz, 2006). They are not experienced as discrete and isolated phenomenon but are integrated and intertwined in a myriad of ways to impact on health and well-being.

Health inequalities produced by these social factors are often manifested through preventable or treatable clinical conditions, both communicable, such as HIV infection, and non-communicable, such as heart disease or diabetes. In Ontario, nearly one in three low-income women report fair or poor health compared to less than one in 10 women in the highest income category (see Figure 17.2). Advances in medical care have resulted in a growing armamentarium of effective interventions that can prevent premature mortality and morbidity resulting from many medical illnesses common and uncommon. Access to quality health

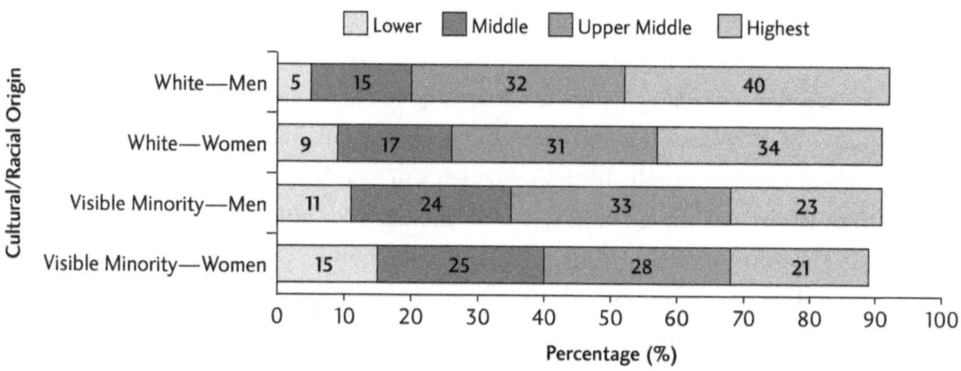

FIGURE 17.1: Income distribution of men and women age 25 and older in Ontario (age-standardized)

Source: A. Bierman, 2008, *The Burden of Chronic Illness and Disability in Ontario: Report to the Ontario Ministry of Health and Long-Term Care* (Toronto: Ministry of Health and Long-Term Care.

care can therefore improve the health of population groups of lower socio-economic position, whereas poor access and quality of care can compound these inequalities (Bierman & Dunn, 2006). Socio-economically disadvantaged individuals are placed in "triple jeopardy" for poor

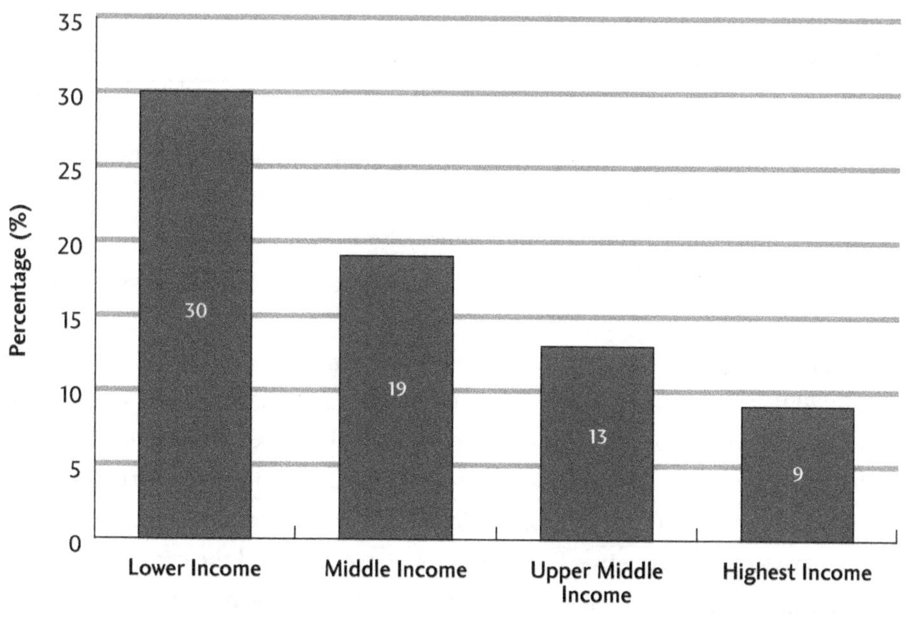

FIGURE 17.2: Fair or poor self-perceived health among Ontario women age 25 and older by income (age-standardized)

Source: A. Bierman, 2008, *The Burden of Chronic Illness and Disability in Ontario: Report to the Ontario Ministry of Health and Long-Term Care* (Toronto: Ministry of Health and Long-Term Care).

health outcomes. The social determinants of health produce a higher illness burden, multiple barriers to accessing make it harder to access needed care, and when care is received they are at increased risk for receiving care of suboptimal quality. Thus, a coordinated approach that addresses the social determinants as well as access to and quality of health care services is most likely to result in sustainable improvements in health outcomes.

Health care is a determinant of health and a mediator between the social determinants of health and health outcomes. Health policies that strengthen primary care are associated with better levels of health and with better preventive care (Starfield, Shi, & Macinko, 2005). In a study of 18 member countries of the Organisation for Economic Co-operation and Development (OECD), the strength of a country's primary care system was associated with lower rates of all-cause mortality, all-cause premature mortality, and cause-specific premature mortality from asthma and bronchitis, emphysema and pneumonia, and cardiovascular disease (Macinko, Starfield, & Shi, 2003). In Canada, the Canadian Institute for Health Information health indicator framework incorporates both the social and medical determinants of health. Men have lower life expectancies than women and higher age-specific mortality rates, while women experience a higher burden of chronic illness, disability, and co-morbidity—factors that are amenable to health care intervention. Coordinated efforts that address the social determinants of health and the quality of health care services could optimize health outcomes in women.

Quality of Care and Health Equity

> Quality is the degree to which health services for individuals and populations increase the likelihood of desired health outcomes and are consistent with current professional knowledge.
>
> (INSTITUTE OF MEDICINE, 1990)

Two landmark studies by the U.S. Institute of Medicine, *Crossing the Quality Chasm*, released in 2001, and *Unequal Treatment*, released the following year, have focused attention internationally on gaps in health care quality as well as inequalities in quality of care associated with race and ethnicity. The Institute of Medicine, in the report *Crossing the Quality Chasm*, concluded that there are serious and pervasive problems in the quality of health care services so that between the health care we have and the care we could have lies not just a gap but a chasm. They added that because the problems come from poor systems and not bad people, the solution requires health system redesign and transformation (Institute of Medicine, 2001).

Sizable gaps in the quality of health care have been well documented in Canada and internationally. In a U.S. study, McGlynn assessed performance on a comprehensive set of ambulatory care indicators of care for acute, chronic, and preventive services and found that only a little over half (54.9 percent) of recommended care was provided (McGlynn et al., 2003). Gaps in performance in ambulatory care have also been reported in Canada. A report by the Health Council of Canada, which included both a literature review and analysis of the Canadian Community Health Survey, found that only half of Canadians with diabetes get all the recommended lab tests and procedures to monitor blood sugar, blood pressure, cholesterol, kidney health, vision, and foot health, and that more than half of Canadians with diabetes do not achieve recommended levels of blood sugar control (Health Council of Canada, 2007). A 2006 cross-national survey of primary care physicians in Australia, Canada, Germany, New Zealand, the Netherlands, the United Kingdom, and the United States revealed striking differences in elements of practice systems that underpin quality and efficiency, and found that Canada lagged in adopting strategies to improve the quality of ambulatory care (Schoen et al., 2006). Compared to other countries, Canadian doctors were less likely to have electronic records systems in place, making comprehensive patient follow-up difficult and inefficient. Seventy-four percent of Canadian physicians do not receive data about clinical outcomes; less than half (45 percent) conduct audits of care; and barely a third (32 percent) have multi-disciplinary teams in place to work together to treat chronic illnesses. More recent reports show that Canada continues to lag in international comparisons of health system performance (CIHI, 2011; Davis et al., 2014).

In *Unequal Treatment: Confronting Racial and Ethnic Disparities in Health Care*, the Institute of Medicine found a consistent body of research that demonstrated that U.S. racial and ethnic minorities are less like to receive indicated services and experience worse health outcomes. Disparities were found even when clinical factors, such as stage of disease presentation, co-morbidities, age, and severity of disease, were taken into account across a wide range of clinical settings, including public and private hospitals, teaching and non-teaching hospitals. These disparities are believed to result from multiple factors, including socio-economic position, bias and discrimination, and differential access to care and its quality (Smedley, Stith, & Nelson, 2002). This is not surprising. Health care systems mirror the dynamics of the broader society. Thus, discrimination and bias associated with race, gender, and class operating within health care institutions contribute identified inequities in health and health care (Geiger, 2006). Socio-economic, gender, and racial/ethnic disparities in health and health care have also been documented in Canada (Bierman et al., 2012).

Women of colour appear to be at particularly high risk for suboptimal quality and outcomes of care (Rathore et al., 2000; Schulman et al., 1999; Sheifer, Escarce, & Schulman, 2000), reflecting the intersectionality of gender, ethnicity, and socio-economic position. This intersectionality creates "multiple jeopardies" for low-income women of colour that need to be acknowledged, understood, and addressed in research, practice, and policy. A study using data from the Health Survey for England 1993-1996 found substantially poorer health among all minority ethnic groups compared to whites, with higher morbidity for minority ethnic women compared to men in the same ethnic group after controlling for socio-economic factors. The magnitude of gender and socio-economic differences varied by ethnicity (Cooper, 2002). Widely accepted indicators of health care quality, when stratified by race/ethnicity or socio-economic position, have shown that socio-economically disadvantaged individuals may receive lower quality of care even when receiving care from the same health system (Fremont et al., 2005).

Both *Crossing the Quality Chasm* and *Unequal Treatment* were made possible by large bodies of compelling evidence built over years by multiple researchers creating a paradigm shift that allowed previously "blasphemous" views to become mainstream and resulted in the subsequent commitment of resources by policy-makers to address these problems and to support research aimed at finding solutions.

Policy, Practice, and Health Outcomes

Public and health policy influences both individual and population health outcomes. Therefore it is important to objectively assess the impact of specific policies on health outcomes. Understanding the relationships among the multiple factors that influence health outcomes can help us identify opportunities for intervention and improvement. Well-intentioned policy interventions can have unintended consequences and sometimes result in worse health outcomes. Clinicians seek to use the best available evidence in making clinical decisions, in order to practise evidenced-based medicine. There is a growing recognition of the need for policy-makers to apply evidence-informed policy. Population health and health services research can make important contributions to the evidence base to help policy-makers implement more effective policies. Research can build the evidence base as to what policies work in fostering health equity by studying the health impacts of existing policies and by conducting objective evaluations of policy interventions.

A framework for understanding the relationships between policy, the organization and financing of care, clinical practice, and biologic-, individual-, social-, and community-level factors that influence health outcomes is shown in Figure 17.3. It includes a patient-centred rather than disease-specific focus, particularly relevant for women who are more likely than men to have multiple chronic conditions. Patient-centred models recognize the net effect of individual conditions and treatments in the context of psychosocial factors and patient values on overall health and well-being (Stewart & Napoles-Springer, 2000).

Women are concerned about the impact of their physical and mental health on their ability to function and to do what is important to them. Functional status is a meaningful outcome measure because it assesses what matters to individuals. In this framework, functional status is measured using multiple domains, including physical, emotional, cognitive, role, and social functioning. A women's functioning is influenced by her biology (i.e., genetics), individual characteristics (i.e., health beliefs and behaviours), family

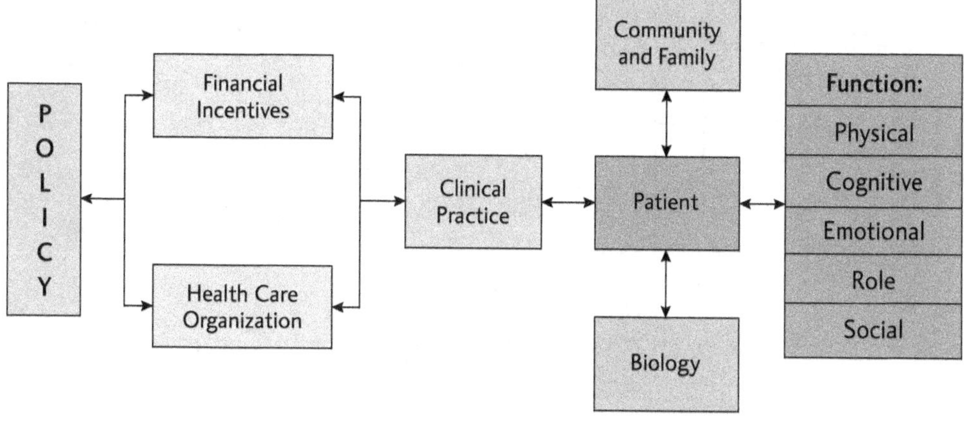

FIGURE 17.3: Policy, organization, finance, clinical practice, patient-level factors, and functional health outcomes

Source: A. Bierman et al., 2008, *Improving the Health Care of Older Americans: A Report of the AHRQ Task Force on Aging* (Rockville, MD: Agency for Health Care Research and Quality).

(i.e., social support), and community (i.e., environmental factors, community services) as well as by her interactions with the health care system. The clinician–patient interaction is influenced by how the clinical setting is organized and the financial incentives created by payment mechanisms, which are in turn influenced by health policy. All of the arrows in the framework are bi-directional, reflecting the multiple, complex interrelationships that influence health and function.

Studying these relationships can provide needed evidence for decision-makers at multiple levels: clinical, community, health system, and policy-makers. Just as evidence is needed for the effectiveness or harms of clinical interventions, research is also needed to provide evidence about the effectiveness or harm of organizational, quality improvement, public health, and policy interventions, as well as evidence for interventions aimed at reducing health inequities.

Access, Quality, and Health Outcomes

The conceptual framework depicted in Figure 17.4 illustrates how access to and quality of care mediate health outcomes (Bierman et al., 1998). This framework can serve as a tool for identifying opportunities for intervention (Bierman & Clancy, 2001). Primary, secondary, and tertiary barriers to access all impede the receipt of effective care. Because men and women have different health care needs, financial and social resources and contexts, and interactions with health care providers, the impact of these barriers and the strategies needed to overcome them can differ by gender.

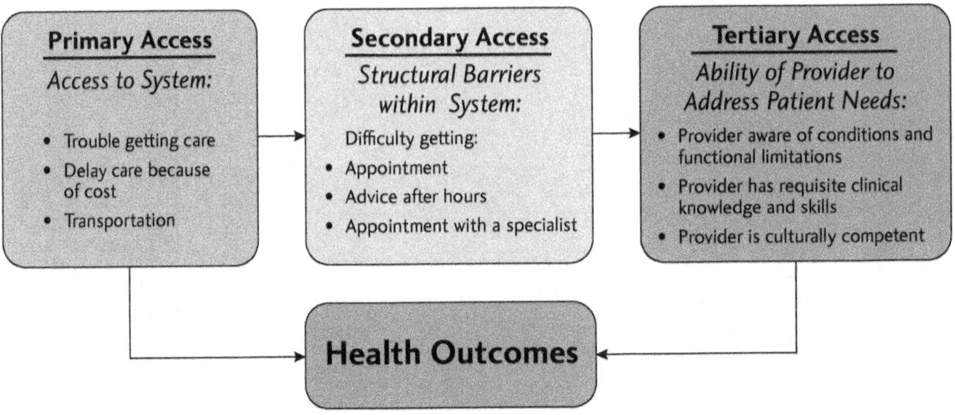

FIGURE 17.4: Access, quality, and health outcomes

Sources: A. S. Bierman, E. S. Magari, A. M. Jette, M. Splaine, & J. H. Wasson, 1998, Assessing Access as a First Step toward Improving the Quality of Care for Very Old Adults, *Journal of Ambulatory Care Management* 21 (3): 17–26; and A. S. Bierman & C. M. Clancy, 2001, Health Disparities among Older Women: Identifying Opportunities to Improve Quality of Care and Functional Health Outcomes, *Journal of the American Medical Women's Association* 56(4): 155–159, 188.

Primary access barriers represent the first obstacle in getting care and include such factors as health coverage, proximity of providers, competing demands such as caregiving, and lack of transportation. Even under Canada's system of universal health insurance, essential services such as drugs or physical therapy may not be covered for everyone. Women who are more likely to be low income and have more chronic illness may be disproportionately affected by these barriers. Secondary barriers are structural barriers within the care delivery system such as difficulty getting appointments, specialty referrals, or advice after hours. Tertiary access is the link between access and quality and reflects the ability of providers and the health care system to understand and address the patient's needs, including the provider's communication skills and cultural competence, knowledge, and clinical skills (Bierman et al., 1998; Weinick, Byron, & Bierman, 2005). Improved access and quality of care for women is dependent upon an understanding of all of these barriers for diverse groups and developing effective interventions to address them.

Sex Matters and Gender Matters

Women's health is determined by sex or the biological differences between men and women as well as by gender, the context of women's lives. Advances in the basic sciences have found that molecular and genetic mechanisms make a much greater contribution to differences in health and illness between men and women than previously believed. Sex differences are observed at the system, organ, tissue, cellular, and sub-cellular levels, and sex hormones are responsible for only a portion of sex differences (Wizemann & Pardue, 2001). Policies have been developed to build our understanding of how sex and gender influence women's health and to develop the evidence base for population health, clinical, social, and policy interventions to improve health and reduce health inequities among women. The U.S. National Institutes of Health mandate the inclusion of women in clinical trials and have developed a policy with respect to the use of both male and female cells in basic biomedical research (Clayton & Collins, 2014). The World Health Organization has a policy of gender mainstreaming in health that requires integrating gender into the formulation, monitoring, and analysis of policies, programs, and projects as a strategy for achieving gender equity (World Health Organization, 2007). The Canadian Institutes of Health Research have a policy for gender- and sex-based analysis in research.

As more studies conduct sex- and gender-based analyses, important differences between men and women are being identified. For example, the Early Lung Cancer Action Project (ELCAP) study found that women who smoke are at greater risk for developing lung cancer than men who smoke. However, when woman develop lung cancer, they are less likely to die from the disease than men (Henschke, Yip, & Miettinen, 2006). Another study looked at differences in the effectiveness of Aspirin in reducing the risk of cardiovascular events. Although Aspirin was protective for both women and men, Aspirin therapy affected risk by reducing the risk of strokes in women and heart attacks in men (Berger et al., 2006).

The INTERHEART Study found that nine cardiovascular risk factors—lipid abnormalities, smoking, hypertension, diabetes, abdominal obesity, psychosocial factors, physical inactivity, low fruit and vegetable intake, and alcohol (moderate alcohol use was protective)—overall accounted for 90 percent of the attributable risk for heart attacks in men and 94 percent in women. The population attributable risk (PAR) is the proportion of cases in the population that can be attributed to a given risk factor. The PAR for heart attack risk factors varies by gender for some risk factors, but not for others. For example, abnormal lipids contributed equally to cardiovascular disease in both men (49.5 percent) and women (47.1 percent), as did abdominal obesity (19.7 percent vs. 18.7 percent, respectively). However, the PAR for smoking was greater in men (42.7 percent vs. 14.8 percent), while the PARs for psychosocial risk factors (28.8 percent vs. 45.2 percent) and hypertension (14.9 percent vs. 29.0 percent) were greater in women (Yusuf et al., 2004). A population-based study in Canada found a high prevalence of modifiable CVD risk factors in the population, with geographic and gender variation in risk factor prevalence (Tanuseputro et al., 2003). Therefore, improving health outcomes in heart disease requires attention to social factors that result in differences in the distribution of risk factors by gender, socio-economic position, and geography, as well as biological differences between men and women.

In reality, when focusing on health outcomes, the effects of sex and gender can be very difficult, if not impossible, to disentangle. For example, while sex influences who will get lung cancer and who will survive it, social factors influence who smokes and is therefore at greater risk and these factors differ by gender and socio-economic position. Social factors may also affect access to care and the quality of care received. In Ontario, 27 percent of low-income women smoke compared to 14 percent of more affluent women (Figure 17.5). Sex- and gender-sensitive tools are needed to facilitate the uptake of new evidence into practice.

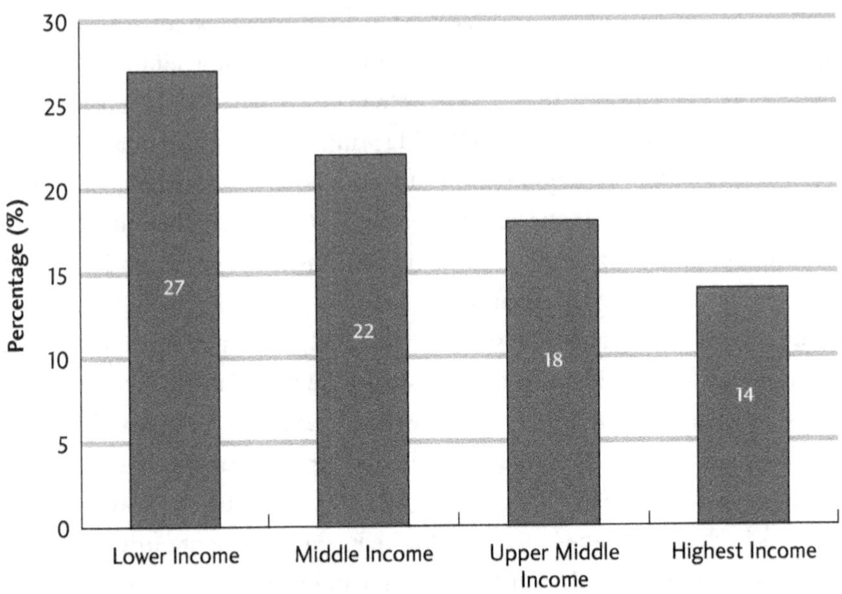

FIGURE 17.5: Percent of women who smoke daily in Ontario (age-standardized)

Source: A. Bierman, 2008, *The Burden of Chronic Illness and Disability in Ontario: Report to the Ontario Ministry of Health and Long-Term Care* (Toronto: Ministry of Health and Long-Term Care).

Performance Measurement: A Tool to Drive Improvement and Equity

The implementation of performance measurement, reporting, and quality improvement using strategically developed quality indicators can lead to improved clinical performance and patient experiences with care, and serve as a tool to accelerate the uptake of evidence into practice. When quality indicators are also used to assess inequities in access, quality, and outcomes of care, they can also serve as a powerful tool to drive equity in health. There are a growing number of examples of health systems that have been able to achieve improvements in health care quality, including the U.S. Veterans Administration, and the National Health Service in the United Kingdom through its Quality and Outcomes Framework (Doran et al., 2006; Singh & Kalavar, 2004). Studies have shown that quality measurement and improvement interventions can result in improved care and reduce disparities for some but not all indicators (Sehgal, 2003; Wells et al., 2004). However, it is also possible to widen disparities if improvement occurs to a greater extent in one group compared to another, although both show improvement, that is, men versus women.

Measurement and reporting by itself does not result in improvement. It must be done in the context of a commitment to change by policy-makers and providers, consensus as to priorities for improvement, measurable objectives, monitoring of progress, and accountability for results. Stratified reporting of performance indicators by gender and for at-risk population subgroups allows us to assess gaps in current practice, target interventions, and monitor progress. However, the design of effective and evidence-based policies and interventions cannot be based on descriptive measures alone since they do not provide a clear understanding of the factors underlying gender, socio-economic, ethnic, and geographic inequities in health. There is a need to complement measurement and reporting initiatives with gender-based analyses to elucidate the underlying pathways and determinants of health that lead to observed health and health care inequities.

Performance measures can be derived from multiple data sources, including administrative data, surveys, disease registries, chart review, or electronic medical records. Well-validated surveys are available that assess multiple domains of patient experiences with care, including doctor–patient communication, care coordination, and access. Large secondary data sets are commonly used both to assess quality and to answer critical research questions about health outcomes, quality of life, and quality of care for specific conditions as well as for populations of interest. Large sample size and inclusion of a large number of variables often provide the statistical power to assess multiple clinical and non-clinical factors associated with health outcomes, as well as variation in outcomes and experiences with care for population subgroups.

Health System Transformation and Equity

The current health care system evolved to meet the needs of acute illness and does a poor job of serving individuals with chronic illness and disability. Without health system transformation it will not be possible to improve health outcomes and/or achieve equity. Wagner and colleagues have developed a Chronic Care Model (CCM) that provides a framework for systems change. This model has been used to improve the quality of care in diverse practice settings (Wagner et al., 2001). The Chronic Care Model, which has guided efforts to improve health care quality using a health systems approach, includes the role of community resources and policy in improving health outcomes. It also recognizes that good health outcomes are dependent upon productive interactions between women and a proactive health care team and empowers patients to take an active role in their care.

Subsequent iterations of the CCM expand upon the role of both communities and the policy environment in fostering health, providing a framework that can be used to address the social determinants of health in the context of system redesign and improvement (Barr et al., 2003; Epping-Jordan et al., 2004). The Innovative Care for Chronic Conditions model (ICCC) adapts the CCM for use in developing nations, includes the community as an equal partner together with providers and patients in improving health outcomes, and identifies critical elements of supportive policies, including resource allocation and consistent financing (Epping-Jordan et al., 2004). In Canada, the province of British Columbia is using the Expanded Chronic Care Model, which emphasizes the role of an activated community as a partner and incorporates a focus on disease prevention and health promotion (Barr et al., 2003). The province of Ontario has adapted this model for its chronic disease strategy. There is growing recognition that successful public health interventions also require community empowerment and participation (Syme, 2004).

Because women in general and disadvantaged women in particular have a higher burden of chronic illness and disability, the current mismatch between the way care is organized and the needs of people with chronic illness disproportionately impacts them. Health system redesign that supports chronic illness care and fosters patient empowerment and community partnership is an important strategy for improving the health of women.

Improving Quality of Care and Health Outcomes for Women

To close the quality gaps for women and thus improve their health and functional status, there are opportunities for improvement across the continuum of care, including: health promotion, clinical preventive services, management of chronic illness, coordination and accountability across different sites and settings of care, and coordination between clinical and community services. In the Framingham study,[1] stroke, depression, hip fracture, osteoarthritis, and heart disease were the major contributors to functional disability among older adults. There are gender differences in the clinical epidemiology and experiences with care for all of these conditions. Women are more likely than men to have the conditions that lead to impaired mobility and functional dependence such as arthritis, osteoporosis, and hip fractures, and are also more likely to suffer from depressive symptoms. Gender disparities in clinical management, use of procedures, and health outcomes for older women with ischemic heart disease and congestive heart failure have been well documented. Women are not only more likely to have chronic conditions that lead to disability, but are also at risk for suboptimal diagnosis and treatment for these conditions.

Clinical interventions can improve functional status by reducing the risk of both acute events, such as stroke and hip fractures, as well as the progressive loss of function from conditions such as arthritis and congestive heart failure. Chronic diseases often produce an insidious decline in functional status over decades. Chronic conditions may be suboptimally managed for decades before affecting an individual's functional status. Examples are congestive heart failure from hypertensive heart disease resulting from poorly controlled hypertension, or peripheral vascular disease leading to claudication and/or limb loss as a complication of poorly controlled diabetes. A hip fracture in a 75-year-old woman with osteoporosis could potentially be related to inadequate calcium intake as an adolescent; failure to recommend calcium supplementation and recommend weight-bearing exercise two decades previously; or failure to diagnose and treat osteoporosis after a previous wrist fracture. Therefore, a life-course approach to optimizing women's health outcomes is required.

Performance measurement and reporting, linked to targeted improvement activities, interventions to address the social determinants of health, and policy-relevant research to increase our understanding of the root causes of suboptimal health outcomes health inequities and what works to address them are all elements for designing and implementing programs and policies that lead to measurable improvements in women's health. In Ontario, the Ministry of Health and Long-Term Care funded the development and implementation of a comprehensive women's health report card, the Project for an Ontario Women's Health Evidence-Based Report (POWER). POWER reported on quality and outcomes of care for the leading causes of illness and death among women, including cancer, heart disease, depression, diabetes, musculoskeletal disorders, and reproductive health as well as overall health of Ontario women, women's access to health care services, and the social determinants of women's health (www.powerstudy.ca). It serves as a tool to help policy-makers and providers improve the health of and reduce inequities among the women of Ontario. Initiatives such as this can inform priority setting; design of population health, health system, and policy interventions; and provide an infrastructure for monitoring progress.

Conclusion: Crossing the Chasm(s)—Research, Policy, Advocacy

Inequities in health are not inevitable. Rather, they are modifiable and amenable to intervention. Population health and health services research can provide the critical evidence needed by providers and policy-makers to improve women's health. By asking meaningful policy-relevant questions, researchers can provide answers that can help drive change. In this context research can serve as a powerful form of advocacy. Researchers can increase the impact of their work not only by communicating the findings of their work clearly to decision-makers, but also by engaging in dialogue to better understand what evidence they need. Community-based advocates can add important context to this dialogue as well as use research evidence to support their advocacy efforts. Policy-makers may be able to increase the likelihood that policies will achieve their stated objectives by building on existing evidence. Performance measurement and quality improvement strategies may not only help drive change, but serve as a mechanism to bridge the chasm(s) between research policy and advocacy.

Note

1. The Framingham Heart Study is a longitudinal project that began in 1948 and continues. It is based in Framingham, Massachusetts. For more information, see www.framinghamheartstudy.org.

References

Barr, V. J., S. Robinson, B. Marin-Link, L. Underhill, A. Dotts, D. Ravensdale, et al. (2003). The Expanded Chronic Care Model: An Integration of Concepts and Strategies from Population Health Promotion and the Chronic Care Model. *Hospital Quarterly* 7(1): 73–82.

Berger, J. S., M. C. Roncaglioni, F. Avanzini, I. Pangrazzi, G. Tognoni, & D. L. Brown. (2006). Aspirin for the Primary Prevention of Cardiovascular Events in Women and Men: A Sex-Specific Meta-Analysis of Randomized Controlled Trials. *JAMA* 295(3): 306–313.

Bierman, A. (2008). *The Burden of Chronic Illness and Disability in Ontario: Report to the Ontario Ministry of Health and Long-Term Care.* Toronto: Ministry of Health and Long-Term Care.

Bierman, A. S., & C. M. Clancy. (2001). Health Disparities among Older Women: Identifying Opportunities to Improve Quality of Care and Functional Health Outcomes. *Journal of the American Medical Women's Association* 56(4): 155–159, 188.

Bierman, A. S., & J. R. Dunn. (2006). Swimming Upstream: Access, Health Outcomes, and the Social Determinants of Health. *Journal of General Internal Medicine* 21(1): 99–100.

Bierman, A. S., E. S. Magari, A.M. Jette, M. Splaine, & J. H. Wasson. (1998). Assessing Access as a First Step toward Improving the Quality of Care for Very Old Adults. *Journal of Ambulatory Care Management* 21(3): 17–26.

Bierman, A. S., A. R. Shack, & A. Johns. (2012, June). Achieving Health Equity in Ontario: Opportunities for Interventions and Improvement. In A. S. Bierman (Ed.), *Project for an Ontario Women's Health Evidence-Based Report: Vol. 2.* Toronto: POWER. Retrieved from http://powerstudy.ca/power-report/volume2/achieving-health-equity-in-ontario/.

Canadian Institute for Health Information (CIHI). (2011, November). *Learning from the Best: Benchmarking Canada's Health System.* Ottawa: Author.

Clark, J. P., & A. S. Bierman. (2009, June). The POWER Study Framework. In A. S. Bierman (Ed.), *Project for an Ontario Women's Health Evidence-Based Report: Vol. 1.* Toronto. Retrieved from http://powerstudy.ca/power-report/volume1/power-study-framework/.

Clayton, J., & F. Collins. (2014, May 15). *Nature* 509(2009): 282-283. doi:10.1038/509282a.

Cooper, H. (2002). Investigating Socio-Economic Explanations for Gender and Ethnic Inequalities in Health. *Social Science and Medicine* 54(5): 693–706.

Davis, K., K. Stremikis, D. Squires, & C. Schoen. (2014). *Mirror, Mirror on the Wall. Update: How the U.S. Health Care System Compares Internationally.* The Commonwealth Fund. Long Beach, CA: Health Resource Centre.

Doran, T., C. Fullwood, H. Gravelle, D. Reeves, E. Kontopantelis, U. Hiroeh, et al. (2006). Pay-for-Performance Programs in Family Practices in the United Kingdom. *New England Journal of Medicine* 355(4): 375–384.

Epping-Jordan, J. E., S. D. Pruitt, R. Bengoa, & E. H. Wagner. (2004). Improving the Quality of Health Care for Chronic Conditions. *Quality and Safety in Health Care* 13(4): 299–305.

Evans, R. G., & G. L. Stoddart. (2003). Consuming Research, Producing Policy? *American Journal of Public Health* 93(3): 371–379.

Fremont, A. M., A. Bierman, S. L. Wickstrom, C. E. Bird, M. Shah, J. J. Escarce, et al. (2005). Use of Geocoding in Managed Care Settings to Identify Quality Disparities. *Health Affairs* 24(2): 516–526.

Geiger, H. J. (2006). Health Disparities: What Do We Know? What Do We Need to Know?

What Should We Do? In A. J. Schulz & L. Mullings (Eds.), *Gender, Race, Class, and Health: Intersectional Approaches* (pp. 261–288). San Francisco: Jossey-Bass.

Health Council of Canada. (2007). *Why Health Care Renewal Matters: Lessons from Diabetes (A Health Outcomes Report)*. Toronto: Author. Retrieved from http://publications.gc.ca/collections/collection_2007/hcc-ccs/H174-5-2007E.pdf.

Henschke, C. I., R. Yip, & O. S. Miettinen. (2006). Women's Susceptibility to Tobacco Carcinogens and Survival after Diagnosis of Lung Cancer. *JAMA* 296(2): 180–184.

Institute of Medicine. (1990). *Medicare: A Strategy for Quality Assurance*. Washington, DC: National Academies Press.

Institute of Medicine. (2001). *Crossing the Quality Chasm*. Washington, DC: National Academies Press.

International Society for Equity in Health. (2007). *Definitions*. Retrieved from www.iseqh.org.

Kawachi, I., B. P. Kennedy, V. Gupta, & D. Prothrow-Smith. (1999). Women's Status and the Health of Women and Men: A View from the States. *Social Science and Medicine* 48(1): 21–32.

Macinko, J., B. Starfield, & L. Shi. (2003). The Contribution of Primary Care Systems to Health Outcomes within Organisation for Economic Co-operation and Development (OECD) Countries, 1970–1998. *Health Services Research* 38(3): 831–865.

Marmot, M. (2006). Health in an Unequal World: Social Circumstances, Biology, and Disease. *Clinical Medicine* 6(6): 559–572.

McGlynn, E. A., S. M. Asch, J. Adams, J. Keesey, J. Hicks, A. DeCristofaro, et al. (2003). The Quality of Health Care Delivered to Adults in the United States. *New England Journal of Medicine* 348(26): 2635–2645.

Mullings, L., & A. Schulz. (2006). Intersectionality and Health: An Introduction. In A. J. Schulz & L. Mullings (Eds.), *Gender, Race, Class, and Health: Intersectional Approaches* (pp. 3–20). San Francisco: Jossey-Bass.

Navarro, V., C. Muntaner, C. Borrell, J. Benach, A. Quiroga, M. Rodriguez-Sanz, et al. (2006). Politics and Health Outcomes. *Lancet* 368(9540): 1033–1037.

Östlin, P., G. Sen, & A. George. (2004). Paying Attention to Gender and Poverty in Health Research: Content and Process Issues. *Bulletin World Health Organization* 82(10): 740–745.

Rathore, S. S., A. K. Berger, K. P. Weinfurt, M. Feinleib, W. J. Oetgen, B. J. Gersh, et al. (2000). Race, Sex, Poverty, and the Medical Treatment of Acute Myocardial Infarction in the Elderly. *Circulation* 102(6): 642–648.

Schoen, C., R. Osborn, P. T. Huynh, M. Doty, J. Peugh, & K. Zapert. (2006). On the Front Lines of Care: Primary Care Doctors' Office Systems, Experiences, and Views in Seven Countries. *Health Affairs* 25(6): 555–571.

Schulman, K. A., J. A . Berlin, W. Harless, J. F. Kerner, S. Sistrunk, B. J. Gersh, et al. (1999). The Effect of Race and Sex on Physicians' Recommendations for Cardiac Catheterization. *New England Journal of Medicine* 340(8): 618–626.

Sehgal, A. R. (2003). Impact of Quality Improvement Efforts on Race and Sex Disparities in Hemodialysis. *JAMA* 289(8): 996–1000.

Sheifer, S. E., J. J. Escarce, & K. A. Schulman. (2000). Race and Sex Differences in the Management of Coronary Artery Disease. *American Heart Journal* 139(5): 848–857.

Singh, H., & J. Kalavar. (2004). Quality of Care for Hypertension and Diabetes in Federal- Versus

Commercial-Managed Care Organizations. *American Journal of Medical Quality* 19(1): 19–24.

Smedley, B. D., A. Y. Stith, & A. R. Nelson. (2002). *Unequal Treatment: Confronting Racial and Ethnic Disparities in Health Care.* Washington, DC: National Academy Press.

Starfield, B., L. Shi, & J. Macinko. (2005). Contribution of Primary Care to Health Systems and Health. *Milbank Quarterly* 83(3): 457–502.

Stewart, A. L., & A. Napoles-Springer. (2000). Health-Related Quality-of-Life Assessments in Diverse Population Groups in the United States. *Medical Care* 38(9 Suppl. II): 102–124.

Syme, S. L. (2004). Social Determinants of Health: The Community as an Empowered Partner. *Preventing Chronic Disease* 1(1): A02.

Tanuseputro, P., D. G. Manuel, M. Leung, K. Nguyen, & H. Johansen. (2003). Risk Factors for Cardiovascular Disease in Canada. *Canadian Journal of Cardiology* 19(11): 1249–1259.

Wagner, E. H., B. T. Austin, C. Davis, M. Hindmarsh, J. Schaefer, & A. Bonomi. (2001). Improving Chronic Illness Care: Translating Evidence into Action. *Health Affairs* 20(6): 64–78.

Weinick, R. M., S. C. Byron, & A. S. Bierman. (2005). Who Can't Pay for Health Care? *Journal of General Internal Medicine* 20(6): 504–509.

Wells, K., C. Sherbourne, M. Schoenbaum, S. Ettner, N. Duan, J. Miranda, et al. (2004). Five-Year Impact of Quality Improvement for Depression: Results of a Group-Level Randomized Controlled Trial. *Archives of General Psychiatry* 61(4): 378–386.

Wizemann, T., & M. Pardue. (2001). *Exploring the Biological Contributions to Human Health: Does Sex Matter?* Washington, DC: National Academy Press.

World Health Organization. (2007). *Integrating Gender Analysis and Actions into the Work of WHO: Draft Strategy.* Geneva: World Health Organization.

Yusuf, S., S. Hawken, S. Ounpuu, T. Dans, A. Avezum, F. Lanas, et al. (2004). Effect of Potentially Modifiable Risk Factors Associated with Myocardial Infarction in 52 Countries (the INTERHEART Study): Case-Control Study. *Lancet* 364(9438): 937–952.

Further Reading

Barr, V. J., S. Robinson, B. Marin-Link, L. Underhill, A. Dotts, et al. (2003). The Expanded Chronic Care Model: An Integration of Concepts and Strategies from Population Health Promotion and the Chronic Care Model. *Hospital Quarterly* 7(1): 73–82.

Bierman, A. S., & C. M. Clancy. (2001). Health Disparities among Older Women: Identifying Opportunities to Improve Quality of Care and Functional Health Outcomes. *Journal of the American Medical Women's Association* 56(4): 155–159, 188.

Institute of Medicine. (2001). *Crossing the Quality Chasm.* Washington, DC: National Academy Press.

Smedley, B. D., A. Y. Stith, & A. R. Nelson. (2002). *Unequal Treatment: Confronting Racial and Ethnic Disparities in Health Care.* Washington, DC: National Academies Press.

Relevant Websites

CIHR Institute of Gender and Health: http://www.cihr-irsc.gc.ca/e/8673.html
International Women's Health Coalition: www.iwhc.org
POWER Study: www.powerstudy.ca
World Health Organization: http://who.int/topics/womens_health/en/

CHAPTER 18

"Our Words, Our Health": The Continuing Value of Including Women in Health Research and Knowledge Translation

Julie Maher and Sara Mohammed

Introduction

The inclusion of women's voices in the determination of their own health and well-being is a strong focus for the Ontario Women's Health Network (OWHN) and has been a long-standing mantra within the women's health field. In the years since the first edition of this book, OWHN's role in helping to ensure that women—especially those from groups who might be considered to be marginalized—have a voice in the issues and policies regarding women's health has not changed, but much has shifted in the political climate and in the funding environments for women's health issues. In this chapter, we use the project Our Words, Our Health to discuss the health concerns and priorities identified by diverse women in Ontario and to reflect upon the constraints of meeting their health care preferences in the current context of cutbacks, constraints, and a general loss of support for women's health initiatives, structures, and programs in the province.

The Ontario Women's Health Network

The Ontario Women's Health Network was founded in August 1997 by several community-based women's health and health promotion organizations through the financial support and encouragement of Health Canada. OWHN was mandated to be a province-wide women's health network, representing the diversity of women in this province and the scope of the health issues they face. While the funding from Health Canada lasted for only a few years, OWHN has continued to be a network of individuals and organizations that promotes women's health. OWHN works with women, health and social service providers, community organizations, and others to support equitable, accessible, and effective health services for all women in Ontario.

OWHN was formed to address major gaps such as the lack of information-sharing, inadequate networking, and poor access to resources for groups and communities working on behalf of women across the province.

OWHN believes that the inclusion of women's voices is critical to informing the development of health policy, research, and service provision, including care and education. OWHN pays particular attention to ensuring the inclusion of women who have experienced marginalization, such as women who are rural, disabled, Aboriginal, of diverse ethnoracial backgrounds, francophone, of low socio-economic status, and at all stages of life. Therefore, a key aspect of OWHN's work is ensuring that women's voices are heard and acted upon. OWHN has developed and used a variety of strategies to achieve this objective, including meeting face to face with women individually and collectively in their community, engaging women in our research to offer them an opportunity to voice their priority issues in health, and strengthening their community networks to address these issues.

Inclusion Research Methodology

OWHN has invested considerable resources in conducting focus groups with diverse women across Ontario who have experienced marginalization. Within these many focus groups, women repeatedly spoke of the importance of coming together in groups to learn from one another and share information. More importantly, though, they expressed how tired they were of organizations, including OWHN, taking information from them but never reporting back on the new knowledge created and what was done with the information as a result of the project. Focus group participants also said they were tired of never personally seeing changes or results based on the solutions suggested during the focus groups. Moreover, they were tired of being asked the "wrong" questions that reflected the interests of the "researcher" but not those participating in the "research."

While expressing their concerns and challenging OWHN to develop a new way of working, the women also indicated their eagerness to be active partners in future projects. Women told us that they wanted to be involved in the creation and implementation of community-based solutions to the barriers to health that they identify while being "consulted" or "researched."

At the same time that OWHN was being challenged by the women participating in our focus groups, we became familiar with the work of Health Nexus (a bilingual health promotion organization that supports individuals, organizations, and communities to strengthen their capacity to promote health) in relation to their definition of inclusion. Health Nexus created a "made in Canada" definition, which OWHN adopted. Accordingly, inclusion is:

> A society where everyone belongs, creates both the feeling and the reality of belonging, and helps each of us reach our full potential. The feeling of belonging comes through caring, cooperation, and trust. We build the feeling of belonging together. The reality of belonging comes through equity and fairness, social and economic justice, and cultural as well as spiritual respect. We build the reality of belonging together by engaging our society to ensure it. (Health Nexus, 2005)

OWHN adopted this concept of inclusion to develop more comprehensive and diverse community engagement strategies and provide a way to generate new knowledge with women in the community. Along with a number of partners, OWHN developed a new approach to community-based research that seeks to reach women facing challenges in relation to the determinants of health to ensure their voices inform the development of health policy, programs, and research. This is Inclusion Research.

The objective of Inclusion Research is to unite researchers from the populations "under study" with professionals (academics, health and social service providers) in order to collectively define research questions, facilitate focus groups, collect and analyze data, and advocate for social change. A strong working principle of Inclusion Research is to move *research to action* in order to transform the root conditions of poverty and exclusion that contribute to health disparities and inequities. With this type of research, the line between the person doing the research and the people being researched is deliberately blurred. Rather than having one expert studying relatively passive objects, everyone is an active participant and an "expert." Thus, Inclusion Research is a meaningful way to engage with women who have experienced marginalization because it is a form of community-based research that necessitates lateral power structures and healthy partnerships to tackle inequities at the source.

"Our Words, Our Health"

In 2010 OWHN undertook a project funded by Echo: Improving Women's Health in Ontario (an agency of the Government of Ontario from 2009 to 2012) to examine how women in Ontario seek and use health information. Echo's mandate was to be the focal point and catalyst for women's health at the provincial level, and to promote equity and improved health for women by working in collaborative partnerships with the health system, communities, researchers, and policy-makers. In this capacity they contracted a number of projects to examine aspects of women's health in Ontario.

The project looked at a number of health issues and their importance to women in Ontario. We were guided by these questions: How do women in Ontario seek and use health information? How can health information be transformed to meet the needs of Ontario women? What are the health issues that are of most interest to women in Ontario, especially in relation to personal experiences with health, services, information, and treatment? Health

Research and Knowledge Translation: Including the Voices of Ontario Women, otherwise known as Our Words, Our Health, engaged over 2,000 women across the province. This project was intended to capture the lived experiences and thoughts of women in relation to health and the health system, as well as how to make health information, services, education, and research more accessible and meaningful.

The significance of Our Words, Our Health is not just its findings and recommendations. With thousands of women in Ontario participating in an online survey and focus groups, Our Words, Our Health strongly demonstrates that women in Ontario are willing to take time out of their busy lives and multiple roles to be actively involved in women's health. It shows that women seek out opportunities to participate in discussions and planning for women's health. It confirms that women are passionate about the health issues that they, their families, and their communities face and that they want to inform the development of health research, policy, education, and services in this province.

The project built on the significant work of OWHN in connecting with women across Ontario to discuss their health needs and concerns. The findings and lessons learned from engaging with women and health and social service professionals in previous projects informed the development of Our Words, Our Health, ensuring we built on the stated desires and needs of Ontario women.[1] With an objective of ensuring the project was meaningful to and inclusive of women in Ontario, the project team adapted the principles of Inclusion Research into the project structure.

While the time frame and budget of this project did not allow for a full Inclusion Research framework, the values of the methodology were respected and, where possible, Inclusion Researchers (peer researchers) participated in the project on the Advisory Committee, as co-facilitators and note takers at the focus groups, as participants in the collaborative data analysis process, and in knowledge-translation activities.

The project team established the Advisory Committee to assist in the project's development, implementation, and dissemination. This provided considerable opportunity to collaborate with diverse organizations that serve women across Ontario. Committee members, representing the community and a broad spectrum of agencies serving women in Ontario, were selected based on their demonstrated capacity and commitment to:

- move research to action;
- work collaboratively with their diverse communities; and
- share knowledge and have a comprehensive understanding of the diverse needs and demographics of women in Ontario.

Study Methods

A concerted effort was made to solicit input from a large number of women in Ontario. A total of 2,062 women participated in the project through either an online survey or focus group.

English- and French-language surveys were posted online and promoted through a variety of avenues (see Table 18.1). While the scope of the project initially allowed only for an English-language survey, following the survey launch, we received multiple requests for a French-language survey. Thanks to a generous volunteer effort to translate the survey data from French into English, we were able to respond to these calls and offer the survey in French. The French-language survey also drew media attention and was the basis of an article in the Sudbury-based online journal *Le Voyageur.*[2]

Fourteen focus groups were also held throughout Ontario. These focus groups concentrated on reaching women who would be less likely to complete an online survey and who represented groups that were less likely to be consulted. These groups focused on rural, Northern, First Nations, lesbian, transgender, and immigrant communities. Thanks to the support and efforts of community-based organizations, the focus groups engaged with diverse women from across the province. The staff at these organizations coordinated all aspects of the focus group, recruited note takers and/or translators, met with the facilitator(s), and were supportive of the project in every possible way. These agencies have strong relationships with women who experience marginalization in their communities and could offer safe, comfortable environments in which to conduct the groups.

We asked women in both the focus groups and the online survey to complete a fairly detailed demographic survey, which, although it included some sensitive questions, had a very high completion rate.

Data Analysis

The data were analyzed using a collaborative process carried out over a day and a half, with 11 participants, including project team members, two inclusion researchers, and members of the advisory committee.

The objective of the process was to identify the similarities (themes) and the differences that emerged in the survey and focus group data and between focus groups. By the end of the collaborative data-analysis session, all of the focus group data had been reviewed and clear themes were emerging.

The project team then used these themes to review the survey data to see how this data supported, challenged, or provided new insights into the questions that were explored. Key recommendations were then developed from these themes.

Study Findings

The ease of recruiting women to participate in the focus groups and the high response rate to the online survey highlighted one of the key findings of this project—that women in Ontario are exceptionally keen to engage in conversation about women's health and that they are looking for opportunities to do so.

	English Online Survey	French Online Survey	Focus Groups
Recruitment	Distribution through the OWHN listserv, Echo newsletter, Ontario Health Promotion E-Bulletin, other networks	Distribution through Le Bloc-Notes, the OWHN listserv, the Echo newsletter, various francophone organizations	In partnership with community-based organizations across the province
Number of respondents	1,800	133	14 focus groups, 129 participants
Data collection tools	Survey Monkey online survey	Survey Monkey online survey	Digital recording, note taking, flip charts
Language conducted	English	French	In English, with some translation of other languages (French, Russian, Spanish)
Location	Ontario-wide, with representative responses from rural and northern areas	Ontario-wide	• Immigrant Women Services, Ottawa • Keystone Child, Youth, and Family Services, Owen Sound • Northern Connections Adult Learning Centre, Sharbot Lake • YWCA of Peterborough, Victoria, and Haliburton, Peterborough • Thunder Bay Indian Friendship Centre, Thunder Bay • Sudbury Women's Centre, Sudbury • Multicultural Council of Windsor-Essex County, Windsor • Sherbourne Community Health Centre, Toronto • Toronto Christian Resource Centre, Toronto • Polycultural Immigrant and Community Services, Mississauga • Working Women Community Centre, Toronto • The Well, Hamilton

TABLE 18.1: Detailed Summary of Data Collection Methods

Critical to this project was ensuring that it did not duplicate previous research and that it added to the current knowledge base. Prior to conducting the survey and focus groups, the project team conducted a scan of research that reviewed academic and grey literature to provide a foundation from which to situate this project and to look for any changes over time. In general, the key findings of this project are very similar to those that were reported in *Turning Up the Volume!*[3] (OWHN, 2006) and other women's health reports that we reviewed (Access Alliance, 2005; Benoit & Carroll, 2001; Bierman et al., 2010; CLGRO, 1997; Daly et al., 2008; Wathen & Harris, 2007). Yet, the value of this project is that in collecting a substantial amount of feedback from women, the project

- allows for a nuanced understanding of the issues;
- builds the current qualitative evidence base;
- provides women with an opportunity to inform priorities and express their concerns, which women indicated not having enough opportunity to do; and
- confirms that there is great consistency in what women are reporting.

The feedback from women participating in the focus groups and the online survey highlights one of the key findings of the report. Women in Ontario are eager to engage in conversations about women's health and are looking for opportunities to do so.

There was a high degree of consistency in the report findings across the diverse populations of women who participated. Where differences occurred, they were primarily influenced by women's experiences of discrimination (i.e., race, class, sexual orientation, gender identity, and the intersections of these identities).

What Is Women's Health?

Two central perspectives on women's health emerged from the project participants. One perspective defined women's health as health issues that are specific to women, such as breast cancer or reproductive health. The other prevailing perspective was that women's health incorporates all factors that impact women's lives, and that health needs to be researched through a gender lens with a comprehensive understanding of the differences between men and women, including how the health issue presents, the treatment, and/or the impacts on women's lives.

When asked about women's health, women also specifically responded that women's health has particular implications for research and/or service delivery.

What Does Women's Health Mean to Women?

The women who participated in the project spoke very eloquently about the importance of women's health, often going far beyond themselves as individuals and incorporating the social determinants of health:

> [Women's health is the] ability to go where I want, when I want; to eat what I want; to live in a safe and friendly community, without fear, pain, or financial straits. It means having access to clean air, water, landscape (whether urban or rural); it

means not worrying about becoming homeless or impoverished in my senior years, and at any age, not dealing with chronic illness in the absence of professional and compassionate support.

It means getting prompt, courteous, accurate and non-patronising medical treatment, advice and medication when necessary, at no cost, and having support for mothering including access to reproductive control, affordable daycare and financial support for in-home caregivers. That's what women's health means to me.

Women's health is about an individual's wellbeing—a woman's mental and physical health—as well as her family's and community's mental and physical health. It is also about women's social, economic and political wellbeing. Finally, women's health is about social justice and the status of women internationally—our autonomy, our freedom of speech, our control over our own bodies, our reproductive choices, our freedom from all kinds of violence.

Where Women Look for Health Information

While women tend to seek information from their doctors and/or other health care providers, it is clear that women use multiple sources when searching for health information. They often use multiple sources to cross-check information and frequently do independent research prior to or following a visit with doctors.

The Internet is widely used by women seeking health information. All focus groups discussed the Internet as a source of information and almost all survey respondents indicated they have used the Internet to look for information.

Facilitators to Finding Credible and Accurate Information

Women generally were able to find the information they were looking for; however, francophone women were slightly less likely to find the information in French and/or francophone services close to home.

Women indicated a high degree of awareness that not all information sources are created equal and not all information is reliable, particularly information found on the Internet. Women were very mindful of the need to find credible sources of information and ensure the information is accurate. Many noted that they find this very hard to do and/or they are unable to gauge the credibility and accuracy of the information.

Overview of Women's Health Priorities

Women identified a wide range of health issues, including priorities for research, information, service provision, and education, which they felt were important to be considered.

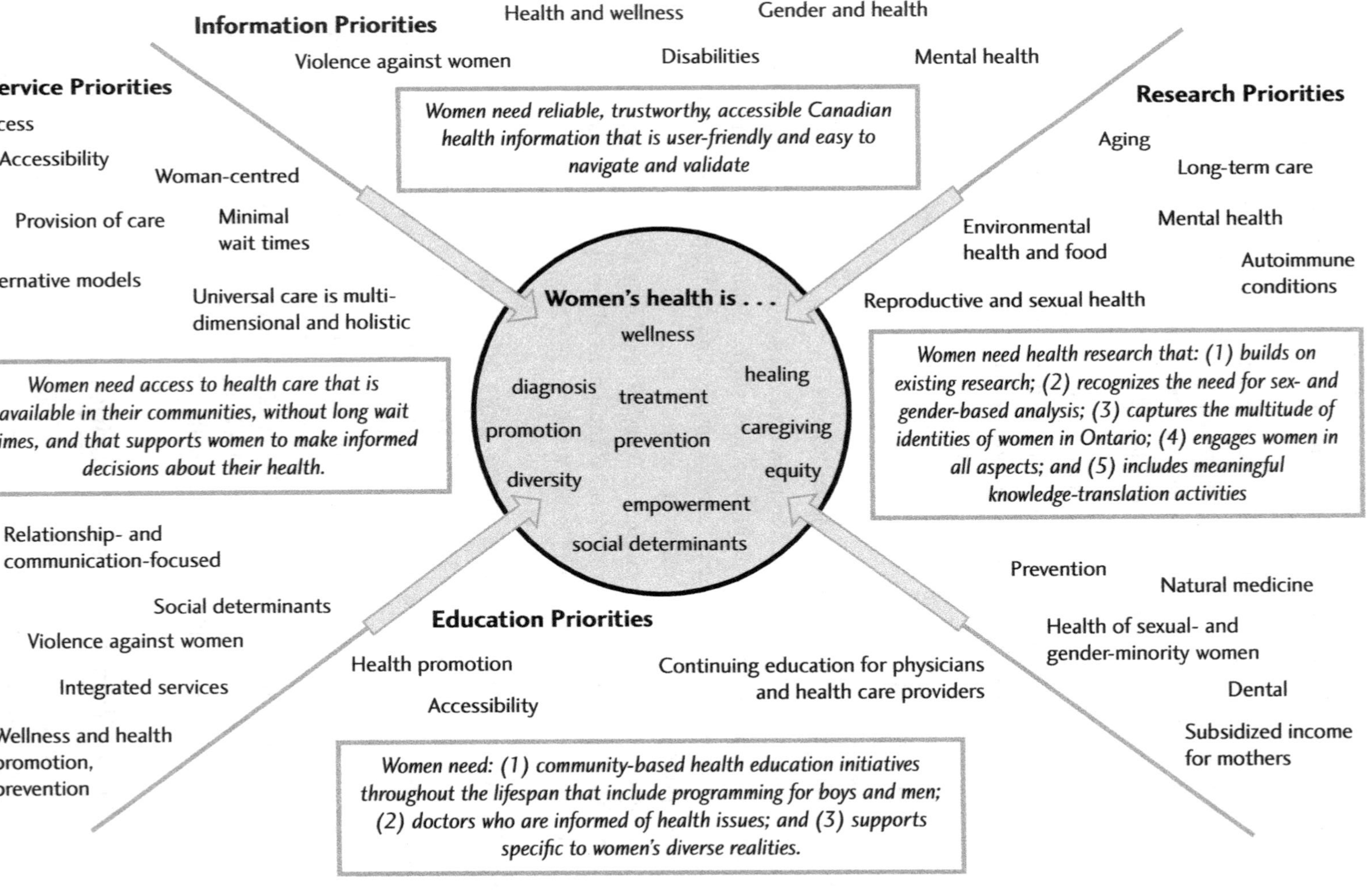

FIGURE 18.1: Women's health priorities

Research Priorities

Women in the study articulated their strong feelings about the importance of conducting research on women's health to impact policy, programs, and service delivery:

> It is very important that women's health be top of mind and that we conduct quality research on a variety of topics to have solid evidence to inform policy and programming.

> I believe that only by producing more research which demonstrates the importance of equitable access to safe abortion and to family planning services will we be able to affect policy change and increase service access.

When asked about their research priorities, the women provided two general directions: (1) how research should be conducted; and (2) what research should be conducted.

How Research Should Be Conducted

Women expressed that women's health is under-researched. They want health research to be woman-focused—that is, they want to see research that recognizes that women and men are different and those differences should have an impact on *how* research is conducted. Women wanted research that was specifically conducted on women as there is research with no women participants, yet the results are extrapolated to women:

> I think Mental Health and Addiction is an issue for every population, but I think that men and women's issues manifest differently and that we cope differently and it's important to look at these issues with as many lenses as possible.

Some women indicated that they wanted research to be conducted in French as well as English within a gender-based analysis framework.[4] In addition to incorporating gender-based analysis, some women thought it was important to connect the medical fields with other fields of study, such as sociology. It was also very important to women that research was transparent, particularly as relating to policy, government, and relationships with drug companies.

As noted earlier, women want to be informed about and involved in research as part of their health system. Women want the opportunity to shape research questions and be a part of conducting research. Among the diverse women of Ontario there was a particular interest in the research being community-specific and accessible to diverse communities. For example, francophone women thought research should be done with a specific focus and outreach to francophone women's community, and trans women expressed strong interest in community-based research. Further, immigrant women pointed to the importance of including newcomers to Canada in research and ensuring that language is not a barrier to participation. Additionally, research should build on the understanding and knowledge of communities, meaning that research has to be shared with women in the community to make a positive difference in the quality of health care received and in the lives of individual women, their families, and their communities.

What Research Should Be Conducted?

As with the breadth of health information that women are seeking, women are also looking for increased research on every health topic imaginable. A high-level overview of some of the topics that women would like to see further researched includes:

- mental health
- environmental health and food
- reproductive and sexual health
- health of sexual- and gender-minority women
- aging
- long-term care
- prevention
- natural medicine
- autoimmune conditions
- dental health
- the benefit of subsidized income for mothers

Discussion: Who Participated in the Project?

An extensive demographic questionnaire was offered to women who participated in both the focus groups and the online survey. While completing this form was time consuming and some of the questions could be construed as sensitive, there was a very high completion rate. There was feedback that a few women were hesitant to indicate their family income due to concerns that this information might be reported to the Canada Revenue Agency or Ontario Works (OW). Some of the questions were open-ended, allowing women to self-identify.

The demographic information collected from the focus groups and online survey shows a large variation in the life circumstances of the women who participated in the project through these different methods. This offers strong evidence of the need for using multiple research methods to reach women to ensure that information from diverse groups is captured and the voices of women who experience marginalization are heard.

Focus group participants included women living in poverty, women with disabilities, and women who are newcomers to Canada. Considerable effort was expended in ensuring women of varying ages were included; each focus group had at least one older woman. In addition, focus groups were held with the lesbian, gay, bisexual, and trans (LGBT) and francophone communities.

Reaching Women Who Experience Marginalization

Given the amount of funding and time for the project, difficult decisions were made by the project team about how much outreach and how many focus groups could be conducted. Focus groups are one of the most effective ways to reach women who are less likely to be represented within research; therefore, there are limitations to the engagement of women from marginalized communities due to the relatively limited number of focus groups held. In addition, the online survey excluded women without access to the Internet. We attempted to mitigate this access issue by providing a paper version of the survey to a number of agencies throughout Ontario; however, we did not receive any completed surveys through this method.

Language

As has already been addressed, the project faced difficulties in conducting outreach, focus groups, and the survey in languages other than English. Where possible and as needed, translation was incorporated into the focus groups and the survey was offered in French. However, we do recognize that the project has been predominantly conducted and presented in English, therefore limiting the participation of women whose first language is not English.

Line of Questioning

The strength of the project was that the open-ended questions enabled women to use their own words to identify priorities and recommendations, and strong themes emerged from their responses that we could determine with confidence were widely shared among the respondents. The limitation of this approach is that due to the specificity of women's priorities and recommendations, we could not validate if that specific recommendation was shared by other respondents. This same benefit and challenge was experienced in the demographic survey, which included an open-ended question asking women to name their ethnocultural background. While this approach offers women the opportunity to self-identify and resulted in a wealth of information about who participated in the project, it is difficult to do a quantitative analysis of this information.

Recognizing the Diversity of Women's Lived Experiences

There was a high degree of consistency in the responses across the diverse populations of women who participated in the focus groups and the survey. The primary areas where there were differences in response were influenced by women's

- experiences of discrimination based on such determinants as race, class, sexual orientation, and gender identity and the intersections of these factors, and
- desire for increased understanding of the issues faced by women in their communities (e.g., trans women requested additional physician training in areas specific to their lived reality).

Reflections

While many issues in women's health have remained constant since the early 2000s, there are areas in which clear changes can be noted. Certainly, the availability of information over the Internet has expanded exponentially over the last few years, providing a rich source of information, but also difficulties in ensuring the reliability and accuracy of the information accessed online and sorting through the volume of information available.

Funding in the non-profit sector has become increasingly competitive and scarce, as economic issues have affected funding bodies throughout the country. Federal funding for women's health has steadily eroded over the past five to 10 years, and there is no evidence that this will improve any time soon. In Ontario, the loss of Echo: Improving Women's Health in Ontario has removed a valuable source of funding for community-based projects. Many organizations focused on women's health have closed or been radically reshaped due to these funding cutbacks.

Funding for community-based research in particular has become less available as more funders are moving to funding models aligned with the Canadian Institute of Health Research (CIHR) guidelines. This makes it more difficult for community organizations to qualify as they need to draw salaries from the projects they conduct. While community-based research adds richness and the validation of various types of knowledge, it is a more expensive and often lengthier process than some other types of research. This has added to its decline as funders are asking researchers to do more with less.

Another change that has had a chilling effect on the women's health sector is the increasing pressure to avoid the word "advocacy," as governments dismiss advocacy as "political," even though this is one of the basic tenets of women's health and the client-centred health care approach that many provinces, including Ontario, have adopted. Self-advocacy and the capacity to advocate and support women to pursue their optimal health and well-being as they define it are necessary for a vibrant, equitable, and inclusive health care system.

While these changes have had an impact on the climate for women's health, women throughout Ontario continue to desire a more responsive and reflexive system to ensure that their voices, issues, and preferences are considered by the health care system:

> Women's health means treating me with respect, listening to what I have to say, believing me when I have a concern, understanding that I'm intelligent and articulate and then getting the treatment that I need. (Hendrickson, Kilbourn, & OWHN, 2011, p. 5)

Acknowledgements

We would like to graciously acknowledge Tekla Hendrickson, Barbara Kilbourn, and Christina Lessels, whose tireless efforts, passion, and work on the Our Words, Our Health research project greatly influenced this chapter. All projects referenced in this chapter are a testimony to the successes and accomplishments of what happens when women come together and bring the personal to the political. The work of the Ontario Women's Health Network is the result of fruitful collaborative processes and as such we want to gratefully acknowledge all the funders, project partners, community stakeholders, and especially the participants and inclusion researchers, who have shaped and shifted, formed, and transformed the landscape of research and knowledge translation, thus allowing us to create a more reflexive and inclusive way of working collaboratively. With too many people to name in gratitude, we trust that you will hear their voices echoed in this chapter.

Notes

1. OWHN's research portfolio is available online at: http://www.owhn.on.ca/research_projects.htm.
2. J. Cayouette, Juillet 15, 2010, Prendre le pouls de la santé des femmes ontariennes, *La Voyageur.*
3. In partnership with local community-based organizations, OWHN conducted 30 regional focus groups, from 2002 to 2005 that reached out to marginalized women across Ontario. This project—*Turning Up the Volume!*—summarized the health concerns of women who experience marginalization in rural and urban communities.
4. "Gender-Based Analysis (GBA) is an analytical tool. It uses sex, gender and other factors of diversity to organize principles and conceptualize information. It helps clarify the differences between and among women and men, the nature of their social relationships, roles and responsibilities, and differences in economic and political circumstances" (Women and Health Care Reform website, Centres of Excellence for Women's Health, retrieved from http://www.womenandhealthcarereform.ca/en/work_timelyaccess_workshop.html).

References

Access Alliance. (2005). *Racialised Groups and Health Status: A Literature Review Exploring Poverty, Housing, Race-Based Discrimination, and Access to Health Care as Determinants of Health for Racialised Groups.* Toronto: Access Alliance. Retrieved from http://accessalliance.ca/sites/accessalliance/files/documents/Literature%20Review_Racialized%20Groups%20and%20Health%20Status.pdf.

Benoit, C., & D. Carroll. (2001). *Marginalized Voices from the Downtown Eastside: Aboriginal Women Speak about Their Health Experiences.* Toronto: National Network on Environments and Health. Retrieved from http://www.cewh-cesf.ca/PDF/nnewh/marginalized-voices.pdf.

Bierman, A., et al. (2010). *The POWER Study: Ontario Women's Health Equity Report: Access to Health Care Services.* Retrieved from http://www.powerstudy.ca/the-power-report/the-power-report-volume-1/access-to-health-care-services.

Coalition for Lesbian and Gay Rights in Ontario (CLGRO). (1997). *Systems Failure: A Report on the Experiences of Sexual Minorities in Ontario's Health-Care and Social-Services Systems.* Toronto: Author. Retrieved from www.clgro.org/info.html.

Daly, T., P. Armstrong, H. Armstrong, S. Bradley, & V. Oliver. (2008, October). *Contradictions: Health Equity and Women's Health Services in Toronto.* Toronto: Wellesley Institute. Retrieved from http://www.wellesleyinstitute.com/publication-papers/healthcare-reform-publications/contradictions__health_equity_and_women%E2%80%99s_health_services_in_toronto/.

Health Nexus. (2005). *Count Me In! Tools for an Inclusive Ontario.* Retrieved from www.count-me-in.ca.

Hendrickson, T., B. Kilbourn, & Ontario Women's Health Network (OWHN). (2011). *Our Words, Our Health. Health Research and Knowledge Translation: Including the Voices of Ontario Women.* Toronto: OWHN.

Ontario Women's Health Network (OWHN). (2006). *Turning Up the Volume!* Toronto: Author. Retrieved from http://owhn.on.ca/turningupvolume.htm.

Wathen, C. N., & R. M. Harris. (2007, May). "I Try to Take Care of It Myself": How Rural Women Search for Health Information. Qualitative Health Research 17(5): 639–651.

Further Reading

In addition to the research reports listed in the References, these additional reports and websites are important to the topics of women's health, inclusion, research, and knowledge translation. This is not an exhaustive list but simply a snapshot of useful resources and websites.

The Ontario Women's Health Network

Hendrickson, T., B. Kilbourn, & Ontario Women's Health Network. (2011). *Health Research and Knowledge Translation: Including the Voices of Ontario Women.* Toronto: Women's Health Network. Retrieved from http://owhn.on.ca/Health_Research_and_Knowledge_Translation.htm.

Ontario Women's Health Network. (2009a). *Inclusion Research Handbook.* Toronto: Women's Health Network. Retrieved from http://owhn.on.ca/tools.htm.

Ontario Women's Health Network. (2009b). *Guide to Focus Groups.* Toronto: Women's Health Network. Retrieved from http://owhn.on.ca/tools.htm.

Ontario Women's Health Network and Research Unit, Prevention and Cancer Control, Cancer Care Ontario. (2013). *Putting Solutions in Place: Bridging the Gap between Women and Breast Cancer Screening.* Toronto: Women's Health Network. Retrieved from http://owhn.on.ca/breastcancerscreening.htm.

Canadian Research Institute for the Advancement of Women

Canadian Research Institute for the Advancement of Women (FemNorthNet) & DisAbled Women's Network (DAWN-RAFH) of Canada. (2014). *Diversity through Inclusive Practice—A Toolkit for Creating Inclusive Processes, Spaces & Events.* Ottawa: Canadian Research Institute for the Advancement of Women, FemNorthNet Project. Retrieved from http://criaw-icref.ca/femnorthnet/publications.

The Canadian Facts

Mikkonen, J., & D. Raphael. (2010). *Social Determinants of Health: The Canadian Facts.*

Toronto: York University School of Health Policy and Management. Retrieved from http://www.thecanadianfacts.org/.

Wellesley Institute

Block, S. (2013). *Rising Inequality, Declining Health: Health Outcomes and the Working Poor.* Toronto: Wellesley Institute. Retrieved from http://www.wellesleyinstitute.com/wp-content/uploads/2013/07/Rising-Inequality-Declining-Health.pdf.

Brown, A. (2013). *Action and Research: Community-Based Research at the Wellesley Institute.* Toronto: Wellesley Institute. Retrieved from http://www.wellesleyinstitute.com/wp-content/uploads/2013/07/Action-and-Research.pdf.

Daly, T., P. Armstrong, H. Armstrong, S. Bradley, & V. Oliver. (2008, October). *Contradictions: Health Equity and Women's Health Services in Toronto.* Toronto: Wellesley Institute. Retrieved from http://www.wellesleyinstitute.com/publication-papers/healthcare-reform-publications/contradictions__health_equity_and_women%E2%80%99s_health_services_in_toronto/.

Mahamoud, A. (2014). *Breast Cancer Screening in Racialized Women: Implications for Health Equity.* Toronto: Wellesley Institute. Retrieved from http://www.wellesleyinstitute.com/wp-content/uploads/2014/05/Breast-Cancer-Screening-in-Racialized-Women.pdf.

Roche, B., A. Guta, & S. Flicker. (2010). *Peer Research in Action I: Models of Practice.* Toronto: Wellesley Institute. Retrieved from http://www.wellesleyinstitute.com/wp-content/uploads/2011/02/Models_of_Practice_WEB.pdf.

The POWER Study

Bierman, A., et al. (2010). *The POWER Study: Ontario Women's Health Equity Report.* Toronto: St. Michael's Hospital. Retrieved from http://powerstudy.ca.

Relevant Websites

Access Alliance: http://accessalliance.ca/

Atlantic Centre of Excellence for Women's Health: http://www.dal.ca/diff/Atlantic-Centre-of-Excellence-for-Womens-Health.html

British Columbia Centre of Excellence for Women's Health: http://bccewh.bc.ca/

Canadian Women's Health Network: http://www.cwhn.ca/

Centres of Excellence for Women's Health: http://www.cewh-cesf.ca/

Feminist Alliance for International Action: http://www.fafia-afai.org/

Health Nexus: http://en.healthnexus.ca/

Health Quality Ontario: http://www.hqontario.ca/

National Collaborating Centre for the Determinants of Health Nexus: http://www.nccdh.ca/

National Network on Environment and Women's Health: http://www.nnewh.org/

Native Women's Association of Canada: http://www.nwac.ca/

Prairie Women's Health Centre of Excellence: http://www.pwhce.ca/

Trans PULSE: http://transpulseproject.ca/

Women's College Research Institute: http://www.womensresearch.ca/

Women's Health in Women's Hands: http://www.whiwh.com

CHAPTER 19

Canaries in the Mine: Filming Women Working in Health Care

Laura Sky

Introduction

For a decade during the 1990s, I worked alongside nurses, doctors, social workers, and first responders, researching and producing a series of documentaries and reports about the state of our health care system. I wanted to explore, dialectically, the strengths and gaps in health care systems from the perspective of patients, families, and health care providers.

For more than 30 years, our organization, the SkyWorks Charitable Foundation, has been committed to a participatory model of research and documentary production based on that research. We developed a method of film dissemination built on the principles of contributing to community engagement for purposes of social change. The foundation of our work rests with the long-term relationships we develop with individuals and organizations that are committed to equity and social justice in their workplaces and communities.

From Factories to Hospitals

My earlier and overlapping research and documentary production focused on working conditions in the manufacturing industry and the public service. I was particularly interested in the "working lean" model in the private and public sectors. I explored the effects of new technologies, peer and management expectations of the rate and speed of work, and the clash between human need and workplace productivity. I witnessed the formal and informal role of gender, power, and authority in the workplace. I saw the effects of these changes in physical and psychological workplace injuries, including the haunting consequences of overwork, peer pressure, and conflict.

When my closest friend Cathy became critically ill, I spent eight weeks at her side in a downtown teaching hospital. I was often joined by a mutual friend, Philip, who had recently completed his PhD in ethics, and was currently studying medicine. The three of us were also political buddies, active in social justice organizations. I rarely left Cathy's hospital room and often processed my observations with Philip and, as she improved, with Cathy, too.

I decided to turn my attention to hospitals as workplaces. I wanted to understand how power, gender, class, technology, and the human spirit determined the care that patients could expect and experience. I became particularly interested in what I saw as the collision between the organization of health care work, the ever-changing technology, and the tensions and dilemmas that these elements imposed for front-line staff.

The feature-length documentaries that were seeded by this research process included *The Right to Care, To Hurt and to Heal, Crying for Happiness, Jake's Life*, and *Crisis Call*. In fact, this research has informed most of my documentary work in the years since. These explorations taught me to unpeel the layers and levels of personal and collective values that inform daily workplace activities. In hospitals I learned to question the visible and invisible assumptions that lead to clinical decisions that promote or undermine healing. I learned that moral suffering in the workplace can create trauma and its consequences for patients, families, and providers.

Although unions and workplace leaders have long been committed to advocating for workers who are injured on the job, what I came to see as moral distress or ethical injury

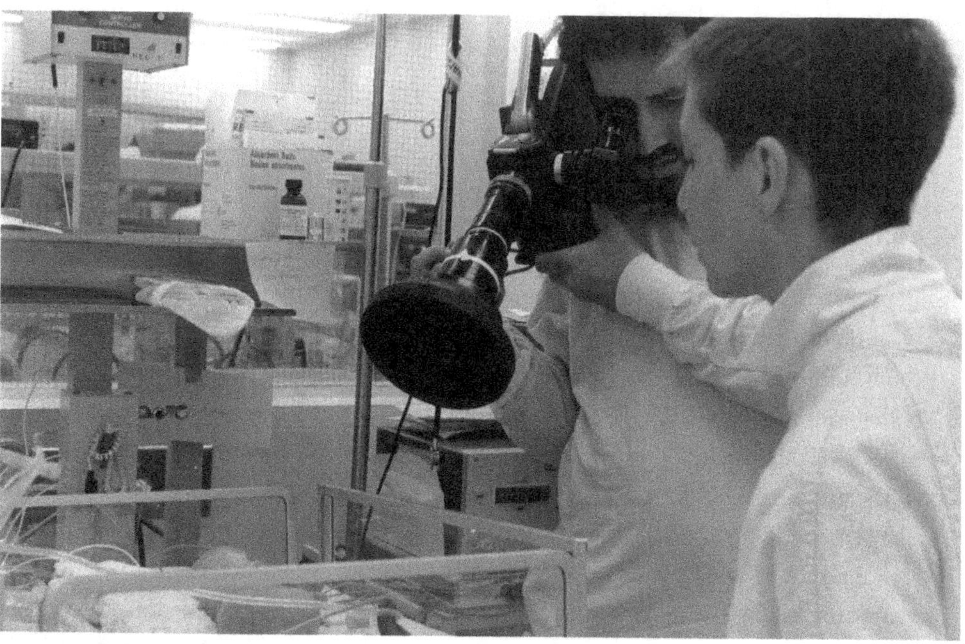

FIGURE 19.1

has been generally under-recognized by health care workers and their union or professional association representatives. At that time, there was little conversation among colleagues about these troubling dilemmas. Staff often suffered in isolation. My chosen mandate was to identify and document these very real issues and their consequences as staff, patients, and families experienced them in hospital and later in their homes.

To prepare my research and to inform the future filming, I rotated through various clinical disciplines in five teaching hospitals. I was usually granted access by clinician-leaders who had their own professional interest in the issues I wanted to explore. I agreed to various conditions in order to research in this way. I committed to maintain patient confidentiality, and to respect the privacy of patients, families, and staff. I agreed to leave the room should my presence impose discomfort for others. I promised to contain my questions or comments, waiting for the opportunity to express these at appropriate times and in appropriate settings. I observed for extended periods of time at various adult and pediatric intensive-care units (ICUs) and neonatal intensive-care units (NICUs). I also teamed up with members of a family practice clinic and followed their work in their emergency department. I worked closely with a neurosurgeon, attending surgeries and daily rounds. I shadowed a director of nursing at a downtown teaching hospital, which took me into executive and management meetings. I studied the consequences of ever-evolving federal and provincial health policies. I spent many nights and days in hospital rooms, by incubators, in surgery, in emergency rooms, following clinical rounds, at presentations and lectures. I observed report during shift changes, family conferences, and countless informal conversations between clinicians of every rank and denomination.

I began this work in a series of pediatric units. These are a series of memories from that time.

Researching and Filming in Pediatric Settings

While researching at various pediatric settings, I can call to memory events during long hours at the bedsides of very fragile children while standing with very capable nurses. I say "standing with" because my relationship with many of the nursing staff involved far more than observation. They permitted me to enter their personal-professional spaces as they processed all manner of experiences, considerations, and dilemmas. I witnessed their struggles, their pride, and their despair.

They cared for critically ill children and their families who were facing intense clinical and emotional needs. The kids were often post-surgical patients as a result of injury or congenital anomalies. Children who were struggling with life-threatening illness required a combination of clinical skills, attentive waiting and watching, interdisciplinary consultation, and definitive action.

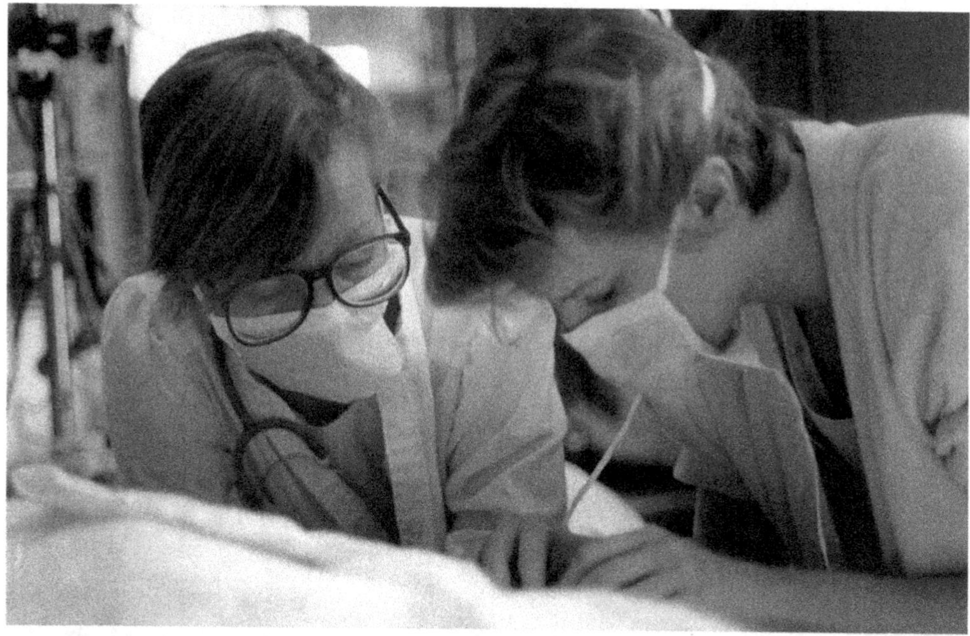

FIGURE 19.2

Establishing Our Rules for Filming, Privacy, and Consent

While filming, our three-person crew created our own protocol in agreement with the hospitals, staff, and families. We carried the most minimal equipment and used no extra lighting. We spent time waiting quietly, away from the bedsides, before we filmed. I would always talk with the patient's parents before we planned to film, discussing with them what we were doing and why we were filming. I would explain that we were producing a documentary that would be a teaching tool for clinicians, medical and nursing students, and one that would be useful for families dealing with similar situations. It was unlikely that the film would be on television, but should that eventuality present itself, we would revisit them for their additional decision about consent. If they agreed to allow us to film, I promised that we would stop at any point if they became uncomfortable with our presence. I also agreed that they could change their minds about participating at any point, no matter how much we had already filmed about their situation.

I promised the front-line health care staff the same opportunities for their participation and their rights of refusal or consent.

I approached these situations as a parent as well as a filmmaker. I cannot imagine a situation more precarious, more intimate, and more demanding than the events that parents were experiencing. The last thing that families stressed to this degree needed, I felt, was the intrusion of a film crew. Similarly, front-line staff were doing the best that they could, devoting their knowledge, skills, and commitment to care to the utmost of their abilities.

If being filmed interrupted their concentration or distracted them from the tasks at hand, we would pull back with no questions or negotiation.

Each of the film's adult participants would have the opportunity to see the footage that we hoped to include in the completed film. This would give them the opportunity to grant or withdraw their final consent.

Given that understanding and agreement, I entered the patient's room first to observe. If events allowed, I would quietly and briefly check in with parents and staff as events unfolded. If they all agreed, I would call in the camera and sound recordist. They would quietly stand back and observe. I would whisper quietly about what was happening and what I hoped we could film. Once filming, they would follow the events from a respectful distance and, if required, stop on a moment's notice.

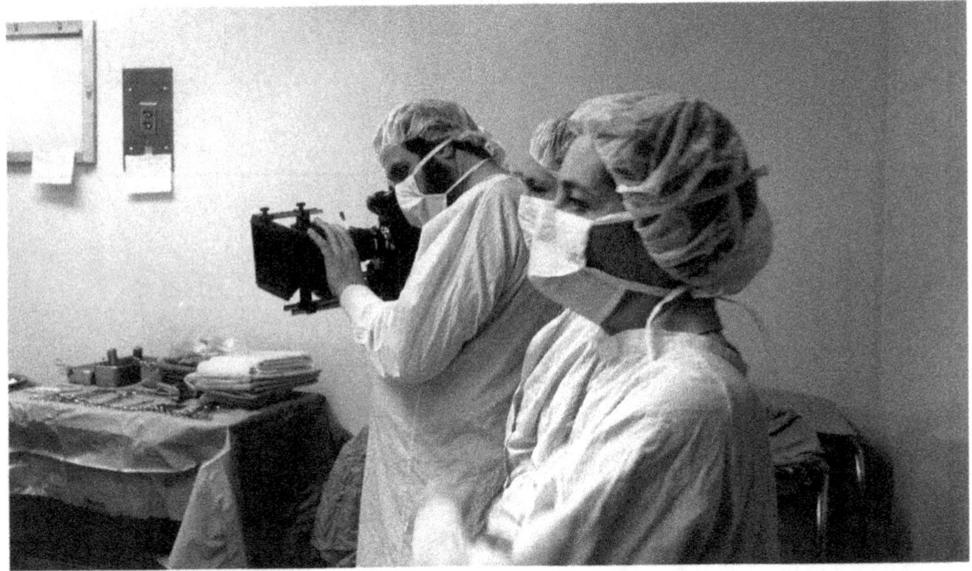

FIGURE 19.3

A Small Boy with a Fragile Heart

One little boy, about three or four, had just had major heart surgery. I will call him Paul. His slender body was long and pale in the pediatric ICU hospital bed. He was intubated, his chest swathed in padding and bandages, and fluorescent with the antibacterial liquid that had protected the surgical site. Paul was silent, but very expressive. His body moved with the rhythm of pain that he was experiencing. His eyes remained closed. The nurse, whom we will call Linda, could read him—she read his pain, his fear, and his need for help. She adjusted his IV pain medication to the prescribed limit and knew when to call for additional help. She was his advocate and his protector.

Linda was also there for his parents. They came to Paul's bedside in a world that was so alien for them. They approached their son's bed as outsiders to this high-tech world that held his fragile life, tethered with tubes, wires, and announced by all manner of alarms. The centre of their focus was their little boy. They could not hold him close; they stroked his cheek with cautious fingers. They were subservient to the technology, alarms, and wires that dominated his small body. Their love was in his room, in his bed, embracing him through this living, breathing struggle. The sounds came from their own murmurs, their silence, the nurse's quiet explanations. They observed, they touched their boy, and they were vigilant, looking for signs of his life in this complex space.

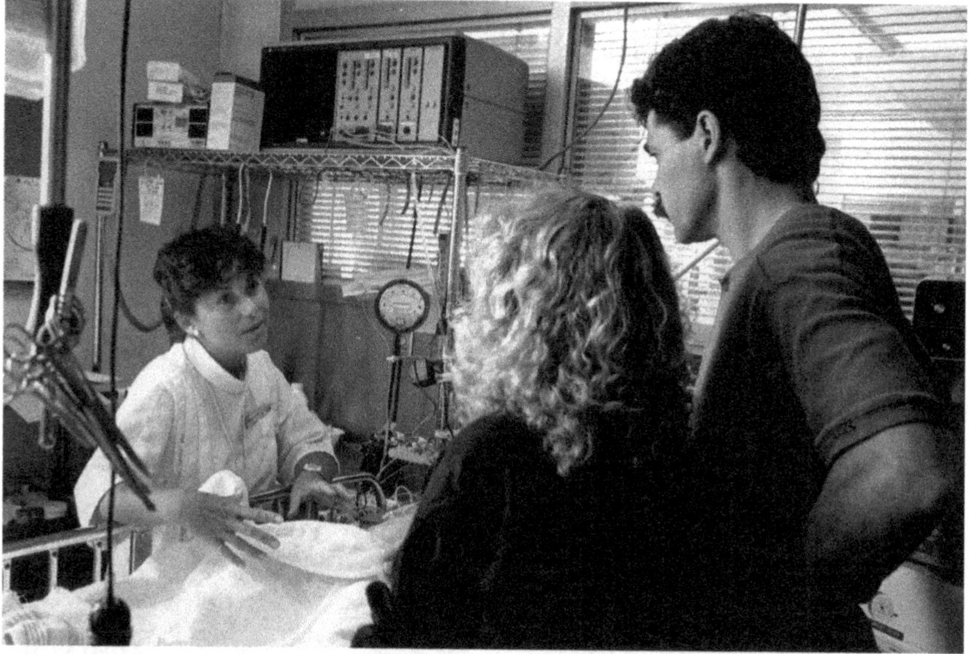

FIGURE 19.4

The pediatric resident came into the room a number of times. David was a young father himself. In fact, he had earlier told me that he and his wife had lost a baby themselves. He knew the pediatric ICU setting as a clinician and as a parent.

The resident paused by the bedside, and spoke softly to the small boy. He stroked the child's face and added another light blanket, avoiding the drainage tubes, IVs, the monitors, and breathing apparatus.

As the child's condition worsened, various doctors attended at his bedside. The conversations became increasingly sombre in tone. Our crew withdrew, leaving the room for discussions between the doctors and the parents. It was decided that the little one would go back into surgery. His situation had become increasingly critical.

Hours passed. Although there were other areas for filming, we were distracted by the medical crisis that we had observed. In fact, each of our crew had young children at home. We observed with the eyes and hearts of vulnerable parents. We felt part of the vigil, awaiting his return from the operation room. Day became night, and finally the child returned. His chest remained open for quick access to his fragile heart should it need to be restarted in another crisis. Staff and parents were now gowned, gloved, and masked. Our crew stayed out of the room, discreetly observing when possible through the large glass window.

The little one survived and slowly recovered. The nursing and medical team went on to the next patient and family. I continued to work beside Linda, the nurse who was the lead with the child and family. The more we worked together, the stronger the bond grew between us. She was my teacher, my guide, and I chose to offer her my support in the hours of care she provided for very ill children.

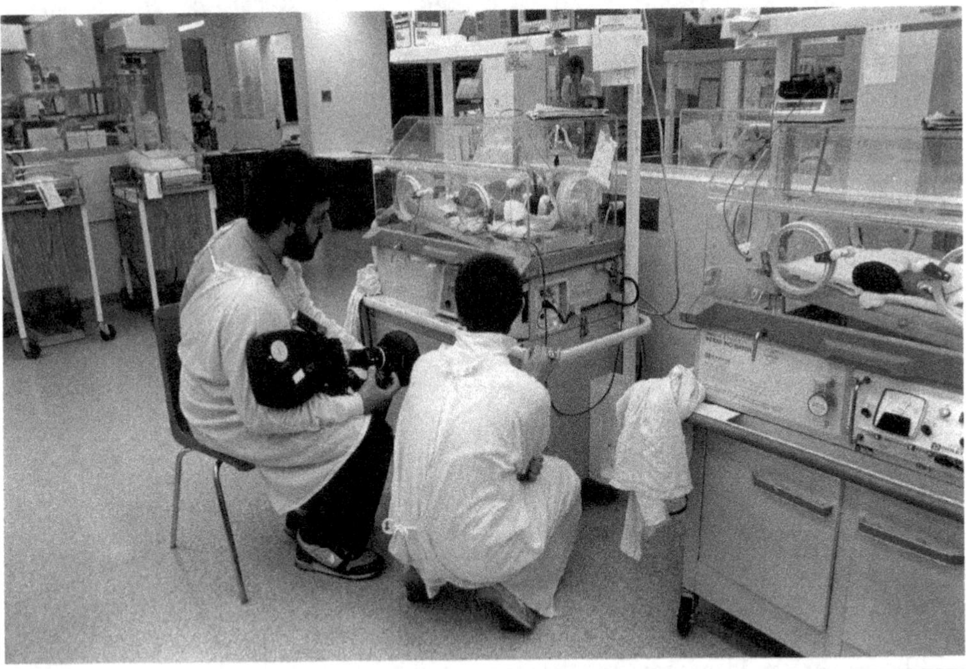

FIGURE 19.5

Working in a Parallel World

As I looked out the windows of this ICU to the streets below, I came to feel that there was a profound distance between the parallel world in the unit and the ordinary day and night activities in the city. I became aware of how difficult it was to talk about the nature of my observations with my own friends and family. I could not have informal conversations about ill and dying children, especially with friends who were parents. I imagined these realities for nurses who left the universe of intensive care, vulnerable children, and frightened parents, returning to their homes, families, and friends.

I also observed the institutional and collegial support systems that existed and that were scarce, given the intensity of this work. There was evidence of informal supports between nurses while working, on breaks, and, to a lesser degree, in team meetings. These exchanges varied depending on the expressed needs of particular nurses and the capacities of their co-workers. At each bedside, each nurse was dealing with complexities, urgency, predictable and unexpected needs of their young patients and their families. "Normal" was illusive at best.

I felt that it was appropriate to be able to offer my support for their workplace experiences in exchange for their remarkable support for my work in this setting. We built trust.

An 18-month-old child was admitted through the emergency unit, severely injured. It was suspected that he had been beaten by one of the people living in his family home. The child was not conscious, and was severely brain damaged. He never woke up. Linda provided his primary nursing care.

The child's mother, grandmother, and the person who came to be known as "the boyfriend" spent long hours waiting in the family room, going out for frequent smokes. They were interviewed a number of times by staff and the police. I observed a palpable yet undeclared class difference between the clinical staff and these family members. Staff empathy was clouded by their suspicions. The boyfriend was described in team rounds as a "Mediterranean" type—clearly a pejorative designation. The mother and grandmother were tense, sorrowful, defensive—all understandable under these terrible circumstances. The staff believed that the boyfriend was responsible for this beating, but the women were seen as culpable as well. There was a wall of tension between the staff and family.

I encountered this disturbing situation while researching the documentary and had no intention of filming. Even had the cameras and crew been available, I would have decided not to film. Dealing with crew and equipment was the last thing that the family and staff needed in the midst of this terrible time. Although child abuse is a matter of grave public concern, at that time, in this critical-care setting, in the dreadful intimacy of these events, each and all participants had their rights to be protected from the filming process.

The child lingered for a day and night. The clinical staff explained to the family that repeated neurological testing had shown that the baby no longer had brain function. Linda and the other members of the team prepared the family for the moment when they would take the child off life support. Linda sat with the mother and grandmother as this time grew near. She offered them comfort, putting aside judgment and condemnation. Once the breathing tubes were removed and the respirator turned off, the child and the room grew still. Linda handed the blanket-covered child to the women and encouraged them to say goodbye. The family left together, trembling and crying, leaving the baby in Linda's arms.

I stood with her, quietly bearing witness and offering her my presence. Otherwise, Linda would have been alone. For all the sophisticated clinical systems that were in place, there was no support for a nurse enduring this tragedy, this immense sorrow.

Linda washed the child and prepared his small body. And then, together, we began the long walk to the hospital morgue. I could not leave her side at that time. She never asked me explicitly to accompany her, but I felt that the bond between us in sharing this experience allowed me to take this journey with her. We talked infrequently as we walked. We entered the morgue, a still and cold place, and left the child there, so alone. Together, Linda and I returned to the ICU silently.

These events speak to a role of nursing that few people outside the profession see. There is trauma and tragedy woven into this job description, this experience of work. Linda and her colleagues bring strength and integrity to the many layers of their work. This is the space where a nurse's skills are informed and nurtured by her compassion and, at times, her sorrow.

Over my 30 years as a documentary filmmaker, a witness, and an advocate, relationships like the one I developed with Linda provide the heart and soul and the veracity of this work.

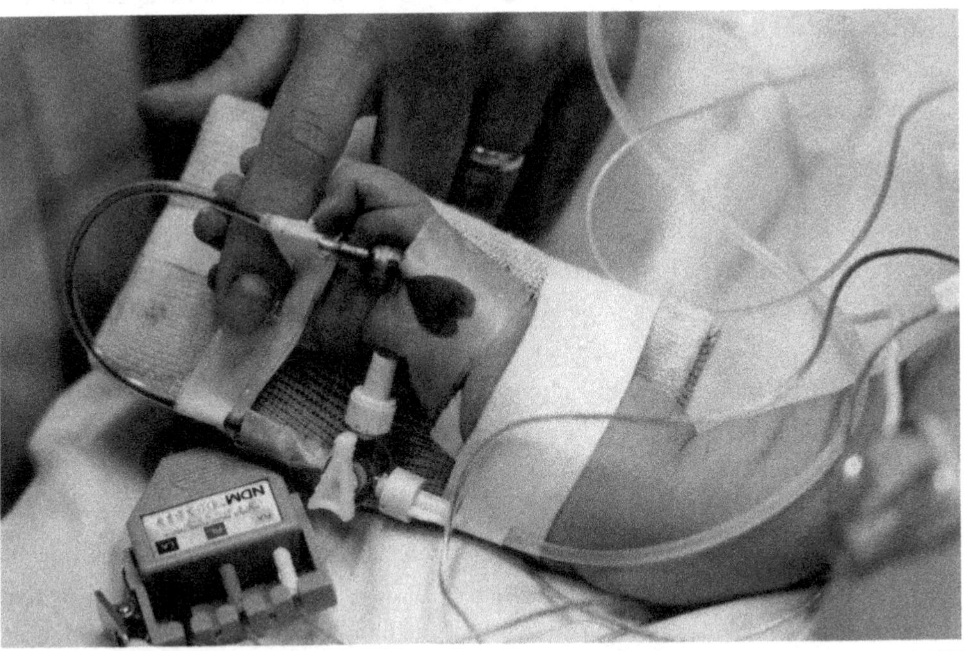

FIGURE 19.6

The Nurse as Truth Teller

These ICU experiences reflected the highest quality of care and skill in clinical nursing and medical care. This is the workspace where compassion and commitment combine to provide patients and families with the best of care while giving nurses the opportunity to be the best that they can be.

I also witnessed the dark side of nursing, which I came to see was the consequence of the industrialization of health care. This included fundamental reorganization of standards, responsibilities, job descriptions, and job security in the pursuit of downsizing and contracting out.

I saw that nurses are the canaries in the mine of the health care system. Delivering nursing services at the hospital or home bedside, they live with the scarcities, the gaps, and the inadequacies of health care policy and practice on a daily basis. They live with the corporate-speak that promises professional satisfaction and excellence, but enshrines cutbacks and scarcity. They work with what is possible and impossible in the delivery of their services. Yet they continue to deliver that care with their heads and their hearts.

I embarked on the research and production on *The Right to Care*, a documentary about how nurses struggle to deliver health care with integrity and commitment to the needs of their patients. As the title implies, the documentary also explores the right of individuals who need health services to receive the care they need.

Donna was a 25-year veteran in the delivery of home care nursing services. I met her through a letter to the editor she sent to the *Toronto Star*, decrying the decline of home health care services in the face of provincial cutbacks. When we met in person, she was fierce and smart. She worked on the front lines of a large national nursing service that she felt was disintegrating in front of her eyes. She believed that her employer was adopting corporate and industrial values that were contrary to the principles of good nursing care, advocacy, and compassion. She felt that this negatively affected the quality of care that patients could expect and the quality of work that front-line nurses could provide. Donna showed me and our audiences the parallel between industrial work systems and the new rules reshaping home and institutional nursing.

We could all count on Donna to tell the truth about health care policies, straight out. Within five minutes of meeting her, I decided to invite her to be filmed for *The Right to Care*.

Donna's clinical and personal skills with her home patients were inspirational—rushing from patient to patient to provide dressing changes, nursing assessments, palliative care, and seamless compassion.

She introduced me to a group of her colleagues at the local coffee shop and to a number of her patients in their homes. I watched, fascinated, as her community nursing colleagues used their lunch breaks to compare the latest information from management, form strategies, complain, buoy each other's spirits, and exchange coveted nursing supplies from the trunks of their cars.

In the *Right to Care*, we watched Donna relate to Edna, an older woman at home recovering from advanced breast cancer surgery. Donna takes a much-needed break, sharing a pot of tea with Edna. "I've been waiting for this cup of tea with you all day. I thought if I could just get to Edna's and have tea with her, I'll be OK. I don't want to bring tears to your eyes, Edna." The warmth and humour of this moment is so authentic and speaks to the spirit of their relationship.

Donna describes preparing Edith, another older patient, to go into a palliative care setting, after having cared for her for a year. "She asked me to get her the cream out of the cupboard so she could get rid of the hair on her chin . . . she was getting ready to die. I wanted to be there when the ambulance came for her, but I couldn't. I had to get to my next person. . . . I was rushing out the door when she called out to me, 'Donna, I just wanted you to know that I loved you.'" Donna savours the memory. "That to me is the meaning of this job."

In contrast, in the film Donna laments the transformation of home care nursing. She analyzes the new language of health care, how "addressing a self-care deficit" is corporate-speak for giving a patient a bath. Referring to her employer, she tells us, "They're making this [organization] into a business. At an administrative level, when I see the work I do treated like a corporation, I get frightened. . . . They laid off 27 of us [full-time nurses], and then advertised in the local paper for 'flexible' staff. What they mean is part-time, casual workers. . . . As a woman I feel angry—for all of us women."

Donna expresses the grief and anger she experienced in being unable to provide the care that has motivated her as a community nurse. She finds herself in the midst of the turmoil created by the reorganization of nursing work, where she is the canary in that mine.

The Toyota System of Health Care

I witnessed with great alarm the work systems based on the Toyota model of workplace organization adopted in our hospitals and community agencies. A few years earlier my documentary *Working Lean* showed the reorganization of factory work in the automotive industry, and the language and work conditions I witnessed in car plants were now appearing in hospitals. I was deeply disturbed that *patient-focused care* appeared to be anything but, and that Toyota's KAIZEN—continuous quality improvement, just-in-time production—was increasingly applied to work policies and practices in health care. The quality of nursing care, which was so important to nurses and patients alike, was being eroded in the name of increased "efficiency" and the "elimination of waste." Cutbacks had become pervasive. The casualization of labour, the reorganization of licensed responsibilities, and increased patient loads reformed training and clinical practices. As health care workforces were depleted, employees were trained and pressured to embrace systems that were to their own detriment and that of their patients.

In the early 1990s, in response to my work with front-line health care staff, I was hired by CUPE to prepare a major report on the erosion of the Canadian medicare system, and the struggles of front-line health care providers to "keep medicare healthy." My research focused on the consequences of policies and practices that enshrine privatization, and the reorganization of work. That research has informed my documentary work in the decades since.

The work took me across Canada and to Newfoundland, Prince Edward Island, and Nova Scotia, where I interviewed nurses, cleaners, and dietary workers—all health care soldiers in the trenches. They had so much to say; they wept, they laughed, and they told their truths.

I witnessed the incursion of private corporations into Canada's public health care system. I followed the progress of large corporations into hospitals large and small: Baxter, Marriot, Johnson, all flourishing, as hospital workers and their patients struggled.

Overcrowding and understaffing, inadequate services, early discharge and readmissions, increased acuity managed by depleted staff and contracting out—all these were key concerns for health care staff and patients alike. I could be documenting this research today—the issues have become the new normal.

I sat with groups of front-line employees, many crying as they talked and listened. They were so deeply troubled about what they witnessed during each shift.

"When there are no beds left on our unit, and we have to admit someone from emergency, we have to send one of our patients to another unit. Often times, the doctor doesn't follow the patient to the new unit and he or she loses the continuity of care. With the pressure to discharge early, they may find themselves home alone, still very sick."

Emergency patients may be invisible in terms of admission statistics. For example, "a patient can come in through emergency for chest pain. Because there are no beds available upstairs, it's in emergency that you stay—for days perhaps. In fact, you can be in emerg for any number of days, and be discharged home directly from there and never been admitted at all. The stats look like business as usual."

Another concerned CUPE member described a still familiar situation, when a parent brings an ill child to hospital and is sent home with medication and instructions for the child's care. "You can just imagine, their child is getting sicker and sicker and the mum is just thinking, 'the doctor said that she should just be at home, all I need to do is give her this medication. . . .' This one mum came in with her little one six times before she could get her admitted."

Listening to their stories, I felt then, and do now, that the economic crunch behind the reorganization of health care leads to the ethical tension that health care providers experience in their workplaces. Many described ethical and moral injuries—traumatized by feelings of professional and personal helplessness in the face of impossible working conditions.

At the conclusion of my research period in Newfoundland, as I was leaving for the airport at five in the morning, I agreed to share a taxi with the Baxter director of operations for Atlantic Canada. At that time, Baxter, an American multinational company, was the largest health care supplier in North America. The morning was dark, foggy, and damp. I was barely awake, but the tears and despair of the health care workers I had interviewed were very much with me. I recognized an unexpected opportunity that this taxi ride offered. I asked the Baxter representative how business was for his company in Newfoundland. "It's never been better," he answered, and I knew there was something terribly wrong in the contrast between the losses felt by health care workers and their patients and the substantial profits enjoyed by these private health care businesses.

When Professional and Personal Experiences Collide

I am a long-time filmmaker and researcher, but also a concerned family member. Five years ago, my husband underwent cancer surgery in one of Canada's most respected teaching hospitals. He endured many complications; some were critical.

Days after his initial discharge, he became increasingly ill at home. An ambulance brought us to that hospital's emergency unit, where he waited in agony for hours. I watched him deteriorate in front of my eyes. He was moved to a hallway waiting space with one frazzled nurse attending to very ill patients. At 2:30 a.m. he began projectile vomiting. He was hot to the touch and in and out of consciousness. The nurse was nowhere to be seen. I roamed the halls frantically, looking for help. Then I saw the sign on the wall from the one of the nursing departments: "Kaizen Workshop Monday at 10am." By that time I was in tears.

I stopped two nurses chatting as they walked. "Please, you have to help my husband. He is so sick." One took my hand and said, "We hear you. Someone will be there soon." They moved on. This was this hospital's version of patient-focused care. Six hours later, just after shift change, my husband was barely hanging on and was finally recognized by a nurse who saved his life. This nurse assessed him and acted immediately. He assembled a team and everything possible was done for my husband on an urgent basis. His kidneys were failing. He had septicemia, his blood pressure spiked, and his diabetes gave way to ketoacidosis. This began a three-month stay in hospital. He underwent a number of surgeries and subsequent stays in the ICU, going from crisis to crisis.

Paradoxically, I was always relieved when Verne was readmitted to the ICU, where he would get the best nursing care the hospital had to offer. When he was finally discharged to go home, he had daily nursing care for dressing changes on a deep post-surgical wound. On a regular basis, the management of the community home care agency tried to cut back on the nursing visits. I strategized with his primary physicians to countermand those attempts. As his advocate and family case manager, I was constantly struggling to stay one step ahead of the agency's version of patient-focused care. I had learned so much from the hospital and community nurses with whom I had researched and filmed.

Verne recovered, but the memory remains. At that time, I was not a filmmaker but a witness to a profound failure of care with dire consequences.

Yes, I have filmed women who work in health care. I have filmed their patients, their working conditions, their strengths, and their suffering. I have served as a witness, a documentarian, and an advocate in my professional life, in my activist activities, and in my family responsibilities. I, too, have become a canary in the mine.

Further Reading

Armstrong, P., H. Armstrong, & K. Scott-Dixon. (2008). *Critical to Care: The Invisible Women in Health Services.* Toronto: University of Toronto Press.

Armstrong, P., A. Banerjee, M. Szebehely, H. Armstrong, T. Daly, & S. Lafrance. (2009). *They Deserve Better: The Long-Term Care Experience in Canada and Scandinavia.* Ottawa: Canadian Centre for Policy Alternatives.

Koren, M. J. (2010). Person-Centered Care for Nursing Home Residents: The Culture Change Movement. *Health Affairs* 29(2): 312–317.

Relevant Websites

Canadian Health Coalition: www.healthcoalition.ca
Skyworks Foundation: http://www.skyworksfoundation.org/about_us/index.html

Conclusions

Ann Pederson and Pat Armstrong

As we describe in the Introduction, this book had its origins in an Ontario Training Centre course on women's health in 2006. By the time this book is published, it will have been almost a decade since that workshop. And as various contributors to this volume have made clear, a number of things have changed in the past 10 years. In particular, we have witnessed a transformation in the infrastructure for women's health research and policy-making that includes the de-funding of the Centres of Excellence for Women's Health, Women and Health Protection, and Women and Health Care Reform. Provinces, too, have cut back support. With the closure of most of the Centres of Excellence and the national working groups, we have lost some of the major mechanisms by which new knowledge across a diverse range of women's health issues has been generated. And with the additional closure of the Canadian Women's Health Network, we have witnessed the erosion of some of the key avenues for knowledge exchange that have been so important to disseminating research findings to practitioners, policy-makers, and women themselves. Without the dedicated research capacity supported by these and other entities, we are likely to see a reduction in the generation of new knowledge about women's health in the years ahead and its translation into programs, services, and policies for girls and women across Canada. This is unfortunate for numerous reasons, not least of which is because, as this book has shown, numerous challenges remain with regard to women's health in Canada.

It is troubling, for example, that many of the issues raised in the focus groups conducted by the Ontario Women's Health Network echo concerns raised more than 20 years ago in British Columbia using a similar process of provincial consultation and by a project conducted by Women and Health Care Reform on what quality health care means to women. Clearly there is still major work to be done on theory, research, and practices.

The reviewers of the first edition identified a number of health topics that are important women's health issues, issues such as sexually transmitted infections; the health of sex workers; violence against women; contraception, abortion, and reproductive health; the menopausal transition and midlife women's health; chronic diseases and conditions; and eating disorders and disordered eating—that warrant their own book-length treatment. Indeed, there is no limit to the list of health topics that still need attention and about which girls and women—and specific groups of them—deserve information, treatment, and support. How do we ensure that these topics remain top of mind in the highly competitive world of academic research? Moreover, what new problems will emerge for women in Canada that have not yet been anticipated?

Demographic changes will continue to transform the health needs of women in Canada. Whether from the aging of the population of post-World War II baby boomers; the influx of newcomers from countries torn apart by civil war, natural disasters, or the legacy of infectious disease; or the movement of the population from the east to the western part of the country, the faces of girls and women in Canada will evolve. It will be important to avoid one-size-fits-all solutions to this growing diversity of the population, to watch out for evidence of inequities in access, treatment, and outcomes, and place these in context.

The tension between the simultaneous pressure for standardization and customization will continue to be a formidable challenge in the provision of care. Meanwhile, there are calls for training health care workers to be skilled in "cultural humility"—a stance that requires being comfortable with not knowing, being open to learning about a person, and working together with a patient to develop an approach to health and illness that is accessible, appropriate, and acceptable. And there are exciting developments in indigenous cultural competency training emerging that may help to change practice and care in relation to First Nations patients and families. These developments also require attending to the diverse needs of care providers, paid and unpaid, and recognizing their skills.

A tension that permeates the field of women's health is the challenge of generalizing about the category of "women" while avoiding essentialism, universalism, and myriad other *-isms*. This dynamic was reflected in this revision to the book as well. Although we have long asked, "Which women?" we were urged by reviewers to expand the number of groups of women that warranted discussion about their unique needs, experiences, or barriers to care. The list was long. We were able to accommodate and engage with some of these additional groups, but we could not cover them all. In doing so, we were reminded of what these diverse groups of women have in common, although less is known about their lives, their health needs, their experiences of care, and their preferences for how they ought to be treated as opposed to how they are treated. And further, we were reminded that it is challenging to embrace an awareness of difference while recognizing some of women's similarities and common experiences when planning and delivering care.

This book recognizes health and social care as work, both paid and unpaid. And the contributors presented evidence about the extent to which this work remains mostly women's work. While there may be movement in some sectors regarding the sharing of familial and domestic labour, there has not been the revolution in household responsibilities that second-wave feminists envisioned. Indeed, we have seen that care work increasingly occurs at home, which means that much of it remains invisible, privately financed, and individually managed. C. Wright Mills wrote in the 1950s that private troubles are often also public problems, yet what is out of sight and deemed to be private is not necessarily individual, and widespread problems arising from the provision of care in the home, for example, deserve to be seen as public policy issues.

In the realm of paid work, we were told about changes in health care labour and the labour force, as well as the extent to which health work remains women's work. Considerable challenges remain for the organization, finance, and delivery of health care in Canada, and governments and health care managers struggle to control costs while incorporating new knowledge, technological innovation, and demand. Workers at all levels are increasingly required to be flexible about embracing change, to manage heavy workloads, and to engage in perpetual professional development.

Bringing all of this together, we asked a few contributors to focus on the links among research, policy, and practice. What we learn is that there are some persistent inequities among and between women that should be put right; that translating research into practice takes time and resources; and that there are myriad forms of knowledge that can, should, and do inform policy-making and program planning. While there remain disciplinary debates about some forms of evidence, we are seeing the emergence of inter- and transdisciplinary research. We have witnessed the rise of participatory methods that embrace newer technical and social technologies, such as digital storytelling, photovoice, and online communities of practice. These transformations in research tools will surely continue as new ways of networking, communicating, and generating information grow. With tools like digital, real-time monitoring of physical activity, sedentary behaviour, and eating, will we see a shift in the issues related to weight? Will fibre optics and computers allow and/or require more people to be cared for at home regardless of where they live? Or will information technologies isolate people from one another, reduce face-to-face interaction, and eliminate social care? What are the implications for health, health care, and equity from such developments?

We argued in the Introduction that it is important to have a book about women's health in Canada because context matters. In this book, contributors have demonstrated in diverse ways how context shapes the resources for health, the meaning of health, and women's priorities for health for themselves and others. We also believe that context matters at a structural and political level. We therefore wonder how developments at a global level will affect women's health in the years to come. How will climate change affect access to food, safe drinking water, and shelter? Will the tobacco epidemic indeed become an epidemic among women? Will the rise of new economic powers challenge Canada's ability to sustain the standard of living that fosters health and health care services as we currently understand them? And will the next generation of women's health researchers, providers, and policy-makers be faced with the same challenges we face today?

In the developing world, education is understood to be a key factor in development and improving women's health. In Canada, Quebec has demonstrated that the availability of daycare is a major poverty-reduction strategy. Despite evidence that affordable daycare has a positive impact on women's education, income, and health, most women in Canada do not have access to such care. Perhaps another "wicked problem" we need to face is not only the challenge of less support for research on women's health but also the challenge of ensuring that evidence informs policy and program development.

Current efforts focus on bringing policy-makers into the very design of research; inviting policy-makers to define research problems; and synthesizing research findings to help identify promising practices. Yet still we see that much of policy-making lacks a sound evidence base. Given the reduction in support for knowledge development in women's health we are currently witnessing, it is perhaps time to discuss how we engage with the political process to ensure that women's health remains a substantive area of scholarship and exploration. Without further attention, we are likely to see the third edition of *Women's Health* reporting that women in Canada not only continue to experience inequities in health outcomes but also face deteriorating health, and that the social investments likely to enhance women's health have not yet materialized.

"Evidence is seldom enough on its own, particularly when operating in an adverse political environment. It's what you do with the evidence that matters" (de Toma, 2011, p. 12). This statement, part of an advocacy tool kit for civil society organizations, is just as true for women's health advocates. Not only is more high-quality sex- and gender-informed research needed, but so, too, are mechanisms for translating that evidence into action. Whether through knowledge synthesis processes, guidance statements such as those generated by the National Institute for Health and Care Excellence (NICE) in the United Kingdom, dialogues, and networking, evidence on women's health needs to be used to improve the lives of girls and women. This entails engagement with advocacy as a central facet of women's health and health promotion, as it is in Australia in organizations such as Women's Health Victoria, a state-funded women's health information clearinghouse for whom advocacy is a mandate, not a cause for investigation and censure as it is becoming here.

Reference

de Toma, C. (2011). *Advocacy Toolkit: Guidance on How to Advocate for a More Enabling Environment for Civil Society in Your Context.* Open Society Forum for CSO Development Effectiveness.

Contributors

Pat Armstrong held a Canada Health Services Research Foundation/Canadian Institutes of Health Research Chair in Health Services, is Distinguished Research Professor in Sociology, and Fellow of the Royal Society of Canada. Her work focuses on the fields of social policy, of women, work, and health and social services. She has published a wide variety of books and articles.

Jennifer Bernier is the Founder and Executive Director of the Centre for Building Resilience for Anti-Violence Education (BRAVE) in Halifax, Canada, which provides services for girls with social and behavioural challenges.

Arlene S. Bierman is an eminent physician and researcher. Her work focuses on improving access, quality, and outcomes of care for older adults with chronic illness, with a special focus on socio-economically disadvantaged populations, inequities in health and health care, and the unique needs of older women.

Caitlin Cassie holds a Master of Public Policy from the University of Toronto and a Bachelor of Arts from the University of British Columbia. She is currently working as a senior adviser in the health policy sector and a community engagement consultant for ThinkFresh Group.

Madeleine Kétéskwew Dion Stout is a Registered Nurse who also has a graduate degree in International Affairs. She has received the Assiniwikamik Award from the Aboriginal Nurses Association of Canada; a Distinguished Alumnus Award from the University of Lethbridge; and Honorary Doctor of Laws from the University of British Columbia and the University of Ottawa. She serves on multiple policy and community boards. She became a member of the Order of Canada on July 1, 2015.

Cheryl Forchuk, RN, PhD, is a Distinguished University Professor and Associate Director of Nursing Research at the Arthur Labatt Family School of Nursing, Faculty of Health Sciences, with a cross appointment to the Department of Psychiatry, Schulich School of Medicine and Dentistry, University of Western Ontario.

Tatiana Fraser is a social entrepreneur and writer. She is co-founder of the Girls Action Foundation, was named an Ashoka Fellow in 2010, and is a Research Associate with the Simone de Beauvoir Institute. She is currently working on a non-fiction title, *Girl Positive*, to be published by Random House in the spring of 2016.

Lorraine Greaves is a medical sociologist and Senior Investigator at the British Columbia Centre of Excellence for Women's Health. She was its Executive Director from 1997 to 2009. Dr. Greaves is an international expert in women's tobacco use, and the use of sex and gender in research, program, and policy development.

Karin Humphries holds the inaugural UBC Heart and Stroke Foundation Professorship in Women's Cardiovascular Health. Dr. Humphries is launching British Columbia's first research program to focus on gender-based differences in cardiovascular disease and developing strategies to improve outcomes in younger women in whom the risk of coronary disease and poor outcomes has increased in the last few years.

Wendy Katherine, among the first regulated midwives in Ontario, has a Master of Business Administration and has led multiple provincial government reports. She is currently Principal Consultant at Phoenix Health Consulting and Chief Executive Officer of Healthmetrix Inc., an international maternal child health quality consultancy.

Katherine Laxer has recently completed a doctorate in Sociology at York University. Her chapter in this book draws on her thesis, "Mapping the Division of Labour in Long-Term Residential Care across Jurisdictions." She also draws on her current post-doctoral work on the comparative perspectives database, with Dr. Leah Vosko. Her published articles focus primarily on issues in counting the labour force.

Beverly D. Leipert is a Professor in the Arthur Labatt Family School of Nursing at the University of Western Ontario. She specializes in rural women's health, innovative qualitative research methods, community health nursing, and health promotion.

Julie Maher is the Executive Director of the Ontario Women's Health Network. She has over 25 years of experience in the health and not-for-profit sectors. She is an advocate for community-based research, and the inclusion of women's voices and experience in health research.

Sara Mohammed works with the Ontario Women's Health Network as their Communications and Social Media Specialist. Her academic credentials include a Bachelor of Science from the University of Toronto and a Master's degree from York University.

Phyllis Montgomery is a Professor in the School of Nursing at Laurentian University in Sudbury, Ontario. Her recent publications include research on men and fathers with mental health issues.

Sharolyn Mossey, RN, MScN, is an Assistant Professor in Laurentian University's School of Nursing. Her clinical research interests include people living with enduring health challenges in a Northern and rural context.

Ann Pederson is the Director, Population Health Promotion, at BC Women's Hospital + Health Centre. She worked for over 17 years at the BC Centre of Excellence for Women's Health and is trained in health promotion and women's health. She is completing a doctorate at the University of British Columbia in sex, gender, and health promotion.

Ito Peng is the Associate Dean, Interdisciplinary and International Affairs, and Professor of Sociology and Public Policy at the Faculty of Arts and Science, University of Toronto (St. George). She is an associate researcher with the United Nations Research Institute for Social Development and a research fellow at the Ontario Ministry of Health and Long-Term Care.

Paula C. Pinto is a researcher at the Centre for Administration and Public Policy in Lisbon, Portugal, and an invited faculty member at the School for Social and Political Sciences, Technical University of Lisbon, and the Department of Sociology, New University of Lisbon.

Robyn Plunkett is Professor of Nursing, Humber Institute of Technology & Advanced Learning. Her areas of specialization include nursing, rural health, women's health, and religion. Most recently she has been writing about health promotion, including curling, in rural areas.

Nancy Poole is the Director of the BC Centre of Excellence for Women's Health and the Prevention Lead for the CanFASD Research Network. Nancy is known for her collaborative work toward improving policy and service provision related to girls and women's substance use and overall health, with governments and organizations in Canada and internationally.

Carol Reichert is a Policy and Research Specialist at the Canadian Federation of Nurses Unions. As a public policy, communications, and research professional, she has had experience in the health care field, on Parliament Hill, as well as in university and non-governmental settings.

Anne Rochon Ford is a long-time women's health researcher, writer, and activist. She most recently served as Executive Director of the Canadian Women's Health Network and is currently a Research Associate with the National Network on Environments and Women's Health.

Linda Silas, RN, has been the President of the Canadian Federation of Nurses Unions, which represents close to 200,000 members and associate members, since 2003. Linda brings years of experience as a nurse-leader, a public speaker, and a negotiator at the local, provincial, and national levels, and is the foremost advocate on behalf of nurses in Canada.

Laura Sky is an independent documentary filmmaker. She founded Skyworks Charitable Foundation in 1983 as a non-profit documentary organization dealing with contemporary social issues to help create strategies for social change.

Ellen Sweeney is a qualitative health researcher and policy analyst. She completed a PhD in the Faculty of Environmental Studies at York University and an MA in Social Anthropology at Dalhousie University. She currently works at the Nova Scotia Health Research Foundation in Halifax.

Christina Talbot has contributed to research studies on girls' and women's health, trauma and substance use, fetal alcohol spectrum disorder, and traumatic brain injury, and currently works with the BC Centre of Excellence for Women's Health. Prior to that, she worked with girls and women, children, and families in school- and community-based programs as well as in child welfare and mental health settings.

Anna Travers is the Director of the Rainbow Health Network Ontario (RHO), Canada's first provincially funded capacity-building resource/network in the area of LGBT health and wellness. She has been involved in LGBT health care for over 15 years and led the development of RHO in 2008.

Sari Tudiver is a cultural anthropologist with a long-standing interest in women's health. Over four decades, she has worked in academic settings, for non-governmental organizations, and for the Canadian federal government. She chairs the board of Inter Pares and works as an independent researcher and writer in Ottawa.

Cheryl van Daalen-Smith is an Associate Professor at York University with appointments in the School of Nursing; the School of Gender, Feminist, and Women's Studies; and the Children's Studies Program. Her work explores girls' and women's health from a feminist critical social theoretical lens.

Bilkis Vissandjée is a Professor in the School of Nursing at Université de Montréal. She is a researcher at the Centre de recherche et de formation du CSSS de la Montagne. Her contributions to the scientific community along with nationally and internationally based partners highlight the importance of accounting for sex, gender, migration, and ethnicity when developing strategies for providing quality and equity-sensitive care within a diversified socio-cultural context.

Copyright Acknowledgements

Section Openers

Section 1: © Steve Design/Shutterstock.com, used under license from Shutterstock.com

Section 2: © DenKuvaiev/iStockphoto.com

Section 3: © Tyler Olson/Shutterstock.com, used under license from Shutterstock.com

Section 4: © monkeybusinessimages/iStockphoto.com

Chapter 4

Figure 4.1: Choi et al. (2014) "Sex-and Gender-Related Risk Factor Burden in Patients with Premature Acute Coronary Syndrome," *Canadian Journal of Cardiology*, 30(1), 113. Copyright © 2014 Canadian Cardiovascular Society. Reprinted with permission from Elsevier.

Chapter 10

Figure 10.3: Intake form and Sherbourne Health Centre logo © 2014 Sherbourne Health Centre. Used with permission.

Table 10.1: Mravcak, Sally. (2006). "Primary Care for Lesbian and Bisexual Women." *American Family Physician* 74(2), 281. Adapted with permission from Laret, Mark. (2004). *Inclusive Language Policy*. San Francisco, Calif.: University of San Francisco Medical Center. © Copyright 2004 University of San Francisco Medical Center.

Chapter 14

Table 14.1: "National and Provincial Data by Selected Characteristics, RNs, 2013" adapted from Canadian Institute for Health Information (CIHI), *Regulated Nurses, 2013*: Data Tables 11, 12, and 13, Available at https://secure.cihi.ca/estore/productFamily.htm?locale=en&pf=PFC2646&lang=en. Copyright © 2014 by the Canadian Institute for Health Information. Reprinted with permission.

Table 14.2: "National and Provincial Data by Selected Characteristics, LPNs, 2013" adapted from Canadian Institute for Health Information (CIHI), *Regulated Nurses, 2013*: Data Tables 33, 34, and 35, Available at https://secure.cihi.ca/estore/productFamily.htm?locale=en&pf=PFC2646&lang=en. Copyright © 2013 by the Canadian Institute for Health Information. Reprinted with permission.

Table 14.3: "Provincial Public Sector Health Care Nurses, Rates of Overtime, Absenteeism, Unionization, 2012" adapted from *Trends in Own Illness or Disability-Related Absenteeism*

Index